CW0073328

Ma

'14

Statistics for Biology and Health

Statistics for Biology and Health

Aalen/Borgan/Gjessing: Survival and Event History Analysis: A Process Point of View

Bacchieri/Cioppa: Fundamentals of Clinical Research

Borchers/Buckland/Zucchini: Estimating Animal Abundance: Closed Populations

Burzykowski/Molenberghs/Buyse: The Evaluation of Surrogate Endpoints

Duchateau/Janssen: The Frailty Model

Everitt/Rabe-Hesketh: Analyzing Medical Data Using S-PLUS

Ewens/Grant: Statistical Methods in Bioinformatics: An Introduction, 2nd ed.

Gentleman/Carey/Huber/Irizarry/Dudoit: Bioinformatics and Computational Biology Solutions Using R and Bioconductor

Hougaard: Analysis of Multivariate Survival Data

Keyfitz/Caswell: Applied Mathematical Demography, 3rd ed.

Klein/Moeschberger: Survival Analysis: Techniques for Censored and Truncated Data, 2nd ed.

Kleinbaum/Klein: Survival Analysis: A Self-Learning Text, 2nd ed.

Kleinbaum/Klein: Logistic Regression: A Self-Learning Text, 2nd ed.

Lange: Mathematical and Statistical Methods for Genetic Analysis, 2nd ed.

Manton/Singer/Suzman: Forecasting the Health of Elderly Populations

Martinussen/Scheike: Dynamic Regression Models for Survival Data

Moyé: Multiple Analyses in Clinical Trials: Fundamentals for Investigators

Nielsen: Statistical Methods in Molecular Evolution

O'Quigley: Proportional Hazards Regression

Parmigiani/Garrett/Irizarry/Zeger: The Analysis of Gene Expression Data: Methods and Software

Proschan/LanWittes: Statistical Monitoring of Clinical Trials: A Unified Approach

Schlattmann: Medical Applications of Finite Mixture Models

Siegmund/Yakir: The Statistics of Gene Mapping

Simon/Korn/McShane/Radmacher/Wright/Zhao: Design and Analysis of DNA Microarray Investigations

Sorensen/Gianola: Likelihood, Bayesian, and MCMC Methods in Quantitative Genetics

Stallard/Manton/Cohen: Forecasting Product Liability Claims: Epidemiology and Modeling in the Manville Asbestos Case

Sun: The Statistical Analysis of Interval-censored Failure Time Data

Therneau/Grambsch: Modeling Survival Data: Extending the Cox Model

Ting: Dose Finding in Drug Development

Vitthinghoff/Glidden/Shiboski/McCulloch: Regression Methods in Biostatistics: Linear, Logistic, Survival, and Repeated Measures Models

Wu/Ma/Casella: Statistical Genetics of Quantitative Traits: Linkage, Maps, and QTL

Zhang/Singer: Recursive Partitioning in the Health Sciences

Zuur/Ieno/Smith: Analysing Ecological Data

For further volumes:
http://www.springer.com/series/2848

Niel Hens • Ziv Shkedy • Marc Aerts • Christel Faes
Pierre Van Damme • Philippe Beutels

Modeling Infectious Disease Parameters Based on Serological and Social Contact Data

A Modern Statistical Perspective

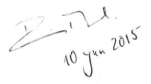

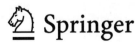 Springer

Niel Hens
Center for Statistics, Interuniversity
  Institute for Biostatistics
  and statistical Bioinformatics
Hasselt University
Diepenbeek, Belgium

Centre for Health Economic Research
  and Modelling Infectious Diseases,
  Vaccine and Infectious Disease Institute
University of Antwerp
Universiteitsplein 1
2610 Antwerpen, Belgium

Marc Aerts
Center for Statistics, Interuniversity
  Institute for Biostatistics and
  statistical Bioinformatics
Hasselt University
Diepenbeek, Belgium

Pierre Van Damme
Centre for the Evaluation
  of Vaccination, Vaccine and
  Infectious Disease Institute
University of Antwerp
Antwerpen, Belgium

Ziv Shkedy
Center for Statistics, Interuniversity
  Institute for Biostatistics
  and statistical Bioinformatics
Hasselt University
Diepenbeek, Belgium

Christel Faes
Center for Statistics, Interuniversity
  Institute for Biostatistics and
  statistical Bioinformatics
Hasselt University
Diepenbeek, Belgium

Philippe Beutels
Centre for Health Economic Research
  and Modelling Infectious Diseases,
  Vaccine and Infectious Disease Institute
University of Antwerp
Antwerpen, Belgium

Please note that additional material for this book can be downloaded from
http://extras.springer.com

ISSN 1431-8776
ISBN 978-1-4614-4071-0   ISBN 978-1-4614-4072-7 (eBook)
DOI 10.1007/978-1-4614-4072-7
Springer New York Heidelberg Dordrecht London

Library of Congress Control Number: 2012941858

Printed on acid-free paper

Springer is part of Springer Science+Business Media (www.springer.com)

To Kelly, Lena and Louisa
To my family
To Els, Anouk and Lauren
To Sven, Hanne and Marte
To Myrjam, Bruno, Tom and Eline
To Conny and Robin

Preface

Mathematical epidemiology of infectious diseases usually involves describing the flow of individuals between mutually exclusive infection states. One of the key parameters describing the transition from the susceptible to the infected class is the hazard of infection, often referred to as the force of infection. The force of infection reflects the degree of contact with potential for transmission between infected and susceptible individuals. The mathematical relation between the force of infection and effective contact patterns is generally assumed to be subjected to the mass action principle, which yields the necessary information to estimate the basic reproduction number, another key parameter in infectious disease epidemiology.

It is within this context that the Center for Statistics (CenStat, Interuniversity Institute for Biostatistics and statistical Bioinformatics, Hasselt University) and the Centre for the Evaluation of Vaccination and the Centre for Health Economic Research and Modelling Infectious Diseases (CEV, CHERMID, Vaccine and Infectious Disease Institute, University of Antwerp) have collaborated over the past 15 years. This book demonstrates the past and current research activities of these institutes and can be considered to be a milestone in this collaboration.

This book is focused on the application of modern statistical methods and models to estimate infectious disease parameters. We want to provide the readers with software guidance, such as R packages, and with data, as far as they can be made publicly available. Please visit www.simid.be for data and code pertaining to this book.

Many persons have contributed either directly or indirectly to this book for which we are very grateful: @ Hasselt University: Steven Abrams, Girma Minalu Ayele, Kaatje Bollaerts, Emanuele Del Fava, Nele Goeyvaerts, Geert Molenberghs, Harriet Namata, and Kim Van Kerckhove, @ University of Antwerp: Mathieu Andraud, Joke Bilcke, Olivier Lejeune, Elke Leuridan, Benson Ogunjimi, and Heidi Theeten, and elsewhere: Kari Auranen, Benoit Dervaux, John Edmunds, Paddy Farrington, Nigel Gay, Janneke Heijne, Daniel Hlubinka, Mark Jit, Peter Kung'U Kimani, Mira Kojouhorova, Andrea Kvitkovicova, Marco Massari, Rafael Mikolajczyk, Joël Mossong, Magdalena Rosinka, Malgorzata Sadkowska-Todys, Stefania Salmaso, Gianpaolo Scalia Tomba, Thierry Van Effelterre, Jacco Wallinga, Andreas Wienke, and James Wood. We also wish to thank the editorial team at Springer, more particularly John Kimmel, Marc Strauss, and Hannah Bracken for their guidance throughout the writing process and the reviewers Piero Manfredi, James Wood, Jacco Wallinga, and Gianpaolo Scalia Tomba whose identity was revealed to us and whose suggestions improved the book considerably.

The authors would appreciate being informed of errors and may be contacted by electronic mail: niel.hens@uhasselt.be.

Hasselt and Antwerp   Niel Hens
                                                                             Ziv Shkedy
                                                                            Marc Aerts
                                                                           Christel Faes
                                                                      Pierre Van Damme
                                                                      Philippe Beutels

Acknowledgements

This book would not have been possible without the strategic basic research project SIMID funded by the agency for the Promotion of Innovation by Science and Technology in Flanders (IWT project number 060081). We further gratefully acknowledge the chair in evidence-based vaccinology, which was sponsored by a gift from Pfizer. Some of the material in this book was developed based on earlier work funded by the Flemish fund for scientific research (FWO project number G039304), EC's sixth framework project POLYMOD, and the IAP research network nr P6/03 of the Belgian Government (Belgian Science Policy). We thank the production team at Springer for their support at the final stage of the publication process.

Contents

Part I
Introducing the Concept of the Book

Chapter 1
Why This Book? An Introduction

1.1 Terms for Germs

For the sake of simplicity, let us start by naming an infectious agent a "germ." There are countless germs that can infect human, animal, and plant hosts. Germs can be transmitted directly between hosts via respiratory air droplets or bodily fluids (e.g., saliva, blood, or secretions from sexual organs). Germs can also be transmitted indirectly through an intermediary source, for instance via mosquitoes, ticks, rodents, environmental particles (e.g., contaminated water and food) or contaminated blood products. Germs evolve and transform while new germs emerge regularly, implying their supply can be considered infinite. A broad distinction is often made between microscopically small germs with relatively short life spans, which replicate within their hosts (often called microparasites such as viruses, bacteria, and fungi), and much larger germs with relatively longer life spans (often called macroparasites such as parasitic worms). Many germs live inside or on the surface of their hosts' bodies without causing illness or even discomfort. In fact, hosts even depend for their survival on germs (e.g., bacteria in the human gut). However, when germs cause disease in their hosts they are often referred to as pathogens. So when we talk about infectious *diseases* we imply that these are caused by pathogens, which are transmissible between hosts, either directly or indirectly. Infectious diseases have been an important cause of sickness and death throughout the history of mankind. With the agricultural revolution, the world population grew and concentrated in clusters. The density of human hosts thus reached levels that allowed continued local (endemic) transmission of a number of lethal pathogens. It seems therefore that diseases like plague, smallpox, measles, and cholera slowed population growth after the initial high growth rates between 10,000 and 5,000 years ago. Most pathogens in humans emerged and spread out from a local community, as they travelled along with their hosts. Nowadays, they quickly establish anywhere environmental conditions allow them to.

N. Hens et al., *Modeling Infectious Disease Parameters Based on Serological and Social Contact Data*, Statistics for Biology and Health 63, DOI 10.1007/978-1-4614-4072-7_1, © Springer Science+Business Media New York 2012

1.2 Models of Infectious Diseases

Mathematical models can take many forms, but essentially they describe a system through mathematical equations. They allow studying how a system changes from one state to the next, as well as the relation between variables used in the equations that define the system. There is a difference with statistical models, which are used to study relations between different variables based on data and to make inferences based on these relations.

The field of infectious disease modeling has been the focus of ever increasing research activity over the last 30 odd years. Figure 1.1 illustrates this by showing the evolution over time of retrieved publications using the search string "model* AND (mathematic* OR statistic* OR simulat*) AND (infect* OR communicable OR epidemic* OR vaccin* OR immuni* OR virus OR viral)" in topics of the Scientific Citation Index (SCI expanded, in ISI Web of Science).

It can be seen that the quantity of publications jumped up in the early 1990s, an observation which holds for many fields of science, likely because in this period access to personal computers and the use of the internet became widely established.

The continuing rising interest in the specific field of infectious disease modeling since the 1990s was likely fueled by various evolutions and events, amongst which we single out the following:

1. Increasing research and computing capacity in multidisciplinary fields, such as mathematical epidemiology and biology, biostatistics, and health economics.

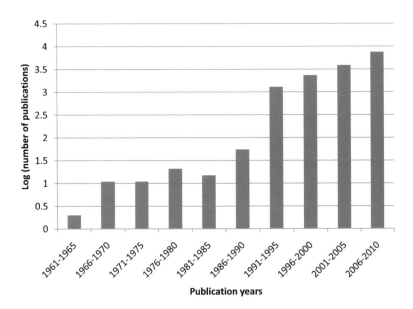

Fig. 1.1 Evolution of publications on models of infectious diseases (on a log-10 scale)

2. Expanded use of mathematical models as part of new standard procedures for evidence-based health policy, often as an implicit part of economic evaluation of pharmaceutical products.
3. New or expanding public health emergencies of international concern (e.g., HIV/AIDS since the 1980s, SARS in 2003, and pandemic influenza A (H1N1)v in 2009).
4. Increasing knowledge base for measuring and categorizing relevant information at both the pathogen and the host level (e.g., genomics, testing of cellular immunity, social contact patterns).

These observations are by no means to imply that infectious disease modeling hardly existed prior to the 1990s. In fact, the central concepts and the foundations for the main techniques used in this field were developed over a century ago and can be traced back to seminal work by d'Alembert (1761), Bernoulli (1766), Ross (1916), McKendrick (1926), Kermack and McKendrick (1927, 1932, 1933), and Muench (1934). Yet the application of these techniques remained much more rare and less internationally dispersed than we can observe today.

While many of the publications in this field are about improving model methodology, by far most of the publications apply a certain modeling approach to a specific problem.

In the application of models of infectious diseases, we distinguish two general aims of such models: forecasting and understanding. By forecasting we mean that projections are made of infections and their consequences under various scenarios of interest (e.g., the time evolution of the number and age distribution of people infected with measles using various scenarios for vaccination schedules and vaccine uptake rates). In relation to forecasting, models are increasingly applied in the slipstream of evolutions 1, 2, and 3 described above. By understanding we mean that models are used that mimic a particular process for infectious disease development or transmission with the aim to improve our knowledge of the process itself, rather than produce estimates of outcomes of this process. In such models the qualitative form and order of magnitude of the results are more important than the exact quantity they represent. Evolutions 1 and 4 above would have been strong drivers for more research on models in relation to understanding the underlying mechanisms of infectious disease transmission, evolution, and development.

1.3 Where Does This Book Fit in the Field?

There have already been many textbooks on infectious disease modeling. Probably the best known and most influential the book written by Anderson and May (1991), who, like Kermack and McKendrick (1927, 1932, 1933), approached the subject from an epidemiologist's angle, using intuitively appealing and elegant mathematical derivation. Their text book has had a major influence on the application of deterministic transmission models, to a wide range of infections. Other textbooks that followed in the same tradition have extended the mathematics and the range of models considered. Examples here include Farrington (2008) and Keeling and Rohani (2008). The recent book by Vynnycky and White (2010) also fits within that tradition. Their book is elaborate in scope, covering many modeling techniques on a very diverse range of infections and populations. They also provided program code so that the avid reader could apply the techniques and models they discussed. Other types of textbooks in this category are provided by Isham and Medley (1996) and Krämer et al. (2010), who edited and bundled contributed papers covering a variety of specific topics in infectious disease modeling by many different authors.

Notwithstanding that many authors of the above textbooks are mathematicians or statisticians to begin with, other textbooks have approached the subject of modeling infectious diseases or epidemics more from a mathematical rather than an epidemiological viewpoint. The pioneering text book that we consider to fit this bill was produced in 1975 by Bailey (1975). More recent examples are provided by Becker (1989), Daley and Gani (1999), Diekmann and Heesterbeek (2000), and Capasso (2008).

Additionally, there have been textbooks focusing on much more specific subjects and their associated specific challenges. For instance, Andersson and Britton (2000) focused on stochastic models of epidemic data, whereas Halloran et al. (2010) covered the design and analysis of observational vaccine studies.

The book you are reading now aims at filling a gap in the latter tradition of textbooks by zooming in on a specific subject. Our book presents a range of modern statistical and mathematical techniques to estimate parameters that are of pivotal importance in infectious disease modeling. The applications we show in this book are on microparasitic pathogens (with a strong focus on viruses), causing infectious disease in humans. We provide model syntax, as well as R code, with which the statistical and modeling analyses can be applied. We also provide datasets to enable exploration of the techniques. Although it is generally recognized that parameters like the force of infection and the transmission rates between infected and susceptible persons are of very high influence, especially in applications of forecasting, relatively little attention has been given to estimating these parameters to the best of our ability. In view of intensified research in this specific area over the past decade, we considered it the right moment to summarize these developments in this book. We strive not only to explain what to do, given the nature of the data, but we also show how to do it. In that sense this text book is hands-on.

1.4   A Road Map for This Book

The book starts well and truly in Part II, by introducing pivotal epidemiological parameters, describing their properties as well as those of different prevailing mathematical models that mimic the spread of microparasitic pathogens between human hosts. Readers already familiar with these rather basic concepts can press on to Part III.

Part III describes the various datasets used throughout the book. This should give the reader clear insights into the kind of data that are used. The most commonly used data throughout the book are age-specific seroprevalence data and social contact frequencies (to which we also refer as social mixing patterns). Some techniques are also illustrated on incidence data. In Part IV, a wide range of statistical methods is explained and illustrated to derive the force of infection from seroprevalence and incidence data. We describe and illustrate parametric, semiparametric, and nonparametric techniques that use serological test results in their traditional sense (as categorical variables), as well as in their crude form (as antibody levels). Part V shows how to estimate a matrix of transmission probabilities from serology or social mixing pattern data alone or by using the combination of these data. Furthermore, methods to estimate the basic reproduction number are also shown. Here too, various methods are proposed and illustrated. The final part, Part IV, integrates the statistical estimation methods for the pivotal infectious disease parameters (as described in Parts IV and V) in the mathematical model framework described in Part II. Thus at the end, we've come full circle: the modern methods for statistical derivation and inference are integrated in and applied to the mathematical model frameworks we introduced at the very beginning of the book.

We endeavored to demonstrate the methods on a good mix of different applications. These include airborne close contact infections (such as mumps, parvovirus B19, rubella, tuberculosis, and varicella), feco-oral infections (such as hepatitis A), and sexually transmitted and/or blood borne infections such as hepatitis B, hepatitis C, and HIV/AIDS.

We included a short appendix in which we introduce the software package R and several statistical concepts such as maximum likelihood, bootstrap-methods, etc.

We hope you will find this book a useful source of information and inspiration and—perhaps less desirable—transpiration.

Part II
Mathematical Models for Infectious Diseases: An Introduction

In this part we introduce several basic concepts. We introduce the Theory of Happenings by Sir Ronald Ross in Chap. 2. In Chap. 3 the SIR model is introduced and several of its aspects discussed including the dynamic properties, the impact of vaccination programs, the time homogeneous SIR model and the SIR model in a population constructed from different subpopulations according to age.

Chapter 2
A Priori and A Posteriori Models for Infectious Diseases

2.1 The Theory of Happenings

Sir Ronald Ross (1916) suggested the name *The Theory of Happenings* for the solution of the following problem. Suppose that a population P is divided into two groups. One part of the population (Z) is affected by something and the other part (A) is not affected. In the context of infectious diseases the population is affected by an infection and therefore Z is the part of the population of infected individuals (the infected class) while A is the susceptible part of the population (the susceptible class). Note that each individual in the population belongs only to one part of the population. At each time unit dt a proportion $h \times dt$ in the susceptible class becomes infected and a proportion $r \times dt$ of the infected individuals recovers and becomes susceptible again. Ronald Ross (1916) assumed that there are three different processes that act simultaneously on the population. The first is the *variation* process which corresponds to demographic changes in the population such as births, deaths, immigration, and emigration. The variation process acts on both A and Z and consequently on P. The second process is the *reversion* process, i.e., the rate at which individuals move from the infected class of the population to the susceptible class. The third process is the *happening* process and it represents the rate at which individuals become infected and move from the susceptible class to the infected class. The main question is to determine the number of infected individuals, number of new cases, and the population size at each time unit. The flow of individuals in the population was formulated by Ross as a set of three differential equations, given below, which represent the population dynamics, the change in the susceptible class, and the change in the infected class. Note that the first equation in (2.1) is the sum of the two last equations:

N. Hens et al., *Modeling Infectious Disease Parameters Based on Serological and Social Contact Data*, Statistics for Biology and Health 63, DOI 10.1007/978-1-4614-4072-7_2, © Springer Science+Business Media New York 2012

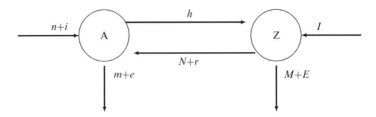

Fig. 2.1 A flow diagram illustrating the model of Ross (1916). Note that in Ross' model immigration and emigration are possible from both A and Z

$$
\begin{cases}
\frac{dP(t)}{dt} = (n - m + i - e)A(t) + (N - M + I - E)Z(t), \\
\frac{dA(t)}{dt} = (n - m + i - e - h)A(t) + (N + r)Z(t), \\
\frac{dZ(t)}{dt} = hA(t) - (M + E + r - I)Z(t).
\end{cases}
\tag{2.1}
$$

The rates n, m, i, e, N, M, I, and E are the variation rates representing births, deaths, immigration, and emigration acting on the susceptible and infected class, respectively. The reversion rate (or the recovery rate) is r while h is (in Ross' own words) the most important rate, the happening element. Note that the term NZ should appear in the third equation. Ross (1916) assumed that this part will generally be born not affected and therefore included this term in the second equation. An illustrative flow diagram of Ross' model is shown in Fig. 2.1.

The number of individuals in each compartment of the model can be calculated by solving the set of differential equations (2.1). The main problem is that some of the parameters are unknown. The solution proposed by Ross was to iterate between two modeling frameworks:

*"The whole subject is capable of study by two distinct methods which are used in other branches of science, which are complementary of each other, and which would converge towards the same results—the **a posteriori** and the **a priori** methods. In the former we commence with observed statistics, endeavor to fit analytical laws to them and so work backwards to the underlying cause (as done in much statistical work of the day); and in the latter we assume a knowledge of causes, construct our differential equations on that supposition, follow up the logical consequences, and finally test the calculated results by comparing them with the observed statistics."*

Today we often use the terminology of mathematical and statistical models for infectious diseases for the a priori and a posteriori methods, respectively. Although the modeling framework of Ross was established in 1916, it still remains the central framework for dynamic models of infectious disease transmission.

In this part of the book we introduce the main concepts about transmission models for infectious diseases and their corresponding application to infectious disease data. We do not aim to discuss all the mathematical details behind the models and throughout this part we introduce modeling concepts in an intuitive way rather than in a formal way. For readers who wish to have an additional insight about the models and the mathematical derivation of some of the results we refer to the books of Anderson and May (1991); Keeling and Rohani (2008), and Vynnycky and White (2010). For readers more familiar with mathematics we refer to the books of Daley and Gani (1999); Diekmann and Heesterbeek (2000), and Capasso (2008).

2.2   An Example: A Basic Model for HIV/AIDS

In what follows we illustrate the modeling framework of Ross using a mathematical and statistical model for HIV/AIDS.

2.2.1   A Mathematical Model for HIV/AIDS

We closely follow Anderson and May (1991), Chap. 11, page 263–269, who used—in hindsight—a too simplistic model to describe the transmission of HIV among homosexuals. Anderson (1988); Isham (1988), and Capasso (2008) discussed similar versions of this model. The flow diagram for the model is shown in Fig. 2.2. It should be clear that this simplistic model is merely used for illustrative purposes here and that it doesn't reflect the current knowledge about the HIV/AIDS epidemic.

The model distinguishes between two groups of infected individuals, those who developed clinical AIDS and those who are HIV infected but do not develop clinical AIDS. For the model discussed below we use the notation of Capasso (2008). Let S be the number of susceptibles in an open homosexual population at time t. The element of happening, i.e., the force of infection, λ, is the rate at which susceptible individuals are infected. We assume that one part of the population, p, will develop clinical AIDS, i.e., this part will become HIV infected (I) and will then transfer to the AIDS class (A) at rate v_1. The other part of the population, $(1 - p)$, will get infected (Y) but will not develop the disease; this part is assumed to move into a noninfectious class (Z) at rate v_2. A deterministic approximation for such

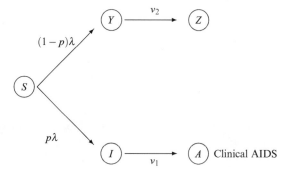

Fig. 2.2 Flow diagram for a very crude transmission model of HIV/AIDS. Note that, for the sake of simplicity, the demographic parameters and disease-related mortality have been dropped from this diagram

a transmission model is given by the following set of differential equations that describes the transmission process

$$
\begin{cases}
\frac{dS(t)}{dt} = B - (\lambda + \mu)S(t), \\
\frac{dI(t)}{dt} = p\lambda S(t) - (\mu + v_1)I(t), \\
\frac{dY(t)}{dt} = (1 - p)\lambda S(t) - (\mu + v_2)Y(t), \\
\frac{dA(t)}{dt} = v_1 I(t) - (\mu + \alpha)A(t), \\
\frac{dZ(t)}{dt} = v_2 Y(t) - \mu Z(t).
\end{cases}
\tag{2.2}
$$

Note that B is the recruitment rate into the population under consideration, i.e., homosexuals, and μ is the natural rate of death. The AIDS related mortality rate (α) is an additional death rate which exists only in the compartment of individuals who develop clinical AIDS (A). Anderson (1988), Anderson and May (1991), and Capasso (2008) assume that the force of infection λ is a function of the number of sexual partners c, the probability (or the risk) of infection per (sexual) partnership β, and the population of infective individuals in the population. More specifically, the force of infection is given by

$$
\lambda = \frac{c\beta}{N}(I + Y).
$$

Here, $N = S + I + Y + A + Z$ is the total population. The factor $(I + Y)/N$ is the probability that a given contact for a susceptible individual will be with an infectious person assuming contacts take place in a random fashion. It is important to realize that a contact as described here refers to having sexual intercourse resulting in the transmission of HIV given the contact occurs between an infectious and a susceptible individual.

Figure 2.3 shows numerical solutions of differential equation system (2.2) for a hypothetical population of size $N(0) = 10,000$ from which five were infected at $t = 0$, i.e., $I(0) = 5$. We assume $p = 20\%$ of the population develops AIDS. The life expectancy of individuals who developed AIDS is assumed to be 1 year ($\alpha^{-1} = 1$ year). We assume that on average an individual in the population has ten sexual partners per year ($c = 10$) and the probability of transmission is $\beta = 0.1$, such that $c\beta = 1$ per year. The life expectancy in the general population is 75 years (μ^{-1}), the recruitment rate is assumed to be equal to $B = N(0)\mu$, and the incubation period (v_1^{-1} and v_2^{-1}) is set to 8 years (Anderson 1988; Anderson and May 1991). We emphasize again that given current knowledge about the HIV-epidemic, the model, its assumptions, and the parameters used in this example are not realistic and merely used to illustrate the framework of Ross.

As graphically displayed in Fig. 2.3, the number of seropositive individuals decreases after the peak at around 12 years due to the high mortality rate for individuals who developed clinical AIDS. We will now show how to obtain these results using the program R.

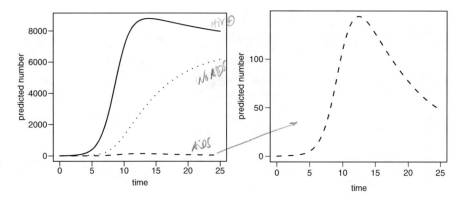

Fig. 2.3 Solution of the AIDS model obtained by numerical integration of (2.2) in R. The *full*, *dashed*, and *dotted lines* correspond to, respectively, the predicted number of seropositives, clinical AIDS cases, and nonclinical AIDS cases

Implementation in R

Throughout the book, we use free software such as R and Winbugs to fit models. Winbugs is free software for hierarchical Bayesian modeling using Markov Chain Monte Carlo (MCMC) methods that can be downloaded from http://www.mrc-bsu. cam.ac.uk/bugs/ (Lunn et al. 2000). R is an open environment for data manipulation, graphical display, and interactive data analysis. We refer to Appendix A for more information about how to use R.

The R package *deSolve* (see e.g., Soetaert et al. 2010) is a package developed for solving initial value differential equations in R which is called within R using *library(deSolve)*. The R function that integrates systems of ordinary differential equations is *ode* and has a general call of the form:

```
ode(y=vector containing state variables,
        times=vector containing the time units for integration,
        func=function containing the model equations,
        parms=vector containing the model parameters)
```

The transmission model (2.2) can be implemented in R in the following way. In our example $S=9995$, $I=5$, $Y=0$, $A=0$, and $Z=0$ correspond to the initial conditions while the time units for integration (*times*) and the model parameters (*parameters*) for the AIDS model can be defined as follows:

```
state = c(S=9995,I=5,Y=0,A=0,Z=0)
times = seq(0,25,by=0.01)
parameters = c(N0=10000,mu=1/75,nu1=1/8,nu2=1/8,p=0.2,alpha=1)
```

Next, the user-defined function *AIDS* is used to define the differential equations of the model in (2.2).

```
AIDS=function(t,state,parameters)
{
with(as.list(c(state, parameters)),
{
B = N0*mu
lambda = (I+Y)/N0
dS = B-(mu+lambda)*S
dI = p*lambda*S-(mu+nu1)*I
dY = (1-p)*lambda*S-(mu+nu2)*Y
dA = nu1*I-(mu+alpha)*A
dZ = nu2*Y-mu*Z
list(c(dS,dI,dY,dA,dZ))
})
}
# Note that we use the total population N0 in the definition
# of lambda, and that it can be replaced by S+I+Y+A+Z,
# i.e. the population still alive.
```

The R function *AIDS* receives as an input the three vectors (time, state variables, and the parameters of the model) specified above. We can integrate the model using the function *ode* and in order to process the output we create an R object (the data frame *out*) which contains the results.

```
require(deSolve)
out=as.data.frame(
ode(y=state,times=times,func=AIDS,parms=parameters)
)
```

The data frame *out* contains six numerical vectors: the time and the number of individuals in each of the five compartments. For example, the vector *S* defined in the *AIDS* function by *dS = B-(mu+lambda)*S* contains the number of individuals in the susceptible class. The first six lines of the output are shown below.

```
> head(out)
   time        S        I         Y          A             Z
1  0.00 9995.000 5.000000 0.00000000 0.000000000 0.000000e+00
2  0.01 9994.950 5.003119 0.04012504 0.006220433 2.507653e-05
3  0.02 9994.901 5.006321 0.08054144 0.012382080 1.004847e-04
4  0.03 9994.850 5.009606 0.12125181 0.018485638 2.265837e-04
                                                     (continued)
```

```
(continued)
5  0.04  9994.799  5.012974  0.16225841  0.024531710  4.036902e-04
6  0.05  9994.748  5.016427  0.20356433  0.030521095  6.322298e-04
```

Note that we can change the integration step by changing the grid of the timescale. A timescale that is too large will produce nonsensible results. It is therefore advised to explore different timescales and assess the impact on the results (see e.g., Chap. 3 in Vynnycky and White 2010).

Figure 2.3 shows the solution of the model for the infected, clinical AIDS (A), and infected but non-clinical AIDS (Z) compartments for an increment in time of 0.01 years. The R-code used to obtain Fig. 2.3 is given by

```
plot(times,out$I+out$Y+out$A+out$Z,type="l",main="  ",
    xlab="time", ylab="predicted number",lwd=2)
lines(times,out$A,lty=2,lwd=2)
lines(times,out$Z,lty=4,lwd=2)
```

2.2.2   A Statistical Model for the Initial HIV/AIDS Outbreak

In the previous section we used a (simple) deterministic model to describe the transmission of HIV/AIDS in a specific population. The model predicts a rapid increase in the number of AIDS cases $(A(t))$ followed by a decline after a peak at 10–12 years.

In this section we focus on the initial stage of the epidemic and use three datasets containing information on the number of reported AIDS cases (shown in Fig. 2.4) to model the initial outbreak of AIDS. The data considered are quarterly data on the newly reported number of cases in the USA (1982–1990, reported by Lindsey 1997), monthly data of newly reported AIDS cases from the UK (1982–1986, reported by Healy and Tillett 1988), and quarterly data of new AIDS diagnoses from Australia (1982–1990, reported by Daley and Gani 1999). All these data consist of individuals in the A compartment in (2.2).

Let $A(t)$ be the number of AIDS cases at time t. We assume that

$$A(t) \sim \text{Poisson}(\delta(t)). \tag{2.3}$$

Here, $\delta(t) = E(A(t))$ is the mean number of cases per time unit. At the beginning of the epidemic $A(0) \approx 0$ and $S(0) \approx N$. We assume that in the initial stage of the epidemic, the number of new cases follows an exponential growth model of the form

$$\delta(t) = A(0)e^{\theta t}.$$

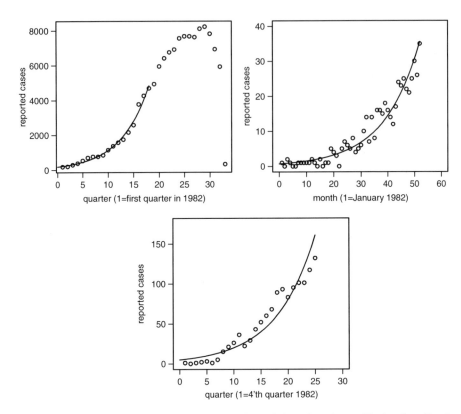

Fig. 2.4 AIDS in the USA, the UK, and Australia. Recorded number of cases (*dots*) and predicted number of cases based on the initial stage of the epidemic (*line*). *Top left panel*: quarterly number of reported cases in the USA (Lindsey 1997). *Top right panel*: monthly number of reported cases in the UK (Healy and Tillett 1988). *Lower panel*: quarterly number of reported cases in Australia (Daley and Gani 1999)

Note that for $t > 0$, the initial number of cases $A(0)$ is a constant and is used as a parameter in the model. The parameter θ represents the growth rate of the epidemic. The model for the number of cases in (2.3) can be formulated as a generalized linear model (GLM, see, e.g., McCullagh and Nelder 1989) with Poisson distribution for the response and log link function

$$\log(\delta(t)) = \log(A(0)) + \theta t.$$

This model can be fitted as a GLM with Poisson distribution and log link function using the function *glm()* in R.

```
fit.aidsUS=glm(cases~t.quarter,family=poisson(link="log"))
```

Data and fitted models are shown in Fig. 2.4. Below, the R output from the analysis for the AIDS data from the USA is presented. Both Healy and Tillett

(1988) and Lindsey (1997) discussed the problem of reporting delays, the difference between the date of report and date of diagnosis, for these types of data. Following Lindsey (1997), in order to avoid the problem of reporting delays in the data, we use the data until middle 1986.

```
> summary(fit.aidsUS)

Call:
glm(formula = cases ~ t.quarter, family = poisson(link
                                              = "log"))

Deviance Residuals:
    Min        1Q     Median        3Q        Max
-4.6738   -2.8327    -0.9165    2.8039    6.9488

Coefficients:
            Estimate Std. Error z value Pr(>|z|)
(Intercept) 5.208901   0.020799   250.4  <2e-16 ***
t.quarter   0.181999   0.001454   125.1  <2e-16 ***
---
Signif. codes:  0 *** 0.001 ** 0.01 * 0.05 . 0.1   1

(Dispersion parameter for poisson family taken to be 1)

    Null deviance: 19960.03  on 17  degrees of freedom
Residual deviance:   231.21  on 16  degrees of freedom
AIC: 393.00
```

The estimated number of initial cases $\hat{A}(0) = \exp(5.2089) = 182.89$ (95% C.I.$175.58 - 190.50$). The growth rate is $\hat{\theta} = 0.1820$ ($0.1791 - 0.1848$) slightly higher than the quarterly growth rate in Australia $\hat{\theta} = 0.1394$ ($0.1292 - 0.1496$). Notice that for all datasets, the predicted number of cases based on the initial outbreak reveals similar patterns because of the assumed exponential model (Fig. 2.4.)

Indeed, the underlying assumption behind the exponential model is that in the initial stage of the epidemic the number of infected individuals appears at an exponential rate.

Alternatively, other growth models, such as Weibull, Gompertz and logistic models, can be fitted to the data as well. For these models the mean structure is given by

$$
\delta(t) = \begin{cases}
A(0)e^{\theta t} & \text{exponential linear growth,} \\
A(0)e^{\theta_1 t + \theta_2 t^2} & \text{exponential quadratic growth,} \\
A(0)t^{\theta} & \text{Weibull model,} \\
A(0)[1 - \exp(-\alpha \exp(\beta t))] & \text{Gompertz growth,} \\
A(0)[\alpha \exp(\beta t)]/[1 + \alpha \exp(\beta t)] & \text{logistic growth.}
\end{cases}
$$

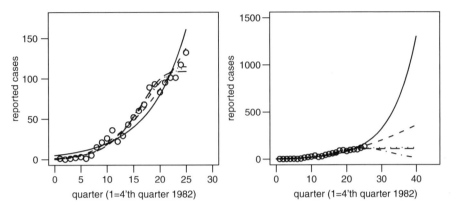

Fig. 2.5 AIDS in Australia. Predicted number of AIDS cases for 40 quarters based on exponential linear growth (*solid line*), exponential quadratic growth (*short-dashed line*), Weibull model (*dotted line*), Gompertz model (*dot-dashed line*), and logistic growth model (*long-dashed line*). *Left*: prediction within the range of the data. *Right*: long-term prediction for a period of 40 quarters

Figure 2.5 shows the AIDS data in Australia with the predicted means obtained from different models. We notice that long-term prediction based on data from the initial stage of the epidemic is problematic and should be interpreted with caution. The fact that a certain model has a good fit within the range of the data does not itself justify the use of this model for long-term prediction.

The Poisson distribution we have used in the GLM has the property that the mean equals the variance. This property is often not fulfilled. In that case distributions such as the negative binomial distribution allowing for overdispersion can be used (Agresti 2002).

2.3   The Mechanism that Generates the Data

The transmission model discussed in the previous section can be interpreted as the mechanism that generates the observed data. Thus, if our assumptions about the transmission model are correct, the observed data should reflect the underlying mechanism. Furthermore, when modeling the data we should take into account the mechanism in the background and, as Ross (1916) argued, we should compare the results obtained from the assumed mathematical model to those which are obtained from the data modeling approach. The two modeling frameworks (mathematical and statistical models for infectious diseases) are complementary and model building within both modeling frameworks can be improved if information from the complementary framework is used. Indeed, almost 100 years after Ross' paper the idea of interaction between mathematical and statistical models, the idea to evaluate the assumptions behind the transmission model using a statistical model, remains central in current day modeling of infectious diseases.

2.4   The Basic Epidemiological Parameters

Before we continue, we need to introduce some of the basic epidemiological parameters often used in infectious disease epidemiology. We will mainly follow Diekmann and Heesterbeek (2000) and Vynnycky and White (2010). Denote S and I the number of susceptible and infectious individuals. Define N the population size and let us assume we have a closed population (no births, no deaths, no migration).

The Mass Action Principle and the Force of Infection

In its simplest form, the mass-action principle states that the number of new cases in generation $g + 1$ is proportional to all possible contacts between infectious and susceptible people in generation g. Mathematically this can be expressed as

$$I_{g+1} = bI_g S_g, \tag{2.4}$$

where b is a proportionality coefficient often referred to as *contact rate* or *transmission parameter* whereas it actually represents the probability per susceptible person of having a contact which leads to a transmission event and therefore the term *effective contact rate* is often preferred. In general, the Greek letter beta, β, is used when referring to the effective contact rate per unit of time. The mass-action principle can then be written as $\beta I(t)S(t)$ which provides the rate at which newly infected individuals emerge.

The force of infection $\lambda(t)$ is defined as $\beta I(t)$. It expresses the rate at which susceptible individuals become infected and depends on the effective contact rate and the number of infectious individual at time t.

The Basic Reproduction Number

Diekmann and Heesterbeek (2000) defined the basic reproduction ratio R_0 as *the expected number of secondary cases per primary case in a "virgin" population.* Nowadays, people tend to prefer the use of the term *number* instead of *ratio* and so will we throughout the text. In general, R_0 can take any value on the positive real line.

When considering the epidemic on a generation basis, the basic reproduction number R_0 can be related to the mass-action principle (2.4) as follows (Vynnycky and White 2010). Consider a totally susceptible population in generation $g = 0$. This means that $S_0 = N$, i.e., the number of susceptible individuals in generation 0 equals the population size. If one infectious person enters the population, $I_0 = 1$, i.e., there is only one infectious individual in generation $g = 0$, the mass-action principle implies that the number of newly infected cases in the next generation ($g = 1$) is given by bN. In continuous time, the number of newly infected cases is given by βND, where D denotes the mean duration of infectiousness. Indeed, in continuous time β is a rate and expresses the effective contact rate per unit of time. Consequently, the generation time during which the introductory case is infectious, i.e., the duration of infectiousness, needs to be taken into account.

If R_0 is larger than 1, the expected number of newly infected individuals is larger than 1 and the infection will spread in the population. Whenever R_0 is smaller than 1, and thus the expected number of newly infected individuals is smaller than 1, the infection will die out. Therefore the threshold of interest for R_0 is 1. The estimation of R_0 will be discussed in part V of the book.

Herd Immunity Threshold and the Critical Vaccination Coverage

Let us consider a continuous time setting. If we assume that after infection people recover and gain lifelong immunity, the number of susceptibles decreases during the course of an epidemic. The expected number of newly infected individuals produced by a primary case is then given by $\beta s(t)ND$, where $s(t)$ is the proportion susceptible at time t. In other words, the effective reproduction number $R(t)$ at time t is given by $s(t)R_0$. Again if $R(t) > 1$ the infection will continue to spread in the population whereas if $R(t) < 1$ the infection will die out. The threshold value $R(t) = 1$ yields that $s(t) = 1/R_0$. In other words, if the proportion susceptible in the population is smaller than $1/R_0$ or if a proportion $1 - 1/R_0$ is immune or immunized either by natural infection or by vaccination, the incidence of infection should decrease. This threshold criterion is known as the *herd immunity threshold*. The concept of *herd immunity* refers to the fact that a fraction of the population escapes infection since in the limit not everyone is infected. Given the herd immunity threshold it suffices to immunize a proportion $1 - 1/R_0$ of the population to stop the infection from spreading in the entire population. We will give a mathematical derivation for this result in Sect. 3.1.2 within the context of the basic SIR model. The proportion $1 - 1/R_0$ is referred to as the critical vaccination coverage.

The Average Age at Infection

A final concept which we need to introduce is the average age of infection which is defined as the average age at infection among individuals who ever experience infection in their lifetime.

2.5 Discussion

In this chapter, the basic concept of a priori and a posteriori models as described by Ross (1916) has been introduced and exemplified using a simple mathematical and statistical model for HIV/AIDS and some basic epidemiological parameters have been defined. In the following chapter we will revisit discussing these basic epidemiological parameters in the context of an SIR model. Furthermore we will show how serological data provide a valuable source of information to estimate some of these parameters in several settings. Readers familiar with the SIR model and its dynamics can skip the following chapter and proceed with Chap. 4 in which the data used throughout this book are introduced.

Chapter 3
The SIR Model

3.1 Introduction

In this chapter, we introduce the basic SIR model and its properties. In this first section, we introduce the SIR model and review its dynamic properties assuming homogeneous mixing. In Sect. 3.2 the SIR model in endemic equilibrium is discussed whereas the link to serological data is made in Sect. 3.3. A short description of additional compartments often added to the SIR model is given in Sect. 3.4. The extension of the SIR model for populations consisting of subpopulations (for instance by age) is discussed in Sect. 3.5. We end this chapter with a discussion in Sect. 3.6.

3.1.1 The SIR Model

Let us consider a transmission model consisting of three compartments: susceptible (S), infected (I), and immune or recovered (R). An underlying assumption of this SIR model is that individuals are born into the susceptible class. Hence the exposure time is the age of the individual. After infection, the individuals transfer to the infected class and after clearing the infection individuals are transferred to the immune/recovered class. It is assumed that, after recovery, individuals gain lifelong immunity and therefore do not take part in the transmission process other than that they represent the complement of those that do (i.e., the more immune people, the fewer there can be infectious and susceptible people in the population). The SIR model is one of the basic compartmental models in infectious disease epidemiology, which is widely used and well suited to model many viral infections in childhood. Given its structure, the SIR model is likely too simplistic for a number of infections, e.g., it is unsuited to model the transmission of infectious agents against which the

N. Hens et al., *Modeling Infectious Disease Parameters Based on Serological and Social Contact Data*, Statistics for Biology and Health 63, DOI 10.1007/978-1-4614-4072-7_3, © Springer Science+Business Media New York 2012

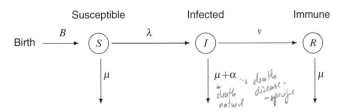

Fig. 3.1 Flow diagram for the SIR model. The individuals enter the susceptible class, then move to the infected class (at rate λ), and after recovering they move into the immune class (at rate v)

host does not acquire permanent immunity after infection (a state which is explicitly represented by the R compartment).

Although the exposure time in the SIR model is age, individuals who were born in different calendar years may participate in the transmission process with different parameters, at least if the transmission parameters depend on the calendar time. Therefore the SIR model can be described using a system of three partial differential equations in age and time given by

$$
\left\{
\begin{array}{l}
\dfrac{\partial S(a,t)}{\partial a} + \dfrac{\partial S(a,t)}{\partial t} = -(\lambda(a,t) + \mu(a,t))S(a,t), \\[2mm]
\dfrac{\partial I(a,t)}{\partial a} + \dfrac{\partial I(a,t)}{\partial t} = \lambda(a,t)S(a,t) - (v(a,t) + \alpha(a,t) + \mu(a,t))I(a,t), \quad (3.1) \\[2mm]
\dfrac{\partial R(a,t)}{\partial a} + \dfrac{\partial R(a,t)}{\partial t} = v(a,t)I(a,t) - \mu(a,t)R(a,t),
\end{array}
\right.
$$

where $S(a,t), I(a,t)$, and $R(a,t)$ are the age- and time-specific number of susceptibles, infected, and recovered, respectively; and with boundary conditions given by $S(0,t) = B(t)$, the number of births in the population at time t, $I(0,t) = R(0,t) = 0$, meaning that we rule out vertical transmission of infection. The initial conditions are given by $S(a,0) = \tilde{S}(a), I(a,0) = \tilde{I}(a)$ and $R(a,0) = \tilde{R}(a)$ where $\tilde{S}(a), \tilde{I}(a), \tilde{R}(a)$ are prescribed functions of age such that $\tilde{S}(a) + \tilde{I}(a) + \tilde{R}(a) = N(a,0)$ with $N(a,0)$ the age-specific population size at time 0. In these equations, $\mu(a,t)$ and $\alpha(a,t)$ denote the natural and disease-related death rate, respectively. It is often assumed that both $\mu(a,t)$ and $\alpha(a,t)$ possibly depend on age but not on time: $\mu(a,t) = \mu(a)$ and $\alpha(a,t) = \alpha(a)$. The force of infection $\lambda(a,t)$ is the rate at which individuals are infected and it is assumed to be both age- and time-dependent whereas $v(a,t)$ is the recovery rate which is often assumed to be constant: $v(a,t) = v$. Figure 3.1 shows the flow diagram for such a model.

We will now focus on the SIR dynamics. To simplify the presentation, we will do so by assuming homogeneity with respect to age meaning that the parameters in (3.1) are assumed constant with respect to age. Throughout the text we will refer to the age-homogeneous model as the basic SIR model.

3.1.2 The Basic Model Dynamics

Assuming age homogeneity and the aforementioned assumptions, model (3.1) simplifies to

$$
\begin{cases}
\dfrac{dS(t)}{dt} = B(t) - \lambda(t)S(t) - \mu S(t), \\[2mm]
\dfrac{dI(t)}{dt} = \lambda(t)S(t) - vI(t) - \mu I(t), \\[2mm]
\dfrac{dR(t)}{dt} = vI(t) - \mu R(t),
\end{cases}
\tag{3.2}
$$

where $\lambda(t) = \beta I(t)$ as given by the mass-action principle discussed in Sect. 2.4. Further, we assume $B(t) = \mu N(t)$ and no disease-related mortality $\alpha = 0$ which results in $B = \mu N$. Indeed (3.2) and $B(t) = \mu N(t)$ yields a constant population $N(t) = N$ because of equal birth and death rates:

$$
\frac{dS(t)}{dt} + \frac{dI(t)}{dt} + \frac{dR(t)}{dt} = \mu\left[N(t) - S(t) - I(t) - R(t)\right] = 0.
$$

Note that (3.2) can be derived by integrating (3.1) over age.

Let $s(t) = S(t)/N(t)$, $i(t) = I(t)/N(t)$, and $r(t) = R(t)/N(t)$ denote the fraction susceptible, infected, and recovered, respectively. The differential equation system (3.2) can be rewritten in terms of these proportions as

$$
\begin{cases}
\dfrac{ds(t)}{dt} = \mu - \tilde{\beta}i(t)s(t) - \mu s(t), \\[2mm]
\dfrac{di(t)}{dt} = \tilde{\beta}i(t)s(t) - vi(t) - \mu i(t), \\[2mm]
\dfrac{dr(t)}{dt} = vi(t) - \mu r(t),
\end{cases}
\tag{3.3}
$$

where $\tilde{\beta} = \beta N$. Note that the population size in a deterministic model is no more than a scaling factor but that the interpretation of β and $\tilde{\beta}$ is different. Whereas β refers to the density dependent or "pseudo" mass-action principle as first used by Hamer (1906) and doesn't depend on the population size, $\tilde{\beta}$ refers to the frequency dependent or "true" mass-action principle (de Jong et al. 1995). For a more elaborate discussion on the difference between these two versions of the mass-action principle we refer to Keeling and Rohani (2008) and Vynnycky and White (2010). We note that since we assume no disease-related mortality and a constant population both versions equivalent here.

The transmission model defined by the differential equation system (3.3) implies that the disease can spread as long as $di(t)/dt > 0$ (or equivalently because of a constant population, $dI(t)/dt > 0$). This allows us to derive the threshold condition by equating the differential equation in the infected compartment to zero:

$$\tilde{\beta}i(t)s(t) - vi(t) - \mu i(t) = 0 \rightarrow i(t)(\tilde{\beta}s(t) - v - \mu) = 0$$

and therefore:

$$s(t) = \frac{v + \mu}{\tilde{\beta}},$$

or equivalently the disease can spread as long as

$$s(t) > \frac{v + \mu}{\tilde{\beta}}. \tag{3.4}$$

The quantity $\tilde{\beta}/(v + \mu)$ is the basic reproduction number R_0 and it represents the number of new infections introduced by one infectious individual in a completely susceptible population (see Sect. 2.4 and, e.g., Dietz 1993; Diekmann and Heesterbeek 2000 (Chapter 3)). Equation (3.4) implies that the disease can spread as long as $R_0 > 1$ while for $R_0 < 1$ the infection will die out.

Indeed, in Sect. 2.4 we have shown that the basic reproduction number $R_0 = \beta ND$ in a closed population and that the threshold of interest is 1. Assuming $\mu = 0$, $R_0 = \tilde{\beta}/(v + \mu) = \beta N/v$, where $1/v = D$ is the mean infectious period, yields the same result. The inclusion of nonzero mortality ($\mu > 0$) lowers the mean infectious period yielding a lower R_0-value. Note that (3.4) implies that the disease can spread as long as the proportion susceptible is larger than $1/R_0$ or equivalently for the reproduction number $R(t) = s(t)R_0 > 1$ (see Sect. 2.4).

A disease is said to be in equilibrium whenever $ds(t)/dt = di(t)/dt = dr(t)/dt = 0$. Equating the differential equation for infectives to zero results in

$$\frac{di(t)}{dt} = 0 \rightarrow i(t)(\tilde{\beta}s(t) - (v + \mu)) = 0 \rightarrow i(\infty) = 0 \text{ or } s(\infty) = \frac{v + \mu}{\tilde{\beta}}.$$

Here $i(\infty) = 0$ implies what is called a disease free equilibrium in which the equilibrium values $(s(\infty), i(\infty), r(\infty))$ are equal to $(1,0,0)$ while $s(\infty) = (v + \mu)/\tilde{\beta} = 1/R_0$ implies what is referred to as the endemic equilibrium. In order to derive the endemic equilibrium value for $i(\infty)$, we substitute $s(\infty)$ in the differential equation for the fraction susceptibles and get

$$\frac{ds(t)}{dt} = 0 \rightarrow \mu - \tilde{\beta}i(t)\frac{1}{R_0} - \mu\frac{1}{R_0} = 0 \rightarrow i(\infty) = \frac{\mu}{\tilde{\beta}}(R_0 - 1).$$

Thus, the endemic equilibrium values are given by

$$s(\infty) = \frac{1}{R_0}, \quad i(\infty) = \frac{\mu}{\tilde{\beta}}(R_0 - 1), \quad r(\infty) = 1 - s(\infty) - i(\infty). \tag{3.5}$$

3.1.3   The Basic Model in R

Let us consider a population of size $N = 5,000$ with $S(0) = 4,999, I(0) = 1$, and $R(0) = 0$. We assume $v^{-1} = 1$ year, a life expectancy μ^{-1} of 75 years, $\mu = 1/75$, and $\beta = 0.0005$. With this parameter setting $R_0 = 2.4671$ and according to (3.5): $(s(\infty), i(\infty)) = (0.4053, 0.0078)$ or $(S(\infty), I(\infty)) = (2,026.67, 39.12)$. A possible R program for system (3.2) consists of a function *SIR* in which we define the set of differential equations. The model as implemented here allows for a disease-related death rate, α.

```
parameters = c(mu=1/75,beta=0.0005,nu=1,N=5000,alpha=0)
state = c(S=4999,I=1,R=0)

SIR=function(t,state,parameters)
{
with(as.list(c(state, parameters)),
{
dS = N*mu-beta*I*S - mu*S
dI = beta*I*S - (nu+alpha+mu)*I
dR = nu*I - mu*R
list(c(dS, dI, dR))
})
}
```

Note that, although the R model is formulated in terms of numbers, its transformation to fractions is straightforward. In the R program we specified $\alpha = 0$ and thus consider the model without disease-related mortality. We define an R object, *res.scen1*, which contains the solution of the integration over a period of 1000 years by 10,000 time units (0.10 years each).

```
times=seq(0,1000,by=0.1)
require(deSolve)
res.scen1=as.data.frame(ode(y=state,times=times,func=SIR,
    parms=parameters))
```

Figure 3.2 (upper row) shows the fractions of susceptible and infected individuals at each time point, and how the numbers of susceptible and infected individuals in the population reach their equilibrium values for the first 250 years. Notice that indeed the equilibrium values for S and I are 2,026.67 and 39.12, respectively (according to (3.5)). The damping effects in $s(t)$ and $i(t)$ over time have a slightly different pattern: $s(t)$ oscillates around the equilibrium value (symmetric oscillations) and as time passes the magnitude of the oscillations decreases up to the point at which $s(t)$ reaches the endemic equilibrium fraction. For $i(t)$ the oscillations

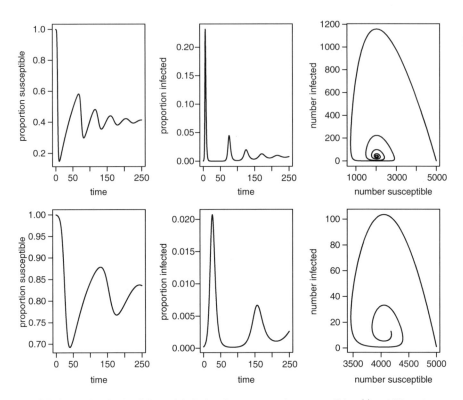

Fig. 3.2 Dynamics in the SIR model. *Left column*: proportion susceptible $s(t)$; *middle column*: proportion infected $i(t)$; *right column* $S(t)$ versus $I(t)$. Parameter setting $N = 5{,}000$, $I(0) = 1$, $\mu = 1/75$, and $\nu = 1$. *Upper row*: $\beta = 0.0005$ and thus $R_0 = 2.47$; *lower row*: $\beta = 0.00025$ and thus $R_0 = 1.23$

exhibit a different pattern with recurrent epidemics for which the peaks decrease over time (damping oscillations). Note that the (time-dependent) force of infection is proportional to $I(t)$ since $\lambda(t) = \beta I(t)$.

Figure 3.2 (second row) shows the solution for a second scenario in which $\beta = 0.00025$ and $R_0 = 1.2336$ ($1/R_0 = 0.8107$). We notice that in addition to the new equilibrium values, $S(\infty) = 4053.33$ and $I(\infty) = 12.46$, the time at which the susceptible class builds up is longer and as a result the interepidemic period, i.e. the time interval between two successive peaks, is longer.

Next, we investigate the influence of the recovery rate ν on the transmission process. We start from the first scenario as defined above and change the value of ν to 2 (reflecting a mean time to recovery of approximately 6 months) by changing the value of the third element of the vector *parameters*. Figure 3.3 shows the number of susceptibles for the two scenarios and shows that $S(\infty)$ is higher for the second scenario with $\nu = 2$ while the interepidemic period is longer compared to the scenario where $\nu = 1$. This is due to the fact that in the second scenario individuals on average spend less time in the infected class and therefore less contacts are

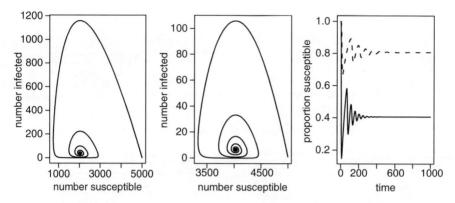

Fig. 3.3 SIR-dynamics in continuous time. Parameter setting: $S(0) = 4,999$, $I(0) = 1$, $R(0) = 0$, $\mu = 1/75$, $\beta = 0.0005$, and $v = 1$ (*left panel*) or $v = 2$ (*middle panel*). *Right panel*: $s(t)$ for the two scenarios: *solid line* $v = 1$ and *dashed line* $v = 2$

made between susceptible and infectious individuals. As a result, at equilibrium $S_{v=2}(\infty) > S_{v=1}(\infty)$ and $I_{v=2}(\infty) < I_{v=1}(\infty)$ as can be seen from both the R output presented in the panel below and Fig. 3.3.

```
# Output
# nu=1
> res.scen1[10001,]
        time        S        I        R
10001 1000 2026.667 39.12279 2934.211
# nu=2
> res.scen2[10001,]
        time        S        I        R
10001 1000 4026.688 6.456782 966.8547
```

Figure 3.4 shows the influence of v on R_0 for a wider range of v-values. The threshold value of $R_0 = 1$ corresponds to the point $(S(\infty), R(\infty)) = (N, 0)$ in Fig. 3.4.

3.1.4   Vaccination in the Basic Model

Let us now discuss the basic reproduction number and the impact of vaccination programs on the infectious disease epidemiology. In this section, focus is on the dynamic changes and we introduce the critical vaccination proportion needed to eradicate the disease.

There are different ways to incorporate a vaccination program in a deterministic model (Halloran et al. 2010). Here we incorporated a vaccination program in the

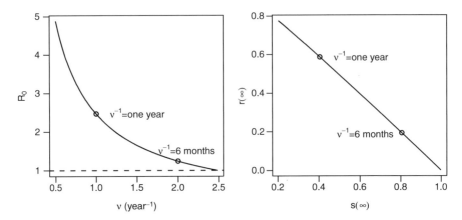

Fig. 3.4 *First panel*: ν versus R_0. *Second panel*: equilibrium values $s(\infty)$ versus $r(\infty)$ for different values of ν

basic SIR model by adding a transition from the susceptible compartment to the immune compartment by assuming that a proportion p of newborns is effectively vaccinated at birth. (i.e., p can be thought of as the product of vaccine uptake, the proportion of vaccine recipients, and vaccine efficacy, the probability that the vaccine is efficacious in a vaccine recipient). We will ignore the issue of efficacy throughout the remainder of the book and refer the interested reader to Halloran et al. (2010). The basic SIR model (3.2) can be rewritten to include vaccination as

$$\begin{cases} \dfrac{dS(t)}{dt} = N\mu(1-p) - (\lambda(t) + \mu)S(t), \\[2mm] \dfrac{dI(t)}{dt} = \lambda(t)S(t) - (v + \mu)I(t), \\[2mm] \dfrac{dR(t)}{dt} = N\mu p + vI(t) - \mu R(t). \end{cases} \qquad (3.6)$$

The SIR model (3.6) implies that a proportion p of newborns enters directly in the immune class. Figure 3.5 shows the prevaccination setting while Figs. 3.6 and 3.7 show the model in which 40% and 80% are vaccinated at birth. Two main patterns can be observed. First, the interepidemic period is longer when the proportion of vaccinated individuals increases. This implies that the average age at infection (which is equivalent to the average duration in the susceptible class) is 10 years and 5 years, respectively. This implies that individuals spend, on average, more time in the susceptible class and as a result the average age at infection increases (Sect. 2.4). Second, in the long run, after vaccination, a new endemic equilibrium will be reached.

Notice that although the prevaccination force of infection $\lambda(0) = \lambda_0$ is equal under all scenarios, in the new equilibrium the force of infection decreases as the proportion of vaccinated individuals increases. Indeed, since $S(t)$ decreases as p increases so does $\beta S(t)I(t)$ and thus the rate at which individuals leave

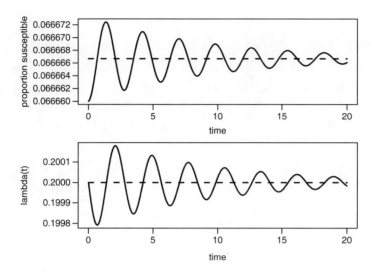

Fig. 3.5 Dynamic aspects of vaccination in the SIR model. Numerical solution for the basic SIR model (3.6) with the parameter setting $\lambda_0 = 0.2$, $\frac{1}{\mu} = 70$, $R_0 = 15$ and $\frac{1}{\nu} = 25$ and without vaccination

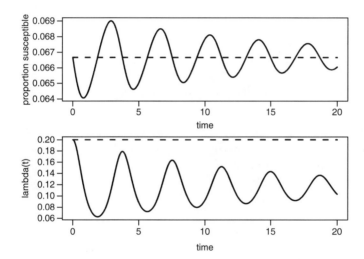

Fig. 3.6 Dynamic aspects of vaccination in the SIR model. Numerical solution for the basic SIR model (3.6) with the parameter setting $\lambda_0 = 0.2$, $\frac{1}{\mu} = 70$, $R_0 = 15$ and $\frac{1}{\nu} = 25$ and 40% vaccination

the susceptible class and become infected decreases. Consequently, $\lambda(t) = \beta I(t)$ decreases. As a result, as shown in Figs. 3.5–3.7 the interepidemic period is longer as p increases. This implies that a vaccination program has two effects on the population. The direct effect is the transfer of a proportion p from the susceptible

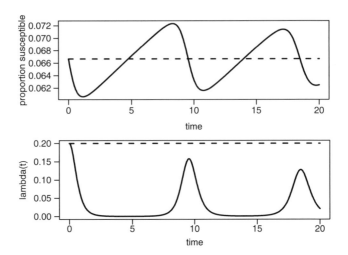

Fig. 3.7 Dynamic aspects of vaccination in the SIR model. Numerical solution for the basic SIR model (3.6) with the parameter setting $\lambda_0 = 0.2$, $\frac{1}{\mu} = 70$, $R_0 = 15$ and $\frac{1}{\nu} = 25$ and 80% vaccination

class directly to the immune class while the indirect effect is related to the decline of the force of infection and its effect on unvaccinated individuals. The latter effect is the herd immunity effect introduced in Sect. 2.4.

3.1.5   The Basic SIR Model with Vaccination in R

In order to include vaccination in the model we need to change the first and the third differential equation in the function *SIR* discussed in Sect. 3.1.3. In the function below p is the proportion vaccinated at birth as in (3.6).

```
SIR=function(t,state,parameters)
{
with(as.list(c(state, parameters)),
{
dS = N*mu*(1-p)-beta*S*I  -  mu*S
dI = beta*S*I - nu*I - mu*I
dR = nu*I -mu*R+N*mu*p
list(c(dS, dI, dR))
})
}
```

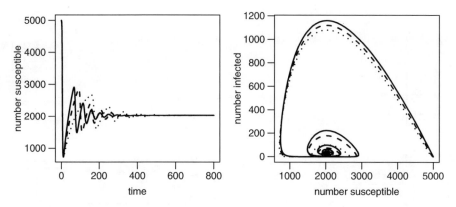

Fig. 3.8 Vaccination in the SIR model. *Left panel*: number of susceptibles for different proportions vaccinated. *Right panel*: $S(t)$ versus $R(t)$ for $p = 0, 0.2, 0.4$ (*solid, dashed*, and *dotted line*, respectively)

Note that the parameter vector and the state variables remain the same as before but we need to specify the proportion vaccinated. For a population of size 5,000, $\beta = 0.0005$, $v = 1$ year^{-1}, life expectancy of 75 years, and vaccination coverage of 40% of newborns we use

```
parameters = c(mu=1/75,beta=0.0005,nu=1)
state = c(S=4999,I=1,R=0)
times=seq(0,1600,by=0.01)
p=0.4
N=5000
```

Figure 3.8 shows the number of susceptibles over time for three scenarios with $p = 0$, 0.2, and 0.4, respectively. Figure 3.8 and the R output below show that in equilibrium the number of susceptibles for $p = 0$ and $p = 0.4$ will be the same (2,026.67). However, the number of infectious individuals for the case where $p = 0.4$ (12.81) will be smaller than the number of infectious individuals for $p = 0$ (39.12).

```
>#number of individuals in equilibrium
>#p=0
> outp0[160001,]
        time        S         I         R
160001  1600  2026.667  39.12281  2934.211
>#p=0.2
> outp02[nnn,]
        time        S         I         R
```

(continued)

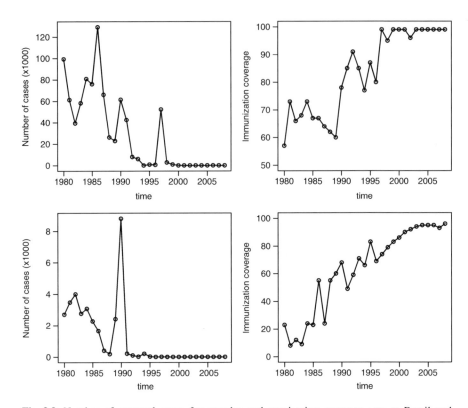

Fig. 3.9 Number of reported cases for measles and vaccination coverage rate at Brazil and Guatemala. Source: World Health Organization: immunization surveillance, assessment, and monitoring. *Top two panels*: Brazil. *Lower two panels*: Guatemala

```
(continued)
160001 1600 2026.667 25.96491 2947.368
>#p=0.4
> outp04[nnn,]
        time         S         I         R
160001 1600 2026.667 12.80705 2960.526
```

An Example: Measles Incidence Data from Brazil and Guatemala

We illustrate the impact of vaccination programs using measles incidence data from Brazil and Guatemala. Figure 3.9 presents the number of reported cases of measles and the coverage rate of vaccination against measles in Brazil and Guatemala (1980–2008). In both countries the yearly incidence decreases as the vaccination coverage increases. Figure 3.9 reveals a second pattern of a possible threshold effect of the proportion of vaccinated individuals on the number of cases (Sect. 2.4).

Note that in Guatemala the number of reported cases from 1999 to 2008 equals zero while the coverage rate increases from 83% in 1999 to 96% in 2008. Similarly, in Brazil, the number of reported cases from 2000 to 2008 equals zero while the coverage rate increases from 87% to 100%.

3.1.6 The Critical Vaccination Coverage

The direct effect of the vaccination program as previously introduced implies that at birth a proportion p of newborns is transferred directly to the immune class. This means that in the new equilibrium after vaccination the proportion of the population in the susceptible class is at most $1 - p$. Recall that in Sect. 3.1.2 we showed that the basic reproduction number at equilibrium is given by $R_0 = 1/s(\infty)$.

Hence, at equilibrium in a vaccinated population $R_0 s(\infty) = R_0(1 - p)$. For $R_0(1 - p) < 1$ the infection will not be able to maintain itself. Therefore, the critical proportion of individuals that has to be vaccinated in order to eliminate the disease, p_c, is the one satisfying $R_0(1 - p_c) = 1$ or

$$p_c = 1 - \frac{1}{R_0}. \tag{3.7}$$

Anderson and May (1991) showed that for such a vaccination program (p vaccinated at birth) the postvaccination force of infection at the new equilibrium decreases linearly with p and is given by

$$\lambda' = \mu R_0(p_c - p),$$

and the postvaccination reproduction number is equal to

$$R = \frac{\lambda' + \mu}{(1 - p)\mu}.$$

As $p \to p_c$ it follows that $\lambda' \to 0$ and the disease will be eliminated.

Let us now turn back to the SIR model as first introduced in Sect. 3.1.1 and discuss how prevaccination serological data can be used to estimate parameters such as the force of infection and the basic reproduction number. To do so we rely on the assumption of endemic equilibrium.

3.2 The SIR Model in Endemic Equilibrium

The starting point in this section is model (3.1) where we assume no disease-related mortality ($\alpha = 0$) and a constant age distribution $N(a)$ which in turn implies constant births as: $B(t) = \int_0^{+\infty} \mu(a)N(a,t)da$. Note that the preceding formula is a

Fig. 3.10 Illustrative figure
of a cross-sectional sample
taken at time $t^\star$

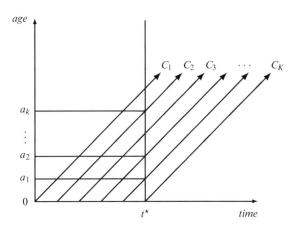

necessary condition to obtain stationarity and does not imply that the age-specific
fertility is the same as the age-specific mortality rate as is evident from, e.g.,
empirical data. Doing so we turn to an age-heterogeneous setting in contrast to the
one of Sects. 3.1.2 and 3.1.4 and further we assume the system to be in endemic
equilibrium. Under endemic equilibrium, also referred to as the steady state of the
model (see e.g. Anderson and May 1991, Chapter 4), there is no time dependence
in the variables resulting in the following set of ordinary differential equations:

$$\begin{cases} \dfrac{dS(a)}{da} = -(\lambda(a)+\mu(a))S(a), \\[2mm] \dfrac{dI(a)}{da} = \lambda(a)S(a)-(v+\mu(a))I(a), \\[2mm] \dfrac{dR(a)}{da} = vI(a)-\mu(a)R(a), \end{cases} \qquad (3.8)$$

and $B(t) = B = \int_0^{+\infty} \mu(a)N(a)da$ is constant. The system of ordinary differential
equations (3.8) is called the time homogeneous model or the static model (Anderson
and May 1991). It assumes that a cohort of individuals is born to a nonvaccinated
population and that the disease is in an endemic equilibrium.

Suppose that the cohort size is $N(0)$ and that at birth all the individuals in
the cohort are susceptible, i.e., $(S(0),I(0),R(0)) = (N(0),0,0)$. The time homogeneous model (3.8) describes how the cohort changes disease stages with age.
Figure 3.10 illustrates this for a population in which cohorts of individuals, marked
by $C_1,\ldots,C_K$, are born at different time points into the population. Note that since
each cohort moves along the 45° line in the age-time plane, age and calendar time
are equivalent given that we take the time of birth as origin.

The calendar time is not of primary interest since the disease is in an endemic
equilibrium and all the derivatives with respect to time are equal to zero. Knowledge
about $\lambda(a)$ and v can give us an indication of how fast individuals in the cohort pass
from the susceptible to the infected class and from the infected class to the immune
class, respectively.

Fig. 3.11 Age-stratified cross-sectional serological sample of hepatitis A from Bulgaria with dots proportional to sample size

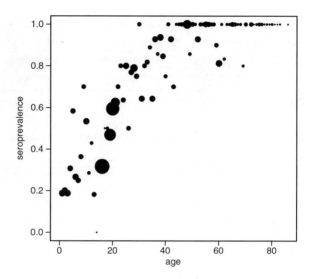

In theory, we could estimate the unknown parameters using a follow-up study in which we follow a cohort from birth to death. In Fig. 3.10, a follow-up study means that we follow a cohort along a single arrow (e.g., C_1) from birth to death and identify the time of infection for the disease of interest. However, conducting such a follow-up study is often not feasible due to the long timescale.

Since the disease is in an endemic equilibrium, the parameters $\lambda(a)$ and v are equal for any two cohorts. The property that $\lambda(a)$ and v are fixed given endemic equilibrium implies that taking a random sample from the population at any point in time $t^\star$ is sufficient to estimate the parameters from that sample.

Suppose that we take a cross-sectional random sample from the population at time $t^\star$, measuring the proportion susceptibles can then be done using markers of past infection. Serological tests use the antibodies as markers of past infection and thus, given that the disease induces lifelong immunity, individuals can be classified according to their status of being immune (seropositive, antibody levels above a predefined cutoff level) or susceptible (seronegative, antibody levels below a predefined cutoff level). We expect the proportion immune to increase with age because of an increase in exposure time with age.

Figure 3.11 shows an age-stratified cross-sectional serological sample of hepatitis A from Bulgaria anno 1964 for which the time-equilibrium assumption is tenable. This figure illustrates the increase of the proportion immune, i.e., the seroprevalence with age (Keiding 1991).

The connection between the time homogeneous representation of the SIR model, serological data, and the estimation of the force of infection is made in Sect. 3.3. A discussion on how one can use antibody levels directly to estimate the force of infection can be found in Chap. 11. In the following section we first elaborate on the time homogeneous model.

3.2.1   Compartments in the Time Homogeneous SIR Model

Before turning to the compartments in the time homogeneous SIR model, we introduce two assumptions often made when including natural mortality in a model. Let $N(0)$ denote the cohort size at birth and $\ell(a)$ the survival function. The number of individuals in the cohort who are still alive at age a is given by

$$N(a) = N(0)P(\text{survival until age a at age } a) = N(0)\ell(a).$$

The two mortality functions often used in the literature are usually referred to as Type I mortality resulting in a population with rectangular age distribution and Type II mortality resulting in a population with exponential age distribution (see, e.g., Anderson and May 1991). For Type I mortality, the survival function is assumed constant up to age L (the life expectancy) after which all individuals promptly die. Hence, for Type I mortality we have

$$N(a) = \begin{cases} N(0) & a \le L, \\ 0 & a > L. \end{cases}$$

For Type II mortality, the probability to survive up to age a is assumed age-dependent, $\ell(a) = e^{-\mu a}$, where μ is a constant mortality rate. For Type II mortality, the life expectancy equals $L = 1/\mu$ and the number of individuals in the cohort still alive at age a is given by $N(a) = N(0)e^{-\mu a}$.

Note that the age distribution in the population is given by $L^{-1}\ell(a)$ which for Type I mortality equals L^{-1} for $a \le L$ and 0 otherwise (rectangular distribution); and for Type II mortality equals $L^{-1}e^{-\mu a} = \mu e^{-\mu a}$ (exponential distribution).

The Type I mortality assumption is sometimes used to approximate the mortality function for developed countries whereas the Type II mortality function is used for most developing countries (Anderson and May 1991). Note that almost any real population has an age-structure in between these two extremes. Assuming Type I or Type II mortality is used because of modeling simplicity and computational ease but not strictly necessary. The impact of the assumptions on models could be substantial when focus is, e.g., on estimating zoster (Brisson et al. 2000) incidence.

We will now discuss each of the compartments in the time homogeneous SIR model. For ease of demonstration we will use a constant force of infection λ in this discussion.

Susceptible Class

Taking into account the survival function $\ell(a)$, the number of individuals in the cohort in the susceptible class at age a, $S(a)$, is given by

$$S(a) = N(0)\ell(a)e^{-\lambda a}.$$

Hence, for Type I and Type II mortality we obtain

$$S(a) = \begin{cases} N(0)e^{-\lambda a} & a \le L, \\ 0 & a > L. \end{cases} \quad \text{and} \quad S(a) = N(0)e^{-(\lambda+\mu)a},$$

respectively. It follows that the derivatives of $S(a)$ with respect to age for Type I and Type II mortality are

$$\frac{dS(a)}{da} = -\lambda N(0)e^{-\lambda a} = -\lambda S(a) \text{ if } a \le L \quad \text{and} \quad \frac{dS(a)}{da} = -(\lambda+\mu)S(a),$$

respectively. For both mortality types, the differential equation describes the change in the susceptible class with respect to age and it is the first differential equation of the static model (3.8) without and with demographic processes, respectively.

Instead of the total number of susceptibles we can define the proportion (or the fraction) of susceptible individuals at age a:

$$s(a) = \frac{S(a)}{N(a)} = \frac{N(0)\ell(a)e^{-\lambda a}}{N(0)\ell(a)} = e^{-\lambda a}. \tag{3.9}$$

Note that when λ depends on age, (3.9) becomes

$$s(a) = e^{-\int_0^a \lambda(u)du}. \tag{3.10}$$

Equation (3.10) illustrates the link to survival analysis where the time to event is the age at infection, $s(a)$ is the survival function (with respect to acquiring infection), $\lambda(a)$ is the age-specific hazard of infection, and $\int_0^a \lambda(u)du$ is the cumulative hazard of infection (see e.g. Therneau and Grambsch 2000).

Infected and Immune Classes

The corresponding differential equation, assuming a constant λ, for the change in the infected class is given by

$$\frac{dI(a)}{da} = \lambda S(a) - (v+\mu)I(a).$$

By integrating with respect to age we obtain the total number of infective individuals $I(a)$:

$$I(a) = \frac{\lambda}{\lambda - v}N(0)\ell(a)\left[e^{-va} - e^{-\lambda a}\right],$$

from which the fraction of individuals in the infected class follows as

$$i(a) = \frac{I(a)}{N(a)} = \frac{\lambda}{\lambda - v}\left[e^{-va} - e^{-\lambda a}\right].$$

Due to the fact that $N(a) = S(a) + I(a) + R(a)$ the fraction immune is

$$r(a) = \frac{R(a)}{N(a)} = 1 - \frac{S(a)}{N(a)} - \frac{I(a)}{N(a)} = 1 - s(a) - i(a).$$

We will now show how the time homogeneous SIR model with constant force of infection is implemented in R.

3.2.2   The SIR Model with Constant Force of Infection at Endemic State in R

We consider two examples in which the force of infection equals 0.1 and 0.2 year^{-1}, respectively. This implies that the average age at infection (which is equivalent to the average time spent in the susceptible class) is 10 years and 5 years, respectively. We assume that the duration in the infected class is 10 days, which means that $v = 1/10$ days^{-1} or $1/(10/365) = 36.5$ years^{-1}. We further assume that $(s(0), i(0), r(0)) = (0.999, 0.001, 0)$.

For a model with $\lambda = 0.1$ and $v = 36.5$ year^{-1}, the parameter vector, the state variables, and the age for integration are given by

```
parameters=c(lambda = 0.1, nu=1/(10/365))
state=c(s=0.999,i=0.001,r=0)
ages=seq(0,90,by=0.01)
```

The time homogenous SIR model (3.8) can be implemented in R in the following way:

```
SIR=function(a,state,parameters)
{
with(as.list(c(state, parameters)),
{
ds=-lambda*s
di=lambda*s - nu*i
dr=nu*i
list(c(ds, di, dr))
})
}
```

Figure 3.12 shows the numerical solutions for the two examples. The upper panels show the results of the model with $\lambda = 0.1$ whereas the lower panels show

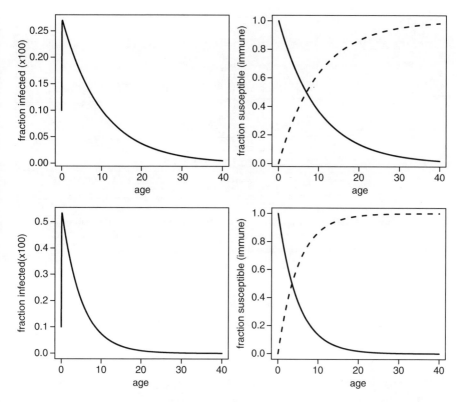

Fig. 3.12 Numerical solution for the static SIR model (3.8). We assume a recovery rate of $v^{-1} = 10$ days. *Upper panels*: $\lambda = 0.1$. *Lower panels*: $\lambda = 0.2$. *Left panels*: fraction of infected individuals. *Right panels*: fraction of susceptible (*solid line*) and immune individuals (*dashed line*)

the results of the model with $\lambda = 0.2$. We notice that for both examples, the fraction infected individuals is relatively small compared to the fraction susceptible and immune. This is due to the differences in average time spent in each compartment. The average duration in the susceptible class is 5 and 10 years for $\lambda = 0.2$ and $\lambda = 0.1$, respectively, and after recovery individuals gain lifelong immunity against reinfection. Compared to an average duration of 10 days in the infected class, we do not expect to observe a high proportion of infected individuals at any age and in fact

$$\frac{R(a)}{N(a)} \approx 1 - \frac{S(a)}{N(a)} \quad \text{or} \quad r(a) \approx 1 - s(a). \tag{3.11}$$

Note that equation (3.11) holds regardless of the assumed age-specific mortality rate as long as there is no disease-related mortality.

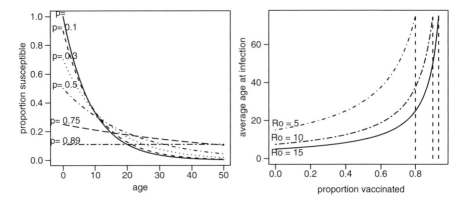

Fig. 3.13 Impact of vaccination programs on the endemic equilibrium after vaccination. *Left panel*: proportion susceptibles by age for different proportions of vaccination with $R_0 = 9.33$ ($p_c = 0.89$). *Right panel*: the average age at infection by proportion vaccinated for different values of R_0. $L = 75$ years

3.2.3 The Critical Proportion of Vaccination in the Time Homogeneous SIR Model

Let us revisit vaccination in the time homogeneous SIR model following Sect. 3.1.4. The proportion susceptible is given by (see Chap. 5, Anderson and May 1991)

$$s(a) \to (1 - p)e^{-(\lambda'a)}.$$

As $p \to p_c$ it follows that $\lambda' \to 0$ and the disease will be eliminated and thus $s(a) = 1 - p_c$.

Let us consider the new equilibrium after vaccination. Figure 3.13 shows the proportion of individuals in the susceptible class at each age value for an infection with $R_0 = 9.33$ ($p_c = 0.89$). Note that for $p = 0.89$ the proportion susceptible in the population is constant and equal to 0.11. For a constant force of infection and Type II mortality with $L = 1/\mu$ (see Sect. 3.2.1), Dietz (1993) showed that at equilibrium $R_0 = L/A = \lambda/\mu$, which means that, for a given value of L, as the average age of infection A increases, R_0 decreases. As $A \to L$, $R_0 \to 1$ and for $A > L$, R_0 is below 1.

Intuitively, we can interpret this as follows: If the average age at infection is higher than the life expectancy, individuals will die before getting infected and therefore the disease cannot spread. At the steady state, after vaccination, the average age at infection of the new equilibrium will be higher than the average age at infection of the steady state before the vaccination program was implemented. Anderson and May (1991) showed that the new average age at infection is $A' = A/(1 - p)$. Figure 3.13 shows the average age at infection, for several values of R_0, as a function of p. Note that as $p \to p_c$ the average age at infection converges to the life expectancy and therefore the disease approaches elimination.

3.3   The Time Homogeneous SIR Model and Serological Data

We now discuss the connection between cross-sectional serological samples and the static model. Let us assume that a cross-sectional sample was taken from the population when the disease is in endemic equilibrium without vaccination. Let Y_i, $i = 1, \ldots, N$, be an indicator variable representing the disease status for the ith individual in the sample

$$Y_i = \begin{cases} 1 & \text{when seropositive (previously infected),} \\ 0 & \text{when seronegative (susceptible to infection).} \end{cases}$$

Let $P(Y_i = 1 | a_i) = \pi(a_i) = E(Y_i | a_i)$ be the probability to be infected before age a_i. It follows that

$$Y_i \sim \text{Bernoulli}(\pi(a_i)).$$

Note that $\pi(a_i) = 1 - s(a_i)$ and using (3.9), which relies on the validity of the SIR assumption for the specific infection under consideration, we obtain

$$\pi(a_i) = 1 - e^{-\lambda a_i}.$$

Hence, in order to estimate the unknown parameter λ, we can define a GLM for the binary response with complementary log–log link function

$$g(\pi(a_i)) = \log(-\log(1 - \pi(a_i))) = \alpha + \log(a_i),$$

where $\alpha = \log(\lambda)$. The model can be implemented in most of the standard software which allows to fit GLMs. For example, a possible implementation using the R procedure function *glm* is given by

```
glmfit=glm(cbind(Pos,Tot-Pos)~1,offset=lAge,
           family=binomial(link=cloglog))
summary(glmfit)
```

Note that *Pos* and *Tot* are the number of seropositives and the sample size at each age value, respectively, and *lAge* is the logarithm of age. Since the linear predictor is $\alpha + \log(a_i)$ we need to use the option *offset* $= lAge$ to ensure that the coefficient of log(age) is 1.

For the Bulgarian hepatitis A data, the estimated force of infection equals $\exp(-2.986) = 0.0505$ with 95% C.I. given by $(0.0459 - 0.0556)$. The solid line in Fig. 3.14 shows the estimated model for the GLM discussed above, together with the data. The dashed line shows a solution for $s(a)$ obtained from the static SIR model (3.8) with $\lambda = 0.0505$ and average duration of 2 weeks in the infected class. Clearly, the dashed line lies almost right on top of the solid line, thus the two

Fig. 3.14 Serological data
and the static SIR model (3.8)
for hepatitis A in Bulgaria:
data, predicted prevalence
(*solid line*) and numerical
solution for the SIR model
with $\lambda = 0.0505$ and v^{-1}
equal to 2 weeks (*dashed line*)

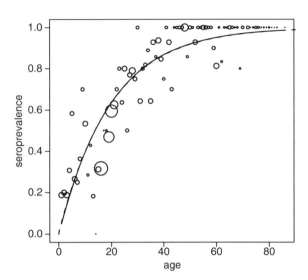

models predict the same pattern for the prevalence. However, there is a fundamental
difference between the two models. The solid line in Fig. 3.14 presents an estimated
model in which the parameters were estimated from the data while the dashed lined
presents a solution of an SIR model in which the parameters were assumed known.

The last point is illustrated graphically in Fig. 3.15. The upper panels show an
example of simulated data generated using the model $\pi(a) = 1 - \exp(-0.0493a)$.
We can clearly see that as the sample size at each age value increases, the variability
of the observed prevalence decreases. The lower panels present the solution of
two SIR models in which the force of infection is assumed to follow a normal
distribution with mean $E(\lambda) = 0.05$ and variance $\sigma_\lambda^2 = 0.02$ and $\sigma_\lambda^2 = 0.01$,
respectively.

The variability in the lower panels is associated with the variance of λ. Note that
as the sample size approaches infinity and $\sigma_\lambda^2 \longrightarrow 0$ both the statistical model and
the mathematical model will predict the same prevalence.

```
Call:
glm(formula = cbind(Pos, Tot - Pos) ~ 1, family =
    binomial(link = cloglog), offset = lAge)

Coefficients:
            Estimate Std. Error z value Pr(>|z|)
(Intercept) -2.98577    0.04866  -61.36   <2e-16 ***
---
Signif. codes:  0 *** 0.001 ** 0.01 * 0.05 . 0.1   1
```

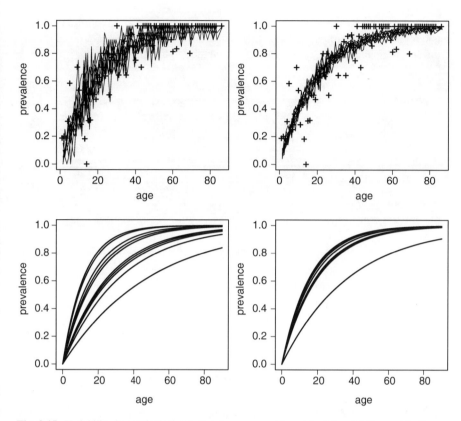

Fig. 3.15 Variability in serological samples (*upper panels*) and in deterministic models (*lower panels*). The *upper panels* present the observed prevalence based on ten samples generated from the true model $\pi(a) = 1 - \exp(-0.0505a)$. Sample sizes at each age group are equal to 20 and 100, respectively. The plusses are the observed prevalence in the Bulgarian dataset. The parameter setting for SIR model is $\mu = 1/75$ for Type I mortality and v^{-1} equals 2 weeks. *Upper left panel:* $n(a) = 20$. *Upper right panel:* $n(a) = 100$. *Lower left panel:* $\lambda \sim N(0.0505, 0.02)$. *Lower right panel:* $\lambda \sim N(0.0505, 0.01)$

This implies that statistical models can be used to estimate the variability that one should incorporate in the transmission model. Furthermore, as Ross (1916) argued, the modeling framework for infectious diseases consists of the interaction between two distinct modeling frameworks which are complementary to each other and which should be used together in order to converge towards the same results.

Estimating the Reproduction Number from Serological Data

Recall that the model for the prevalence (or the probability to be infected before age a) for the serological sample of the Bulgarian hepatitis A data is given by $\pi(a) = 1 - e^{-\lambda a}$. Assuming a constant force of infection, the average age at infection is equal to $1/\lambda$ and $R_0 = \lambda L$ (Dietz 1993). Both the average age at infection, A, and the basic reproduction number, R_0, together with their standard errors can be estimated from serological data by applying the delta method to the *glmfit*-object.

```
> library(car)
> deltaMethod(coef(glmfit),"1/exp((Intercept))",
    vcov.=vcov(glmfit))
                       Estimate        SE
1/exp((Intercept))  19.80182  0.963607
> deltaMethod(coef(glmfit),"75*exp((Intercept))",
    vcov.=vcov(glmfit))
                       Estimate         SE
75*exp((Intercept))   3.78753  0.1843108
```

Assuming that the life expectancy is 75 years, the estimated average age at infection is $\hat{A} = 19.80$ years (95% C.I:17.91–21.69 years) and $\hat{R}_0 = 3.79$ years (95% C.I:3.43–4.15 years). Note that this value equals the estimated value by Keiding (1991) who reported $\hat{R}_0 = 3.8$ using a nonparametric isotonic regression to estimate the prevalence (see Chap. 9 for isotonic regression).

3.4   Models with Maternal Antibodies and Latent Periods

So far all SIR models (without vaccination) assumed that newborns enter the population directly in the susceptible class. In this section we add two additional compartments to the model. The first compartment allows for a maternal antibody period in which individuals are protected and therefore are not yet susceptible. The second compartment describes the latency period, i.e., the period in which the individual is infected but not yet infectious (exposed individuals).

Figure 3.16 shows the observed antibody levels of varicella for individuals below age 18 months in a serological sample taken in Belgium. The antibody level of individuals younger than 12 months starts relatively high and shows a decrease with age up to 1 year. For individuals older than 1 year, the antibody level depends on the infection status and there is a clear separation between individuals who were infected before (and have a high antibody level) and those individuals still susceptible (and who have a low antibody level). More recently, people have used cohort studies to better estimate the decay rate of maternal antibodies (see e.g. Leuridan et al. 2010, 2011).

We can include both a maternal antibody period as well as a latent period in which the individuals are infected but not yet infectious (the exposed class) in the SIR model using the following system of ordinary differential equations while assuming endemic equilibrium:

Fig. 3.16 Antibody levels
(on log scale) for varicella in
Belgium for individuals
younger than 18 months

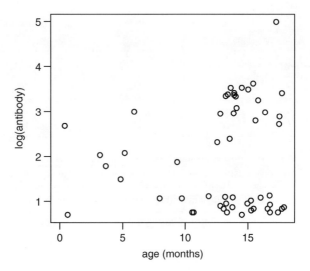

$$
\begin{cases}
\dfrac{dM(a)}{da} = -(\gamma + \mu(a))M(a), \\[2mm]
\dfrac{dS(a)}{da} = \gamma M(a) - (\lambda(a) + \mu(a))S(a), \\[2mm]
\dfrac{dE(a)}{da} = \lambda(a)S(a) - (\sigma + \mu(a))E(a), \\[2mm]
\dfrac{dI(a)}{da} = \sigma E(a) - (v + \mu(a))I(a), \\[2mm]
\dfrac{dR(a)}{da} = vI(a) - \mu(a)R(a),
\end{cases}
\qquad (3.12)
$$

where $M(0) = B$, the number of births in the population, S, I, and R are the number of susceptible, infectious, and immunized or recovered individuals in the population as before, whereas additionally M and E represent the number of maternally protected and infected but not yet infectious individuals, respectively.

Following (3.12), the fraction of individuals protected by maternal antibodies at age a is given by

$$
m(a) = \frac{M(a)}{N(a)} = e^{-\gamma a}.
$$

Figure 3.17 shows the flow diagram for the individuals in the population. Notice that in terms of duration within each compartment, individuals spend few months protected by maternal antibodies and a relatively short time in exposed and infected classes. Longer durations are expected in the susceptible and immune class (assuming lifelong immunity against reinfection).

Figure 3.18 shows an example of an MSEIR model with the following parameter setting: $\gamma = 2$ (average length of the maternal protection is 6 months), $\lambda = 0.2$

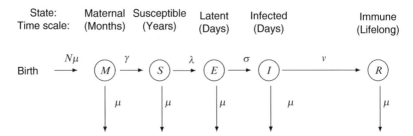

Fig. 3.17 Illustration of the MSEIR model. Individuals enter the population protected by maternal antibodies. After losing maternal immunity individuals move to the susceptible class. When acquiring infection individuals first transfer to the latent or exposed class before becoming infectious, eventually individuals recover and move to the immune class

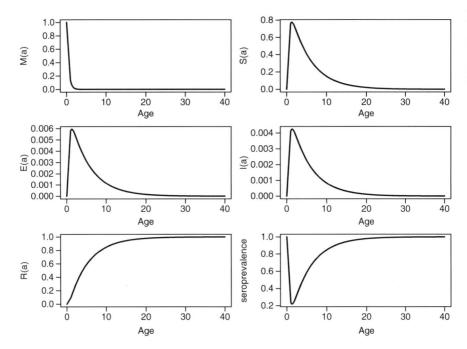

Fig. 3.18 Solution for the MSEIR model (3.12). The average duration in the maternal antibodies class is 6 months, 5 years in the susceptible class ($\lambda = 0.2$), 14 days in the latent class, and 10 days in the infected class

(average age at infection is 5 years), $\sigma = 26.07$ (average duration in the exposed class is 14 days), and $v = 36.5$ (average recovery period is 10 days). It is assumed that after recovery, individuals gain lifelong immunity against reinfection. Note that due to the different timescale for each compartment the fraction of immune individuals is approximately $r(a) \approx 1 - m(a) - s(a)$.

3.5   Transmission Within Multiple Subpopulations

The law of mass action discussed in Sect. 2.4 states that the number of newly infected individuals depends on the current number of infected individuals (I), the number of susceptibles (S), and the transmission rate between these two groups (β). In its simplest form, the mass-action principle states: number of new cases $= \beta IS = \lambda S$ (see Sect. 2.4). The underlying assumption behind the latter equation is that infected and susceptible individuals mix homogeneously and therefore β is age- and time-independent. Note that as a consequence, in endemic equilibrium, the force of infection is constant as we have assumed for the analysis of the Bulgarian hepatitis A data.

The assumption about homogeneous mixing in the population usually does not hold. Most populations do not mix in a random fashion but are made up of subpopulations in and between which individuals mix such as, e.g., different age groups within a school, households within a community, and sexual activity groups within the population. In this section, we discuss transmission settings in which the social structures in the population determine the mixing patterns in the population. We assume that the population is constructed from multiple subpopulations which may or may not interact with each other. As a result, the transmission process is determined by the mixing patterns in the population.

A central characteristic of a model taking into account the mixing patterns in the population is the mixing or "Who Acquires Infection From Whom" (WAIFW) matrix which determines the transmission process (Anderson and Aitkin 1985). For example, considering a population with two subpopulations A and B, the mixing pattern between these two groups can be described by the following WAIFW matrix:

$$C = \begin{pmatrix} \beta_{aa} & \beta_{ab} \\ \beta_{ba} & \beta_{bb} \end{pmatrix}. \tag{3.13}$$

The mixing rate for individuals from group A with those of group B is denoted as β_{ab} and conversely β_{ba} denotes the mixing rate for individuals from group B with those of group A. Individuals can also mix with individuals from the same group. β_{aa} and β_{bb} denote the within-group mixing rates for groups A and B, respectively. Figure 3.19 illustrates the mixing pattern for this simple example.

We now illustrate the behavior of an infectious disease in a population consisting of K subpopulations.

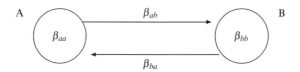

Fig. 3.19 Mixing patterns between two subpopulations: β_{aa} is the mixing rate within group A, β_{bb} is the mixing rate within group B, and β_{ab} and β_{ba} are the mixing rates between the two groups

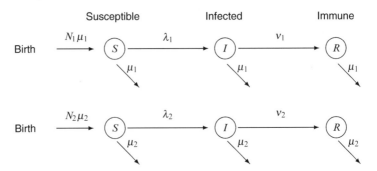

Fig. 3.20 Illustration of an SIR model for two subpopulations

3.5.1 An SIR Model with Interacting Subpopulations

In this section people are assumed to belong to a subpopulation for life. We consider an SIR model in which individuals are assumed to make contact within and across these subpopulations. For a case with K subpopulations the WAIFW or mixing matrix is given by

$$C = \begin{pmatrix} \beta_{11} & \beta_{12} & \cdots & \beta_{1K} \\ \beta_{21} & \beta_{22} & \cdots & \beta_{2K} \\ \vdots & \vdots & & \vdots \\ \beta_{K1} & \beta_{K2} & & \beta_{KK} \end{pmatrix}. \tag{3.14}$$

For each subpopulation, the population size is $N_i = S_i + I_i + R_i$, $i = 1,\ldots,K$. The main difference between the current model and the SIR model discussed in Sect. 3.1.2 is that in the current model the number of new cases in subpopulation i depends on the mixing pattern within and across subpopulations, i.e.,

$$\left(\Sigma_{j=1}^{K}\beta_{ij}I_j\right)S_i = \lambda_i S_i, \quad i = 1,\ldots,K.$$

The system of differential equations for the ith subpopulation is given by

$$\begin{cases} \dfrac{dS_i(t)}{dt} = -\left(\Sigma_{j=1}^{K}\beta_{ij}I_j(t)\right)S_i(t) + N_i\mu_i - \mu_i S_i(t), \\[2mm] \dfrac{dI_i(t)}{dt} = \left(\Sigma_{j=1}^{K}\beta_{ij}I_j(t)\right)S_i(t) - (\mu_i + \nu_i)I_i(t), \\[2mm] \dfrac{dR_i(t)}{dt} = \nu_i I_i(t) - \mu_i R_i(t). \end{cases} \tag{3.15}$$

Figure 3.20 illustrates the flow of $N_i\mu_i$ individuals into the susceptible class for the first two subpopulations.

Implementation in R

Let us consider the special case of $K = 2$ and a symmetric mixing matrix in the population given by

$$C = \begin{pmatrix} \beta_{11} & \beta_{12} \\ \beta_{12} & \beta_{22} \end{pmatrix}. \tag{3.16}$$

Since there are two populations we need to specify six differential equations in the user-defined function *SIRtwo*. The R objects *s1*, *i1*, and *r1* are the proportions corresponding to *S*, *I*, and *R* in the first population and *s2*, *i2*, and *r2* are the proportions corresponding to S, I, and R in the second population. We use the general notation introduced in (3.14) with $K = 2$ where symmetric mixing implies $\beta_{11} = \beta_{22}$ and $\beta_{12} = \beta_{21}$. Since we formulated the model in R in terms of proportions we use $\tilde{\beta}_{ij}$ instead of β_{ij}. Note that $s1+i1+r1 = 1$ and $s2+i2+r2 = 1$.

```
SIRtwo=function(t,state,parameters)
{
with(as.list(c(state, parameters)),
{
ds1 = -(betatilde11*i1+betatilde12*i2)*s1+mu-mu*s1
di1 =  (betatilde11*i1+betatilde12*i2)*s1-nu1*i1-mu*I1
dr1 =    nu1*i1 - mu*r1
ds2 = -(betatilde21*i1+betatilde22*i2)*s2+mu-mu*s2
di2 =  (betatilde21*i1+betatilde22*i2)*s2-nu2*i2-mu*i2
dr2 =    nu2*i2-mu*r2
list(c(ds1,di1,dr1,ds2,di2,dr2))
})
}
```

We run the model using the set of parameters as discussed by Capasso (2008). In the first scenario we assume that both subpopulations are not interacting, i.e., $\tilde{\beta}_{12} = \tilde{\beta}_{21} = 0$. In the second scenario, the model allows for interaction by specifying $\tilde{\beta}_{12} = \tilde{\beta}_{21} = 0.03$. The input parameters for the first scenario are given by

```
parameters=c(betatilde11=0.05,betatilde12=0,betatilde21=0,
             betatilde22=0.05,nu1=1/30,nu2=1/30,mu=0.001)
state=c(s1=0.8,i1=0.2,r1=0,s2=0.8,i2=0.2,r2=0)
times=seq(0,10000,by=0.01)
```

The upper row in Fig. 3.21 shows the infected fraction versus the fraction susceptible individuals in the first subpopulation under the two scenarios. Notice that

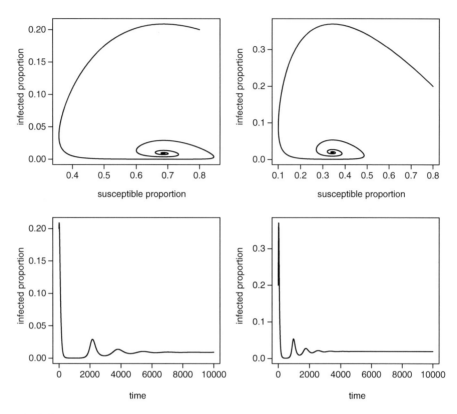

Fig. 3.21 Fraction infected versus susceptible individuals (*upper row*) and the fraction infected individuals versus time (*bottom row*) in an SIR model with two interacting subpopulations for two scenarios. *Left column*: no interaction: $\tilde{\beta}_{12} = \tilde{\beta}_{21} = 0$; *right column*: interaction: $\tilde{\beta}_{12} = \tilde{\beta}_{21} = 0.03$. Parameter setting (Capasso (2008)): $v_1 = v_2 = 1/30$, $s_1(0) = s_2(0) = 0.8$, $i_1(0) = i_2(0) = 0.2$, and $r_1(0) = r_2(0) = 0$

at equilibrium the susceptible fraction is smaller in the second scenario. Although none of the parameters change within the first subpopulation, the first peak occurs earlier in the second scenario as can be seen in the lower row of Fig. 3.21.

In order to investigate the influence of the off diagonal parameter $\beta_{12} = \beta_{21}$ on the endemic equilibrium, we rerun the model for $\tilde{\beta}_{12} = \tilde{\beta}_{21} = 0, 0.025, 0.05$, and 0.075, respectively. We focus the discussion on the first population. The R output in the panel below shows the equilibrium values for susceptible and infected compartments. Figure 3.22 shows that the proportion of infected individuals increases while the proportion of susceptible individuals decreases as a result of the increment in the *between populations* contact rate even though all other parameters in the model remain the same.

Fig. 3.22 Fraction susceptible and infected individuals in the first subpopulation in a SIR model with two interacting subpopulations corresponding with $\tilde{\beta}_{12} = \tilde{\beta}_{21} = 0$ (*solid line*), $\tilde{\beta}_{12} = \tilde{\beta}_{21} = 0.025$ (*dashed line*), $\tilde{\beta}_{12} = \tilde{\beta}_{21} = 0.05$ (*dotted line*), and $\tilde{\beta}_{12} = \tilde{\beta}_{21} = 0.075$ (*dashed–dotted line*). Note that the fraction infected individuals is presented on a log scale

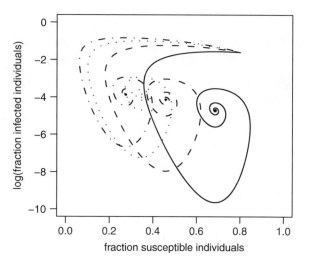

```
>#betatilde12=betatilde21=0.00
> outbeta120[1000001,1:3]
             time         s1              i1
1000001 10000 0.6869925 0.009141676


>#betatilde12=betatilde21=0.025
> outbeta12025[1000001,1:3]
             time         s1              i1
1000001 10000 0.4577859 0.01579231


>#betatilde12=betatilde21=0.05
> outbeta1205[1000001,1:3]
             time         s1              i1
1000001 10000 0.3433333 0.01912617


>#betatilde12=betatilde21=0.075
> outbeta12075[1000001,1:3]
             time         s1              i1
1000001 10000 0.2746667 0.02112621
```

3.5.2 Transmission Over Age and Time

Let us turn to a special case of an SIR model with interacting subpopulations: an age-time dependent SIR model or age-structured SIR model. In such a model the population is divided into a finite number of age groups interacting with each other. Figure 3.23 shows the flow of individuals in an age-structured SIR model.

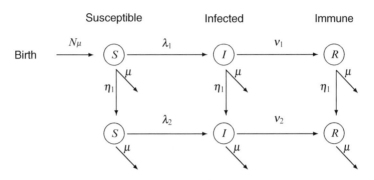

Fig. 3.23 Illustration of an age-structured SIR model with two age groups

An important difference to the model discussed in the previous section is that the flow of individuals into the susceptible class is possible only in the first age class. A second difference is that in the current model, individuals can pass to the same compartment in successive age classes, this means that a susceptible individual in age group i can remain susceptible and transfer (as age passes) to the susceptible compartment in the successive age group, i.e., this individual passes from S_i to S_{i+1}. This model with discrete age compartments represents an alternative strategy to the continuous age-structured model (3.1).

For a population with K age groups, the system of ordinary differential equations for the first age group ($i = 1$) in an age-structured SIR model is given by

$$
\begin{cases}
\dfrac{dS_i(t)}{dt} = - \left(\Sigma_{j=1}^{K} \beta_{ij} I_j(t) \right) S_i(t) + N\mu_i - \mu_i S_i(t) - \eta_i S_i(t), \\[2mm]
\dfrac{dI_i(t)}{dt} = \left(\Sigma_{j=1}^{K} \beta_{ij} I_j(t) \right) S_i(t) - \nu_i I_i(t) - \mu_i I_i(t) - \eta_i I_i(t), \\[2mm]
\dfrac{dR_i(t)}{dt} = \nu_i I_i(t) - \mu_i R_i(t) - \eta_i R_i(t).
\end{cases}
\tag{3.17}
$$

Here, η_i is the rate at which individuals pass from S_i, I_i, R_i to $S_{i+1}, I_{i+1}, R_{i+1}$. From the second age group onwards, the system of differential equations (3.18) is similar to the system in (3.17) but without births into the susceptible class (i.e., without $N\mu_i$) and with the additional flows $\eta_{i-1} S_{i-1}$, $\eta_{i-1} I_{i-1}$, and $\eta_{i-1} R_{i-1}$ corresponding to the susceptible, infected, and recovered compartment from the previous age group, respectively:

$$
\begin{cases}
\dfrac{dS_i(t)}{dt} = - \left(\Sigma_{j=1}^{K} \beta_{ij} I_j(t) \right) S_i(t) + \eta_{i-1} S_{i-1}(t) - \mu_i S_i(t) - \eta_i S_i(t), \\[2mm]
\dfrac{dI_i(t)}{dt} = \left(\Sigma_{j=1}^{K} \beta_{ij} I_j(t) \right) S_i(t) + \eta_{i-1} I_{i-1}(t) - (\nu_i + \mu_i) I_i(t) - \eta_i I_i(t), \\[2mm]
\dfrac{dR_i(t)}{dt} = \nu_i I_i(t) - \mu_i R_i(t) + \eta_{i-1} R_{i-1}(t) - \eta_i R_i(t).
\end{cases}
\tag{3.18}
$$

3.5.3 Estimating the WAIFW Matrix

The age-structured SIR model introduces the challenge of estimating the mixing matrix which, up to this point, was assumed to be known. In practice the mixing matrix is unknown and should be estimated. In order to estimate the WAIFW matrix, Anderson and Aitkin (1985) introduced a framework in which the mixing matrix itself was assumed unknown but its structure, the mixing pattern, was assumed to be known. Let us consider an age-structured SIR model with two age groups, $[0, a_1)$ and $[a_1, L)$, as described above. For each age group there is an age-specific constant force of infection, λ_i, $i = 1, 2$. Using the mixing matrix (3.14) it follows that

$$\begin{pmatrix} \lambda_1 \\ \lambda_2 \end{pmatrix} = \begin{pmatrix} \beta_{11} & \beta_{12} \\ \beta_{21} & \beta_{22} \end{pmatrix} \begin{pmatrix} I_1 \\ I_2 \end{pmatrix}. \tag{3.19}$$

Let us assume that both λ_i and I_i were estimated from prevaccination cross-sectional serological data. In that case we can plug in the estimates in (3.19) and it follows that

$$\begin{aligned} \hat{\lambda}_1 &= \beta_{11}\hat{I}_1 + \beta_{12}\hat{I}_2, \\ \hat{\lambda}_2 &= \beta_{21}\hat{I}_1 + \beta_{22}\hat{I}_2. \end{aligned} \tag{3.20}$$

There are four unknowns (the β's) and two equations in the system (3.20) and therefore the unknowns cannot be determined. The framework as introduced by Anderson and Aitkin (1985) assumed that, although the values of the β_{ij}'s are unknown, the mixing pattern in the population, i.e., the configuration of the WAIFW or mixing matrix C has a specific known structure. For example, consider three possible configurations for the mixing patterns in the population

$$C_1 = \begin{pmatrix} \beta & 0 \\ 0 & \beta \end{pmatrix}, C_2 = \begin{pmatrix} \beta & \alpha \\ \alpha & \beta \end{pmatrix}, C_3 = \begin{pmatrix} \beta & \alpha \\ \alpha & \alpha \end{pmatrix}.$$

The WAIFW matrix C_1 implies an assortative mixing pattern (where people mix only with people of similar age) in which the age groups do not interact with each other. The WAIFW matrix C_2 is symmetric with a common rate parameter on the diagonal, i.e., β is the mixing rate for within age-group contacts and α is the mixing rate for between age-group contacts. In the third WAIFW matrix α is the background mixing rate whereas β is a different within mixing rate for the first age group. Note that these specific structures where the number of unknown mixing parameters is equal to the number of age groups enable the estimation of the mixing parameters.

In Sect. 2.4, it was shown that the basic reproduction number $R_0 = \beta ND$. In the age-heterogeneous SIR model R_0 equals the dominant eigenvalue of the next generation operator, for which the (i, j)th element of the corresponding matrix is given by $\beta_{ij}N_iD$ (here i and j are indices with respect to the age categories, see, e.g., Diekmann et al. (1990)). Note that in an age-homogeneous setting the next generation operator simplifies to βND.

For a more elaborate discussion on estimating WAIFW matrices using prevaccination cross-sectional serological data, we refer to Chap. 14 for an illustration of the traditional approach and Chap. 15 for the approach first introduced by Wallinga et al. (2006) where contact data are used to augment the estimation of the WAIFW matrix from serological data.

3.6   Discussion

In this chapter we introduced the SIR model in terms of its dynamics over time, the impact of vaccination, the time homogenous setting, and the link to serological data. We introduced population structures and mixing patterns in the transmission process. We assumed that the population is constructed from subpopulations that may or may not interact with each other. In part IV of the book we discuss again the problem of the estimation of the basic reproduction number where mixing patterns of individuals in the population are a central characteristic of the estimation procedure. This allows us to obtain more realistic estimates for both R_0 and the associated variability.

Part III
Data Sources

This part introduces the datasets used throughout the manuscript. Three main data sources are being used. The first are serological data, representing the age-specific prevalence of past infection in a population. The second are incidence data such as case reports from passive or active surveillance systems containing the notified counts of disease. The third data source are contact surveys from which contact rates can be estimated. The datasets which we could make publicly available can be found on the web site of the book.

Chapter 4
Data Sources for Modeling Infectious Diseases

In previous chapters, focus was placed on the description of the most important infectious disease parameters. The next chapters will make the connection between the mathematical models and statistical models in order to estimate these parameters from data. In this chapter, we present a range of datasets that are analyzed repeatedly throughout the book. The datasets are used to motivate and illustrate the methods discussed in the text. Three main data sources are being used. The first are serological data, representing the age-specific prevalence of past infection in a population. These are described in Sect. 4.1 including multisera data in which serum samples are tested against multiple diseases (Sect. 4.1.9). The second data source is incidence data such as case reports from passive or active surveillance systems containing the notified counts of disease. Examples of incidence data are listed in Sect. 4.2. The third data source are contact surveys from which contact rates can be investigated, as mentioned in Sect. 4.3. All datasets are available on the web site of this book.

4.1 Serological Data

Serological surveys are commonly used to study the epidemiology of infectious diseases. Serological samples taken at a certain time point provide information about whether or not the individual has been infected before that time point. In practice, antibodies which were formed in response to an infecting organism are identified in the serum. Typically the antibody levels from the serological data are then compared to a predetermined cutoff level to determine whether the individual has been infected before (see Chaps. 5 and 11 for a discussion on this matter). Serological data are usually collected in cross-sectional surveys. Under the assumptions of lifelong immunity and that the epidemic is in a steady state (i.e., at equilibrium), the age-specific prevalence and force of infection can be estimated from such data (Sect. 3.3).

N. Hens et al., *Modeling Infectious Disease Parameters Based on Serological and Social Contact Data*, Statistics for Biology and Health 63, DOI 10.1007/978-1-4614-4072-7_4, © Springer Science+Business Media New York 2012

Table 4.1 Summary of the serological datasets used in this book

Infection	Main transmission route	Time frame	Country	Age range	Multisera companion
Hepatitis A	Feco–oral	1993–1994	Belgium (Flanders)	0–85	–
Hepatitis A	Feco–oral	2002	Belgium (Flanders)	0–65	–
Hepatitis A	Feco–oral	1964	Bulgaria	1–86	–
Hepatitis B	Sexual	1999	St.-Petersburg	0–80	–
Hepatitis C	Blood	2006	Belgium	0–25	–
Mumps	Airborne	1986–1987	UK	1–44	Rubella
Parvovirus B19	Airborne	2001–2003	Belgium	0–82	VZV
Parvovirus B19	Airborne	1996	England and Wales	1–79	–
Parvovirus B19	Airborne	1997–1998	Finland	1–78	–
Parvovirus B19	Airborne	2003–2004	Italy	1–79	–
Parvovirus B19	Airborne	1995–2004	Poland	1–79	–
Rubella	Airborne	1986–1987	UK	1–44	Mumps
Tuberculosis	Airborne	1966–1973	Netherlands	6–18	–
VZV	Airborne	1999–2000	Belgium (Flanders)	1–44	–
VZV	Airborne	2001–2003	Belgium	0–40	Parvovirus B19

In this section we present several serological surveys from less to more severe viral infections like, e.g., the hepatitis A and C virus, mumps, parvovirus B19, rubella, and varicella. For most of these viruses we can assume they govern lifelong immunity after infection. We list these infections in alphabetical order. A summary of the serological datasets used in this book is given in Table 4.1.

4.1.1 Hepatitis A

The hepatitis A virus (HAV) is mainly ($> 95\%$) transmitted through the feco–oral route (e.g., through food and water polluted by faeces containing the virus). Transmission is facilitated by poor hygienic living and housing conditions, and is particularly common in developing countries (Hadler 1991; Beutels et al. 1997). In these countries HAV is mainly a childhood infection, whereas in industrial countries HAV infection occurs during adulthood as well as childhood. In the poorest developing countries, the pattern of high endemicity is characterized by rapid infection at a very young age; over 90% of the children become infected by the age of 5. In this book, the results from two surveys on HAV are used. The first dataset comes from a survey in Flanders (Belgium), the second one from a survey in Bulgaria.

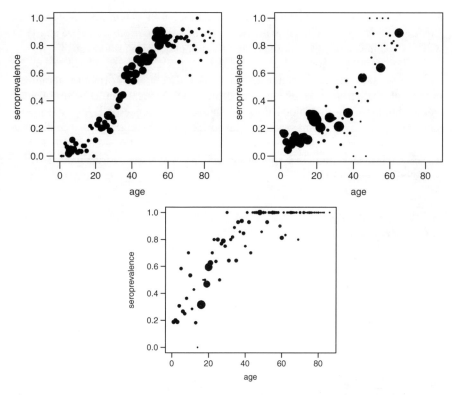

Fig. 4.1 Hepatitis A data. Proportion positive samples based on the cross-sectional survey in Flanders anno 1993–1994 (*upper left panel*), Flanders anno 2002 (*upper right panel*), and Bulgaria (*lower panel*)

In 1993 and early 1994, a study of the prevalence of HAV antibodies was conducted in the Flemish Community of Belgium (Beutels et al. 1997). The purpose of this study was to obtain data on the prevalence of hepatitis A in Flanders and to analyze the epidemiological pattern of HAV. During the study period serum samples were collected from hospitals (noninfectious disease wards) in the Flemish Community. The dataset contains the serological results of 3,161 Belgian individuals together with their age (mostly given in years), ranging from 0.5 to 85 years. The study group was similar in composition to the Flemish population in terms of age. The seroprevalence of Hepatitis A in Belgium is shown in the left panel of Fig. 4.1. The proportion of positive samples per age class is displayed, with the size of the dots proportional to the total number of samples collected. This dataset is used to illustrate parametric modeling approaches in Chap. 6.

A second serological sample of hepatitis A has been collected in 2002. This sample is a subset of the serological dataset of Varicella-Zoster Virus (VZV) and Parvovirus B19 in Belgium where only individuals living in Flanders were selected.

More details about the complete serological dataset are given in Sects. 4.1.5, 4.1.8, and 4.1.9. This dataset together with the hepatitis A data collected in 1993 and 1994 will be used in Chap. 13 to test the assumption of endemic equilibrium.

Keiding (1991) introduced the HAV dataset from Bulgaria. The data consist of a cross-sectional survey conducted in 1964 and contain information about 850 individuals from Bulgaria with age range from 1 to 86 years. Samples were collected from schoolchildren and blood donors. The seroprevalence of HAV in Bulgaria based on this survey is presented in the lower panel of Fig. 4.1. An application of this dataset was already given in Chap. 3, and it is also used in Chap. 6 to illustrate parametric modeling approaches and in Chap. 9 to illustrate models with a monotonicity constraint.

4.1.2   Hepatitis B

Hepatitis B is a major health problem in most parts of the world. The World Health Organization estimates that 350 million people are carriers of the virus and that annually 0.5–0.9 million people die from the disease. Most of the disease burden is due to chronic infection, which can culminate in severe inflammation of the liver, and lead to cirrhosis and hepatocellular carcinoma (HCC). Transmission can occur via a multitude of routes: (1) perinatal transmission from an infected mother to her child; (2) horizontal transmission (mostly from child-to-child) by transfer of blood particles (e.g., in saliva) via small skin wounds; (3) sexual transmission with the rate of sexual partner change and receptive anal intercourse as important risk factors; (4) parenteral transmission by penetration of the skin with an infected object, i.e., by needle stick, mucous membrane splash, tattooing, ear piercing, etc.

Data from a seroprevalence study conducted in St.-Petersburg (Russia) in 1999 are available (Mukomolov et al. 2000). The latter study intended to collect sera from 100 healthy persons (50 males, 50 females) in each of the following age groups: < 1, 1–2, 3–6, 7–10, 11–14, 15–19, 20–24, 25–29, 30–39, and > 40 years of age (total original sample: 1,003 sera). For the youngest age groups, the sample was taken primarily among children in the kindergartens and schools and supplemented with sera from children entering the hospitals with acute noninfectious pathologies (e.g., trauma, emergency surgery, pneumonia). Sera from teenagers and young adults were obtained from a variety of schools (excluding nursing schools) as well as from hospitalized persons requiring urgent surgery. Sera from adults were obtained from primary blood donors, pregnant women, and persons entering the hospitals with acute noninfectious pathologies. All sera were tested for anti-HBc.

The seroprevalence of Hepatitis B in St.-Petersburg is shown in Fig. 4.2. The proportion of positive samples per age class is displayed, with the size of the dots proportional to the total number of samples collected. Based on these serological data, the force of infection of Hepatitis B is estimated in Chap. 5, which is compared with an estimate based on incidence data of Hepatitis B (introduced in Sect. 4.2).

Fig. 4.2 Hepatitis B data. Proportion positive samples based on cross-sectional survey in St.-Petersburg with dots proportional to sample size

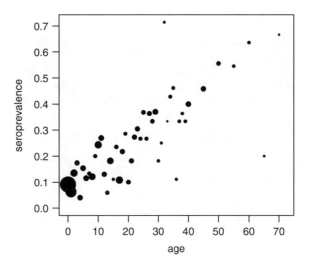

4.1.3   Hepatitis C

The hepatitis C virus (HCV) is the leading cause of known liver diseases in most industrialized countries. It is a common cause of cirrhosis and HCC as well as the most common reason for liver transplantation. At least 170 million people worldwide are believed to be infected with this virus. Following the identification of hepatitis A and hepatitis B, this disorder was categorized in 1974 as "non-A, non-B hepatitis." In 1989, the HCV was discovered and was found to account for the majority of those patients with non-A, non-B hepatitis (Baker 2002). HCV is an RNA virus of the Flaviridae family. There are six HCV genotypes and more than 50 subtypes. These genotypes differ by as much as 30–50% in their nucleotide sequences. The virus also has a high mutation rate. The extensive genetic heterogeneity of HCV has important diagnostic and clinical implications, causing difficulties in vaccine development and the lack of response to therapy (Baker 2002).

HCV transmission occurs primarily through exposure to infected blood. This exposure exists in the context of injection drug users (IDU), blood transfusion, solid organ transplantation from infected donors, use of unsafe medical practices, occupational exposure to infected blood, through birth to an infected mother, multiple sexual partners, and high-risk sexual practices (Baker 2002). Historically, in industrialized countries, blood transfusions and administration of clotting factor concentrates were the most important mode of transmission. However, following the introduction of current blood screening strategies in the early 1990s, HCV infection via these routes has become a rare event in industrialized countries. Hepatitis C seems to be acquired rapidly after initiation of drug injection and many people may have been infected as a result of occasional experimentation with the drug.

Fig. 4.3 Belgian hepatitis C data. Proportion positive HCV samples in injecting drug users as function of the duration of injecting with dots proportional to sample size

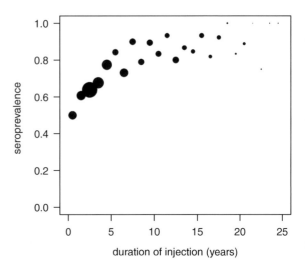

Mathei et al. (2006) presented a study of HCV infection among injecting drug users ($N = 421$). The data consist of IDUs from three areas in Belgium: Charleroi (population: 200,000 inhabitants), Antwerp (a port town with approximately 450,000 inhabitants), and the province of Limburg (a mixed urban–rural population where even the largest cities have no more than 80,000 inhabitants). All injecting drug users were interviewed by means of a standardized face-to-face interview and information on their socio-demographic status, drug use history, drug use, and related risk behavior was recorded. Overall 325 IDUs (77.2%) were found to be seropositive. The timescale used for the analysis is the exposure time or the duration of injection.

The seroprevalence of hepatitis C is presented in Fig. 4.3, with the dots being proportional to the sample size. An application of this dataset appears in Chap. 6 to illustrate some parametric approaches for modeling the seroprevalence and force of infection.

4.1.4 Mumps

Mumps is a childhood disease that occurs worldwide. Mumps is a viral disease caused by a paramyxovirus. The most common symptoms of mumps are bilateral parotid swelling, fever, headache, and orchitis. The symptoms are typically not severe in children, but complications are more common in teenagers and adults. Mumps is a highly contagious disease spread by airborne or droplet transmission.

Before the introduction of the measles, mumps, and rubella vaccine in England in 1988, mumps and rubella occurred commonly in school-aged children, and over 90% of adults had antibodies to mumps and rubella. These results were obtained

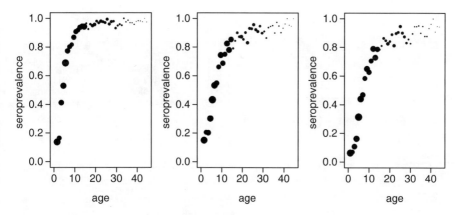

Fig. 4.4 Mumps and rubella data. Proportion of positive samples of mumps and rubella based on a cross-sectional survey in the UK. *Left panel*: proportion infected individuals with mumps. *Middle panel*: proportion infected individuals with rubella. *Right panel*: proportion infected individuals with both mumps and rubella with dots proportional to sample size

from a large survey of prevalence of antibodies to mumps and rubella viruses in the UK (Morgan-Capner et al. 1988). A total of 8,716 samples of serum collected between November 1986 and December 1987 from five public health laboratories in different parts of the UK were tested. The survey, covering subjects from 1 to over 65 years of age, provides information on the prevalence of antibody by age. On average 250 samples were tested for the one-year age categories: 1–14 years; the two-year age categories: 15–34 years; the five-year age categories: 35–44; and the ten-year age categories thereafter.

The age-specific observed prevalences are presented in Fig. 4.4 (left panel), with the size of the dots proportional to the number of samples collected in the corresponding age category. The data on mumps are used in this book to illustrate parametric (Chap. 6) and nonparametric (Chap. 7) approaches to model the prevalence and force of infection and to illustrate Bayesian models for the force of infection (Chap. 10).

4.1.5 Parvovirus B19

Parvovirus B19 is the infectious agent of erythema infectiosum, commonly known as slapped cheek syndrome or fifth disease (Broliden et al. 2006). The disease is usually mild in children and teenagers, but infection during pregnancy has been associated with miscarriage, intrauterine fetal death, fetal anemia, and nonimmune hydrops (Tolfvenstam et al. 2001). The disease is mainly transmitted through the respiratory route, but blood-borne and nosocomial transmissions are reported as

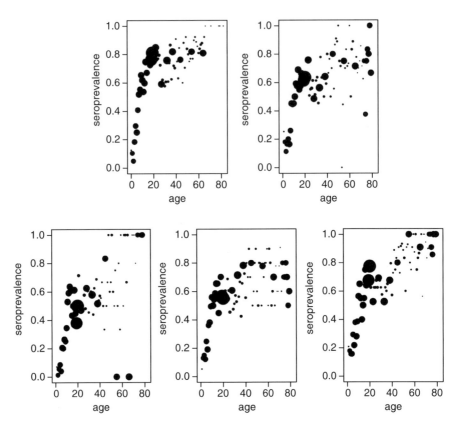

Fig. 4.5 Parvovirus B19 data. Proportion positive samples in Belgium (*left upper*), England and Wales (*right upper*), Finland (*left bottom*), Italy (*middle bottom*), and Poland (*right bottom*) with dots proportional to sample size

well (Young and Brown 2004; Zaaijer et al. 2004). The secondary attack risk for exposed household persons is about 50% and about half of that for classroom contacts.

A seroprevalence survey testing for parvovirus B19 IgG antibody was performed on large representative national serum banks in Belgium, England and Wales, Finland, Italy, and Poland. The sera were collected between 1995 and 2004 and were obtained from residual sera submitted for routine laboratory testing. Sera covered all age groups, were approximately evenly distributed between males and females, and were geographically representative in each country (Mossong et al. 2008b). A total of 3,080, 2,821, 1,117, 2,513, and 2,493 samples from, respectively, Belgium, England and Wales, Finland, Italy, and Poland were tested.

The proportion of positive samples per age class is displayed in Fig. 4.5. The size of the dots is proportional to the number of samples collected. This dataset is analyzed with non- and semiparametric methods in Chaps. 5 and 8. It will be seen that these data lead to an issue of monotonicity, which is described in Chap. 9. Finally, in Chap. 14, the effect of different mixing patterns on the estimation of the force of infection is investigated.

4.1.6 Rubella

Rubella, as mumps, is a childhood disease that occurs worldwide. Rubella, commonly known as German measles, is a disease caused by the rubella virus. It is usually a mild illness causing a rash, sore throat, and swollen glands. However, the symptoms are more severe in adults. Moreover, if a pregnant women gets infected with rubella virus, the virus can cause the potentially sever rubella syndrome in the newborn. Rubella is highly contagious and spreads by airborne or droplet transmission. Before the introduction of mass vaccination, rubella was a common childhood infection spread worldwide. However, since the start of universal vaccination, the incidence of rubella has declined rapidly.

The prevalence of rubella in the UK was obtained from a large survey of prevalence of antibodies to both mumps and rubella viruses (Morgan-Capner et al. 1988) and introduced in Sect. 4.1.4. The age-specific proportions of positive samples are presented in Fig. 4.4 (middle panel) and are analyzed in Chaps. 6 (parametric models), 8 (nonparametric models), and 10 (Bayesian models).

4.1.7 Tuberculosis

Tuberculosis (TB) is a bacterial infection caused by *Mycobacterium tuberculosis*. TB can attack any organ, but most infections are restricted to the lungs. Similar to the common cold, tuberculosis is highly infectious through air droplets via coughing, sneezing, or talking. In many individuals, the infection is asymptomatic, and they cannot spread TB to other people. Approximately 5–10% of the asymptomatic individuals develop active TB at some time during their life. The immunocompromised patients (especially those with HIV infection) are much more likely to develop TB. If left untreated, active TB can progress rapidly to death.

In 1966–1973, a study of tuberculosis was conducted in the Netherlands (Sutherland et al. 1984; Nagelkerke et al. 1999). Schoolchildren, aged between 6 and 18 years, were tested using the tuberculin skin test (purified protein derivative, PPD). If a person is not infected with TB, there is no reaction with the injected PPD. If a person is infected with TB, a raised and reddened area will occur. Indurations larger than 10 mm were considered evidence of previous infections. Since oral BCG vaccination was given to newborns during 1950 and 1951 in the Netherlands, these cohorts have been omitted from analysis (Nagelkerke et al. 1999). The age- and year-specific proportions of positive samples are presented in Fig. 4.6. In Chap. 13, the age- and time-specific prevalence and force of infection are modeled from these data.

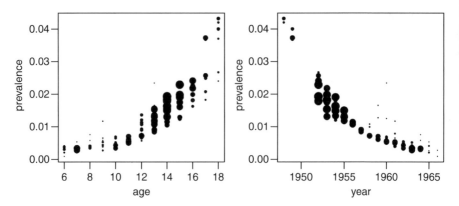

Fig. 4.6 Tuberculosis data. Proportion positive samples of tuberculosis in a survey in the Netherlands as function of age (*left*) and time (*right*) with dots proportional to sample size

4.1.8   Varicella

The VZV, also known as human herpes virus 3, is one of eight herpes viruses known to affect humans (and other vertebrates). Primary VZV infection results in chickenpox (varicella), which may rarely result in complications including bacterial surinfection, encephalitis, pneumonia, and death. It has a two-week incubation period and is highly contagious by air droplets starting two days before symptoms appear. Infectiousness is known to last up to ten days. Therefore, chickenpox spreads quickly through close social contacts. Even when clinical symptoms of varicella have resolved, VZV remains dormant in the nervous system of the host in the trigeminal and dorsal root ganglia.

In this book, we use two cross-sectional surveys which were conducted in Belgium. In the first survey, the age-specific seroprevalence of VZV antibodies was assessed in Flanders (Belgium) between October 1999 and April 2000. Sera from 1,673 individuals, aged 1–44 years, were analyzed. These sera were residual specimens submitted to laboratories for other diagnostic purposes. Sera for the age group 1–12 years were collected from outpatients at a hospital in Antwerp, Belgium. Sera for the age group 12–16 years were obtained from volunteers in vaccine trials (Center for the evaluation of vaccination, Antwerp). Sera for individuals older than 16 years were provided by a medical laboratory in Antwerp. This population was stratified by age in order to obtain approximately 100 observations per age group. Data were reported by Thiry et al. (2002). The second survey is the same as the one used to study the seroprevalence of parvovirus B19 in Belgium, as described in Sect. 4.1.5. In total, 3,080 sera were tested for VZV and 2,657 sera were tested for B19, from which 2,382 sera were tested for both VZV and Parvovirus B19.

Figure 4.7 shows the proportion of positive samples per age class based on the survey in Flanders (left panel) and in Belgium (right panel), with the size of the dots

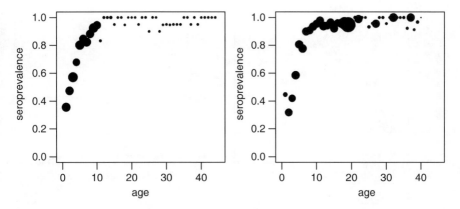

Fig. 4.7 Varicella data. Proportion positive samples of varicella–zoster Virus based on cross-sectional survey in the Flemish population of Belgium (*left panel*) and in the whole population of Belgium (*right panel*) with dots proportional to sample size

proportional to the number of samples collected in the corresponding age category. Based on these data, the force of infection is estimated using parametric models in Chap. 6 and using Bayesian methods in Chap. 10.

4.1.9 Multisera Data

For feasibility and economical reasons, serum samples are often tested for more than one antigen. In this way, the (past) disease status of individuals on multiple diseases is known, and allows studying the association in acquisition between several infections. This is interesting especially when both infections are transmitted through similar routes, i.e., through close contacts. This is the topic of interest in Chap. 12.

In this book, two surveys are being used in which multisera data are collected: mumps and rubella in the UK and varicella VZV and Parvovirus B19 in Belgium. Data from mumps and rubella are obtained from a large survey on the prevalence of antibodies to these infections in the UK, as described in Sects. 4.1.4 and 4.1.6. In this survey, in total 8,179 individuals were tested for mumps, 4,230 were tested for rubella, and of these 4,156 individuals were tested for both mumps and rubella. The age-specific observed prevalences for having had both diseases are presented in Fig. 4.4 (right panel), with the size of the dots proportional to the number of samples collected in the corresponding age category.

Data from VZV and Parvovirus B19 are collected in a survey in Belgium, as described in Sects. 4.1.8 and 4.1.5, respectively. In total, 3,080 sera were tested for VZV and 2,657 sera were tested for B19, from which 2,382 sera were tested for both VZV and Parvovirus B19. Figure 4.8 shows the observed proportion of sera

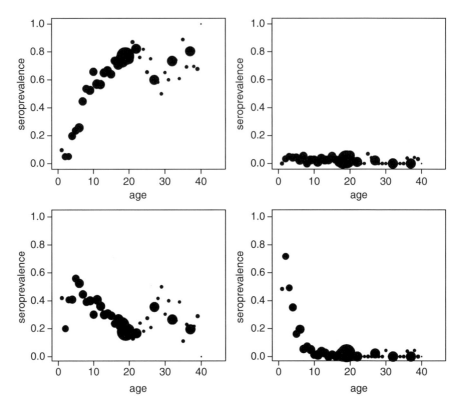

Fig. 4.8 Varicella and parvovirus B19 data. Proportion of samples that tested positive on both varicella and parvovirus (*top left panel*), that tested positive on varicella only (*top right panel*), that tested positive on parvovirus only (*lower left panel*), and that tested negative on both viruses (*lower right panel*), based on a cross-sectional survey in Belgium anno 2001–2003 with dots proportional to sample size

that tested positive for both VZV and B19 (top left panel), that tested positive on varicella only (top right panel), that tested positive on parvovirus only (lower left panel), and that tested negative on both viruses (lower right panel).

4.2   Hepatitis B Incidence Data

Incidence data, also often called case notifications, measure the number of people who get a disease in a certain time period. This is different from the prevalence measured by serological data, describing the number of people who have (had) the disease. Incidence data are commonly obtained from governmental notifications, disease registries or from hospital or physician diagnosis.

The incidence of Hepatitis B in St.-Petersburg (Russia) was estimated from mandatorily reported cases (Beutels et al. 2003). By law, physicians and nurses

Table 4.2 Summary of Hepatitis B incidence data

Year	Reported number of cases	Average age of symptomatic case		Ratio Male/Female	Reported cases per 100,000
		Male	Female		
1994	1,903	24.27	25.49	1.71	39.79
1995	2,167	23.33	26.24	1.77	44.94
1996	1,741	24.11	26.48	1.58	35.81
1997	1,364	25.38	26.43	1.84	27.89
1998	1,611	23.30	25.10	2.15	32.71

have to refer all acute symptomatic (jaundiced) cases to a hospital. Russian health care officials are convinced that non-referral of symptomatic cases is virtually nonexistent. Since 1994, referred cases are diagnosed as caused by hepatitis A, B, or C by means of clinical diagnosis combined with highly sensitive and specific blood tests. All Hepatitis B virus cases are mandatorily reported as regards age (in years), gender, and date (monthly) to a central registrar. A general summary of the findings based on reported incidence between 1994 and 1998 is given in Table 4.2. It shows the yearly number of reported symptomatic cases of Hepatitis B, the average age at notification of the case per gender, the ratio of male to female cases, and the number of reported symptomatic cases per 100,000 inhabitants. Figure 4.9 shows the annual age- and gender-specific number of reported acute symptomatic Hepatitis B cases per 100,000 inhabitants. The full line shows the incidence of symptomatic cases for males, the dashed lines for females. The data over the years seem to show a weak cyclic evolution. A peak of new infections is observed for individuals aged around 20 years, with higher incidence for males as compared to females.

It is well established that acute symptomatic infections present only part of the picture because most Hepatitis B infections evolve asymptomatically or atypically. The probability of showing clinical symptoms upon acute infection ranges from 4% to 11% in children between 1 and 5 years old (McMahon et al. 1985; Shapiro 1993; Edmunds et al. 1993). This probability gradually increases with increasing age at infection. In approximately 3 of 4 infected adults the illness is asymptomatic or presents only flu-like symptoms. The age-dependent ratio of total versus symptomatic infections, derived from McMahon et al. (1985); Shapiro (1993); Edmunds et al. (1993), is presented in Fig. 4.10.

Applying this property to the reported symptomatic cases, we estimated the total number of Hepatitis B infections by age at infection over time. The total number of cases (i.e., symptomatic and asymptomatic infections combined) is estimated as 10,762, 12,271, 9,818, 7,841, and 9,255 for years 1994–1998. Thus, the total incidence is estimated fivefold greater than the reported incidence. Overall, 8,786 symptomatic cases were reported over the 5 years combined and 49,947 number of infections were estimated. The annual age- and gender-specific number of estimated Hepatitis B infections per 100,000 inhabitants is presented in Fig. 4.11. The same trends as in Fig. 4.9 are observed, but the peaks are even more pronounced.

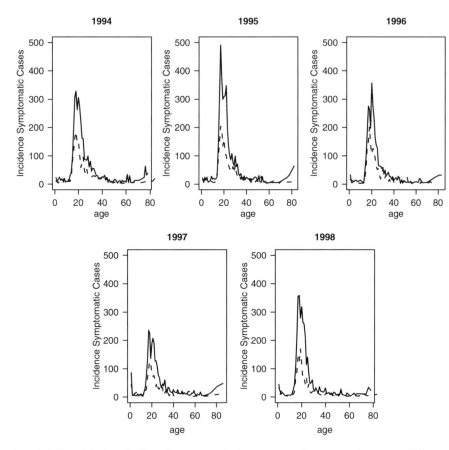

Fig. 4.9 Hepatitis B in St.-Petersburg: yearly incidence rates of symptomatic cases. *Solid line*: males; *dashed line*: females

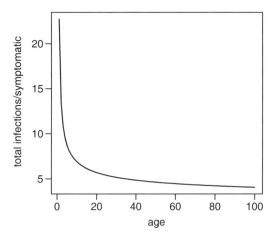

Fig. 4.10 Age-specific proportion of the total number of Hepatitis B cases versus the number of symptomatic Hepatitis B cases

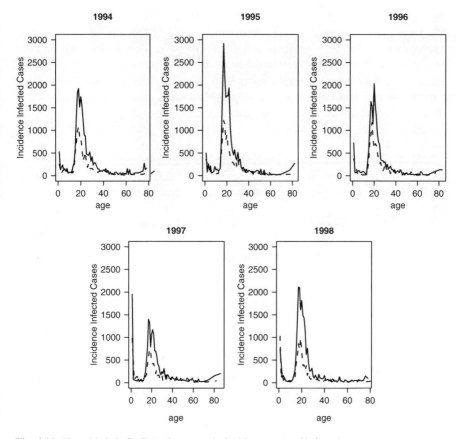

Fig. 4.11 Hepatitis B in St.-Petersburg: yearly incidence rates of infected cases

4.3 Belgian Contact Survey

Mathematical models of infectious diseases require assumptions on the way the disease is spread. These assumptions are typically related to the social interactions of individuals, or how individuals mix with each other. One can impose a certain mixing pattern or estimate the mixing pattern from a contact survey. This is discussed in Chaps. 14 and 15.

The European commission project "POLYMOD" conducted a large multi-country population-based survey, in order to gain insight into social mixing behavior relevant to the spread of close contact infections (Mossong et al. 2008b). These surveys of social contacts were held in eight European countries: Belgium, Germany, Finland, Great Britain, Italy, Luxembourg, the Netherlands, and Poland. Previous to this survey, only small-scale surveys had been conducted to get some idea of the social contacts (Edmunds et al. 1997, Beutels et al. 2006, Edmunds et al. 2006, Wallinga et al. 2006, Mikolajczyk and Kretzschmar 2008). In Belgium, this survey was conducted in a period from March until May 2006. A total of 750 participants, selected through random digit dialing, completed a diary-based questionnaire about their social contacts during one randomly assigned weekday and one randomly assigned day in the weekend (not always in that order). Survey participants were recruited in such a way as to be broadly representative of the whole population in terms of age, sex, and geographical spread. Children and adolescents were deliberately oversampled, because of their important role in the spread of infectious agents. Only one person per household was asked to participate in the study.

The dataset consists of participant-related information such as age and gender and details about each contact: age and gender of the contacted person, and location, duration, and frequency of the contact. In case the exact age of the contacted person was unknown, participants had to provide an estimated age range and the mean value is used as a surrogate. Further, a distinction between two types of contacts was made: non-close contacts, defined as two-way conversations of at least three words in each others proximity, and close contacts that involve any sort of physical skin-to-skin touching. For young children, a parent or exceptionally another adult caregiver filled in the diary. Using census data on population sizes of different age by household size combinations, weights are given to the participants in order to make the data representative of the Belgian population. In total, 12,775 contacts were recorded of which 3 are omitted from analysis due to missing age values for the contact person. For a more in depth perspective on the Belgian contact survey and the importance of contact rates on modeling infectious diseases, we refer to Hens et al. (2009b) and Chap. 15.

Part IV
Estimating the Force of Infection

This part focuses on the estimation of the force of infection. The first chapter introduces basic statistical concepts and notation related to the analysis of serological data and briefly discusses several modeling issues. In subsequent chapters we discuss several statistical models to estimate the prevalence and the force of infection, mainly as a function of age but also as a function of other covariates. We will discuss their pros and cons and will look into more detail at assumptions, complexities, and other issues. Chapter 6 reviews rather restrictive parametric models as well as more flexible parametric models, whereas Chaps. 7 and 8 discuss non- and semiparametric alternatives. In Chap. 9 it is shown how to deal with the constraint of monotonicity. Bayesian models are introduced in Chap. 10. Chapter 11 introduces an alternative approach based on mixture models which allows antibody levels to be directly modeled, without the use of any threshold(s) and corresponding dichotomization. In Chap. 12, models are extended by considering joint estimation of serological data of two or more diseases. In Chap. 13, modeling serial seroprevalence data in terms of both age and time is discussed.

Chapter 5
Estimating the Force of Infection from Incidence and Prevalence

As discussed in Chap. 4, the use of serological surveys is one of the most common ways to investigate the epidemiology of infectious diseases and to estimate important parameters such as the force of infection. This chapter introduces basic statistical concepts and notation related to the analysis of serological and incidence data and briefly discusses several modeling issues.

5.1 Serological Data

Consider an age-specific cross-sectional sample of size N and let a_i be the age and Z_i the antibody activity level (in U/ml) of the ith subject. The antibody activity levels Z_i are quantitative results calculated from the optical densities obtained from commercial IgG enzyme immune-assays (EIAs). The left panel of Fig. 5.1 shows a scatter plot of the logarithm of the antibody activity levels as a function of age for data on the Parvovirus B19 infection. The data shown in Fig. 5.1 result from testing for parvovirus B19 IgG antibodies on a large representative Belgium serum bank and were collected between 1995 and 2004. As there is currently no vaccine available against parvovirus B19 and because immunoglobulin G (IgG) antibodies following infection are thought to persist for a lifetime, these antibody activity level data can be used to derive the force of infection. The right panel of Fig. 5.1 shows a histogram of the antibody levels (on a log scale), clearly showing that the distribution of the log(IgG) in the population can be considered as arising from a mixture of susceptible individuals (left part) and of infected (or immune) individuals (right part). This mixture concept will be further exploited in Chap. 11, where we introduce an estimation method which acts directly on the antibody activity levels.

The coming chapters however take dichotomized data as the starting point for estimating the force of infection. Corresponding to the compartmental mathematical model in Chap. 3, each individual is compartmentalized into the susceptible or a non-susceptible compartment (merging the I and R compartments) according to predefined threshold values. In Fig. 5.1 such threshold values are shown for the

N. Hens et al., *Modeling Infectious Disease Parameters Based on Serological and Social Contact Data*, Statistics for Biology and Health 63, DOI 10.1007/978-1-4614-4072-7_5, © Springer Science+Business Media New York 2012

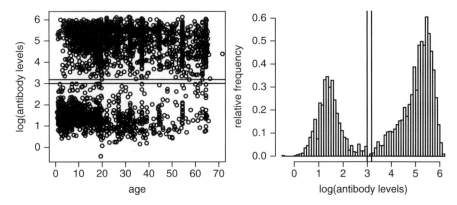

Fig. 5.1 Belgian Parvovirus B19 data. Logarithm of antibody activity levels in U/ml. *Left panel*: as function of the individual's age, with threshold values as *horizontal lines*. *Right panel*: histogram with threshold values as *vertical lines*

Belgian Parvovirus B19 data (as horizontal lines in the left panel and vertical lines in the right panel). Samples with antibody activity levels exceeding 24 U/ml (3.178 on log scale) were considered positive, while samples with antibody activity levels less than 20 U/ml (on log scale 2.996) were considered negative, and samples in between were considered equivocal. In this example the number of equivocal results is limited and therefore excluded from further analyses. But in general the choice of the lower and upper threshold and the treatment of the equivocal cases as missing data are important issues in the analysis of serological data. As compartmentalization is not needed in the direct method, this is one of the main advantages of this approach (Chap. 11).

Define the dichotomized version of Z_i as the binary variable Y_i:

$$Y_i = \begin{cases} 1 & \text{if} \quad Z_i > \tau_u, \\ 0 & \text{if} \quad Z_i < \tau_\ell, \end{cases} \tag{5.1}$$

and missing if $\tau_\ell < Z_i < \tau_u$ where τ_ℓ and τ_u are the lower and upper threshold values (20 respectively 24 U/ml for Parvovirus B19). So, for each individual i we observe whether (s)he has experienced infection before age a_i. We do not observe the age at infection, but rather a censored value: right censored if $Y_i = 0$ and left censored if $Y_i = 1$. This censored data point of view and this link to survival analysis will regularly show up. The left panel of Fig. 5.2 shows the values of Y_i as a function of age a_i as dichotomized version of Z_i in Fig. 5.1.

Denote $\pi(a_i)$ the probability to be infected before age a_i. This probability will be referred to as the so-called seroprevalence. It is important to note that, due to misclassification, the seroprevalence is not exactly equal to the disease prevalence. This brings us to concepts of sensitivity and specificity of diagnostic tests, an important issue which is addressed further in Chap. 11.

In coming chapters different ways to model $\pi(a_i)$ are introduced and discussed, from fully parametric to fully nonparametric models. They are all based on

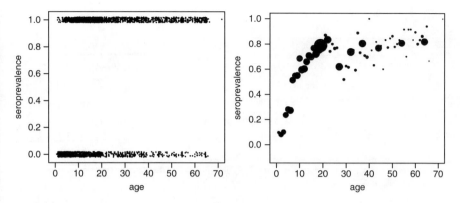

Fig. 5.2 Belgian Parvovirus B19 data. Dichotomized antibody activity levels. *Left panel*: (jittered) individual data as function of age. *Right panel*: proportion positive, as function of the corresponding one-year age categories with dots proportional to sample size

maximizing the loglikelihood as a function of the model parameters (Appendix B.1), based on the data $\{(a_i, Y_i)\}_{i=1}^{N}$, where N denotes the sample size (excluding the equivocal cases). The loglikelihood is given by

$$\ell = \sum_{i=1}^{N} Y_i \log\{\pi(a_i)\} + (1 - Y_i) \log\{1 - \pi(a_i)\}. \tag{5.2}$$

For notational simplicity, the dependence on the model parameters is suppressed here, but will be made explicit in coming chapters. In the terminology of generalized linear models (GLM, see, e.g., McCullagh and Nelder (1989) and Appendix B.2), the age-dependent probability $\pi(a)$ is modeled as

$$g(P(Y = 1|a)) = g(\pi(a)) = \eta(a), \tag{5.3}$$

where $\eta(a)$ is the so-called linear predictor and g is the so-called link function. For binary responses, g is often taken to be a logit link function, $\log(\pi/(1 - \pi))$, but other link functions such as the complementary log–log link, $\log(-\log(1 - \pi))$, and log link, $-\log(1 - \pi)$, can be used as well. In the next section the age-dependent force of infection (FOI), $\lambda(a)$ is derived from the seroprevalence $\pi(a)$, for different link functions g. Strictly spoken, we should use terminology as "sero-FOI," as it is derived from the seroprevalence.

5.2   Age-Dependent Force of Infection

As discussed in Chap. 3 the force of infection can be easily derived from the seroprevalence under assumptions including time homogeneity and lifelong immunity. In terminology of survival analysis, the FOI is nothing else than the hazard function.

Table 5.1 General expressions for the force of infection according to different link functions in a GLM framework

Link function	$\pi(a)$	$\delta(\eta(a))$	$\lambda(a)$
log	$1 - e^{-\eta(a)}$	1	$\eta'(a)$
complementary log–log	$1 - e^{-e^{\eta(a)}}$	$e^{\eta(a)}$	$\eta'(a)e^{\eta(a)}$
logit	$\dfrac{e^{\eta(a)}}{1 + e^{\eta(a)}}$	$\dfrac{e^{\eta(a)}}{1 + e^{\eta(a)}}$	$\eta'(a)\dfrac{e^{\eta(a)}}{1 + e^{\eta(a)}}$
probit	$\varPhi(\eta(a))$	$\dfrac{\phi(\eta(a))}{1 - \varPhi(\eta(a))}$	$\eta'(a)\dfrac{\phi(\eta(a))}{1 - \varPhi(\eta(a))}$

$\varPhi$ denotes the cumulative distribution function and ϕ the density function of the standard normal distribution

Using a so-called catalytic model with log link (i.e., $\pi(a) = 1 - e^{-\eta(a)}$) leads to a simple interpretation of the first derivative of the linear predictor. Indeed, $\eta(a)$ is the cumulative hazard and hence the force of infection is simply the first derivative of the linear predictor:

$$\lambda(a) = \frac{\pi'(a)}{1 - \pi(a)} = \frac{\eta'(a)e^{-\eta(a)}}{e^{-\eta(a)}} = \eta'(a). \tag{5.4}$$

In general, when the link function is not restricted to be the log link, the force of infection can still be derived analogously. Basic calculus shows that for a GLM based on (5.2) and (5.3), the force of infection can be expressed as a product of two functions:

$$\lambda(a) = \eta'(a)\delta(\eta(a)). \tag{5.5}$$

Here, $\delta(\cdot)$ is a known function for which the form is determined by the link function g. Table 5.1 shows the aforementioned four link functions with their corresponding structure for the force of infection.

In the coming chapters we will introduce and discuss several ways to model the predictor $\eta(a)$ in combination with a particular link function g. This will lead to estimates $\hat{\pi}(a) = g^{-1}(\hat{\eta}(a))$ and, according to Table 5.1, to estimates $\hat{\lambda}(a)$ for the force of infection. In the next section we look into important complexities and issues when modeling the FOI.

5.3 Modeling Issues

Figure 5.3 shows the right panel of Fig. 5.2 again, but extended with the proportion positives of the age category from 0 to 6 months (excluded previously) and overlaid with the fits for the seroprevalence and the FOI, based on a local quadratic fit with a (too) small smoothing parameter. Note that the local polynomial estimator will be discussed in more detail in Chap. 7. Here its application with a nonoptimal smoothing parameter will just serve illustrative purposes.

Fig. 5.3 Belgian Parvovirus B19 data. Proportion positive, as function of the corresponding one-year age categories, extended with the proportion positives for the age group from 0 to 6 months (indicated with *open circle*), together with a local polynomial fit for seroprevalence (*upper curve*) and for the force of infection (*lower curve*), using a (too) small smoothing parameter with dots proportional to sample size

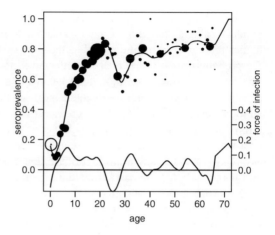

A *first issue* is the definition of antibody activity levels as they truly reflect natural infection, rather than maternal antibodies (inherited immunity) or vaccine induced activity (vaccine immunity). Since there is currently no vaccine available against Parvovirus B19, the latter possibility can be discarded. For the age group from 0 to 12 months the distinction between maternal antibodies and those reflecting natural infection is less clear. It is generally accepted that maternal antibodies fade away during the first 6 months, whereafter naturally acquired antibodies take over (Sect. 3.4). But within the first 12 months the data cover a mixture of two types of antibodies, which is especially difficult to categorize at the (unknown) change point around 6 months. Figure 5.3 includes the proportion positives 0.17 in the age group of 0–6 months. An ad hoc approach commonly applied is to delete the observations which are believed to refer (at least partly) to maternal antibodies (in this case corresponding to the first 6 months).

A *second issue* is the decay of the antibody activity some (longer) time after infection, and related to that, the assumption of lifelong immunity. Of course this depends highly on the infectious disease under consideration. For Parvovirus B19 it is assumed that immunity is lifelong and that antibody levels persist after infection and remain for a long time at a higher level, certainly above the threshold(s). The left panel of Fig. 5.1 does not seem to contradict this assumption. We refer to Goeyvaerts et al. (2011) for a more in depth discussion about this issue for Parvovirus B19.

A *third issue* concerns the already mentioned possibility of misclassifying an individual as susceptible or being infected (using the threshold(s) approach), together with the deletion of the equivocal cases. It is not always clear what consequences are implied by this problem, such as bias in the estimation of the force of infection and consequently in the estimation of the basic reproduction number. Methods to correct for misclassification, based on estimates for the sensitivity and the specificity, can be used, as well as direct estimation avoiding this problem. These methods are discussed in Chap. 11. Depending on the type of infection, this issue is ignored or taken care of. Here, in most chapters, we assume it is reasonable to ignore this issue.

As antibody activity reflects past infection, the seroprevalence $\pi(a)$ should be nondecreasing as function of age a. This *fourth issue* seems an obvious point: the higher the age a of an individual at the time of the (serological) test, the higher the probability that (s)he has been infected in the past. The local quadratic fit in Fig. 5.3 shows some non-monotone behavior, not only partly as a consequence of a too small smoothing parameter, but also through the presence of maternal antibodies (as indicated in the decrease at the very low ages) and by a striking jump downward at about the age of 25 years. Is it an artifact, a confounding factor or a true process related to the disease and contradicting the time homogeneity assumption? Did a new more highly virulent strain of the same disease take over at some point in time in past? Note that a decreasing behavior of the seroprevalence fit is translated into a negative FOI, as shown by the lower curve in Fig. 5.3. We again refer to Goeyvaerts et al. (2011) for a more in depth discussion about this peculiar profile for Parvovirus B19.

The fourth issue brings us in a seamless way to the *fifth issue*: the choice of a model for the predictor function $\eta(a)$. Choosing a too restrictive parametric model might not reveal complications in the data, such as an apparent non-monotonicity. Moreover, a too restricted model might not be able to indicate multiple peaks in the force of infection. It is clear that the fit in Fig. 5.3 is too closely following the data, not only indicating unnecessary areas with a negative force of infection, but also indicating too many local peaks. The optimal selection of the smoothing parameters, as well as the type of smoothing, are intrinsic parts of finding an appropriate flexible model. In the next chapters we will illustrate several approaches, starting with a historical overview on basic parametric models, gradually moving to more flexible parametric, nonlinear, nonparametric, and semiparametric models.

A final *sixth issue* concerns the paradigm for inference. Where most of the methods in this book are formulated in the likelihood framework, we will also look at Bayesian approaches in Chap. 10 (see Appendix B.5). A related point is whether inference is based on a single final model or whether one should opt for multi-model inference (model-averaging).

We conclude this chapter with a brief note on how incidence data can be used to estimate the force of infection.

5.4   Incidence Data

Let X_{ij} be the number of infections in age group i $(i = 1, \ldots, I)$ at time j $(j = 1, \ldots, J)$ and N_{ij} the corresponding population sizes. Based on age-specific incidence data (X_{ij}, N_{ij}), it is straightforward to calculate the age-specific incidence rate, or attack rate, defined as the number of new cases per time unit in a given age class divided by the total number of individuals in that age class in the population

$$X_{ij}/N_{ij}.$$

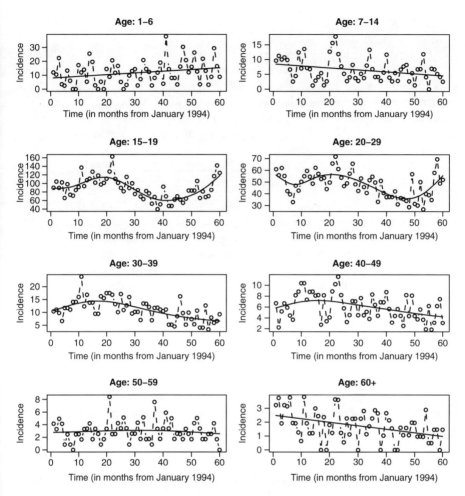

Fig. 5.4 Hepatitis B in St.-Petersburg: age-specific incidence of all infections (symptomatic and asymptomatic) in time, per age group

Figure 5.4 shows incidence estimates of all hepatitis B infections (i.e., symptomatic and asymptomatic infections combined) per 100,000 inhabitants in St.-Petersburg from January 1994 to December 1998. For each age group, a cubic regression spline (see Chap. 8) is used to estimate the trend in time. Figure 5.4 shows a slightly increasing incidence in the 1-6-year old and quasi-status quo for age groups above 40 years. It seems noteworthy that the group aged 50–59 years was born just before or during the second world war. These birth cohorts were very small compared to other cohorts. Furthermore, as a result of the specific circumstances during or in the aftermath of the war, these people may have been exposed to the virus and co-mortality relatively more and earlier in life compared with other age groups (Beutels et al. 2003). In all the intermittent age groups the incidence of infection shows a decreasing effect until the year 1997. Between 1997 and 1998 the incidence increased markedly among the age groups of 15–19- and 20–29-year old.

The attack rate however does not account for the number of individuals that are still at risk for the infection. A decrease in the attack rate with time can be due either to a decrease in the rate at which individuals acquire the infection or to a decrease of the number of susceptible individuals in the population. As a result, the attack rate should be interpreted with care (Grenfell and Anderson 1985).

Assuming time homogeneity (as commonly assumed for serological data), the force of infection $\lambda(a)$ is given by

$$\lambda(a) = X_a/S_a, \tag{5.6}$$

with S_a and X_a the number of cases of age a. Muench (1934) was the first to use a model to estimate the rate at which susceptibles acquire infection, or the force of infection, from summation data. He suggested using a catalytic model to do so. The case notifications can be accumulated to obtain a measure of the rate at which a susceptible acquires infection (and not necessarily disease). Griffiths (1974) and Grenfell and Anderson (1985) extended this approach to encompass a more flexible description of changes in the FOI with age. A common assumption made is that all members of the population are susceptible at birth, a necessary assumption because of the lack of information on the susceptible population in a case notification system. Another option is to start from an assumed percentage of susceptibility for newborns ($S_0 = p_s N_0$) in order to estimate the force of infection, as proposed by Hens et al. (2008a). Note that assuming a fully susceptible birth cohort corresponds to the absence of vertical transmission. Given $S_0 = p_s N_0$, the number of susceptibles for any other age group a can then be calculated recursively as

$$S_a = \frac{S_{a-1} - X_{a-1}}{N_{a-1}} N_a, \tag{5.7}$$

with $X_0 \equiv 0$. Varying the percentage of susceptibility p_s then results in a sensitivity analysis on the estimated force of infection.

Figure 5.5 shows the estimated force of infection based on the incidence data of Hepatitis B in St.-Petersburg. Similar to modeling the incidence rates using cubic regression splines, we model the susceptibility rates calculated from the crude data using (5.6) and (5.7), conditional on the assumed proportion of susceptibility p_s. We let the proportion of susceptibility at birth p_s vary over the interval 0.8 to 1.0 in steps of 0.05 and look at the effect on the estimated force of infection. The full line in Fig. 5.5 shows the estimated year-specific force of infection profile, conditional on $p_s = 1$. When decreasing the susceptibility proportion p_s, the magnitude of the force of infection increases while the shape remains about the same. For most years, the age-specific force of infection profiles give three local maxima which are located around the age of 21, 45, and 78, respectively. The age at the second local maxima varies with the susceptibility rate, when the susceptibility proportion decreases from 100% to 80%, the peak moves from age 45 to age 51. The third peak gets weaker when the susceptibility rate decreases. Note that we assume time homogeneity,

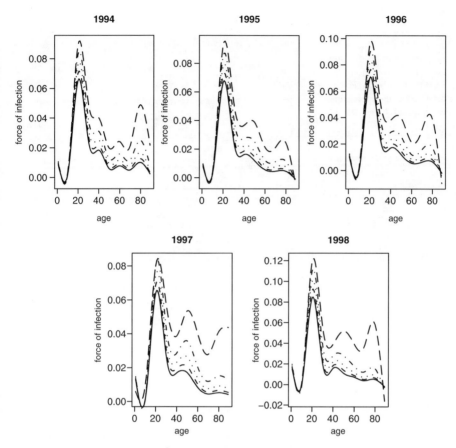

Fig. 5.5 Hepatitis B in St.-Petersburg: force of infection calculated from case notification data, assuming a susceptibility proportion varying from 100% to 80% (in steps of 5%) at birth More specifically: $p_s = 0.8$ (long dashed), 0.85 (dotted-dashed), 0.9 (dotted), 0.95 (dashed), and 1.00 (solid), respectively

i.e., we assume a cohort passes through different age classes ignoring the effect of changes within age classes over time. One could state this to be a too strong assumption.

The estimates based on reported cases were validated by comparing them with data from a seroprevalence study conducted in St.-Petersburg in 1999, as introduced in Sect. 4.1.2. Similar to the methods as applied above, the force of infection was estimated from this seroprevalence survey using cubic regression splines (see Chap. 8). The force of infection rises steadily from birth, peaks at age 21, stays flat until the age 51, and declines thereafter (Fig. 5.6). This shape seems to be a mixture of the two peaks as seen in the estimated force of infection based on incidence data. Based on the seroprevalence data we can get an estimate of the susceptibility proportion at birth p_s. In the sample, there are 99 samples from children <1 year of age, of which nine were Hepatitis B positive samples. As a result, we estimated

Fig. 5.6 Hepatitis B in
St.-Petersburg:
seroprevalence data,
seroprevalence (*solid line*),
and force of infection (*dashed
line*) from seroprevalence
data with dots proportional
to sample size

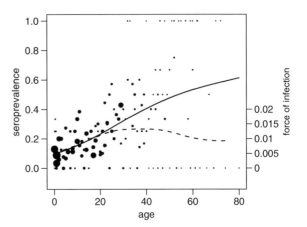

the susceptibility proportion at birth as 91%. This is close to the susceptibility
proportion of 90% as used in Fig. 5.5 (dotted line). Note that these prevalence
data are based on a different year, and thus the comparison between prevalence
and incidence data is only valid given time homogeneity. Nonetheless the results
obtained from the prevalence study seem to confirm the general trends observed
with the incidence data.

Chapter 6
Parametric Approaches to Model the Prevalence and Force of Infection

This chapter discusses several parametric models for the seroprevalence and the force of infection. In the first section we give a brief historical overview of the first parametric models used to model the force of infection, including polynomial and nonlinear models. In the second section we introduce the family of fractional polynomials as a natural extension of polynomial models, circumventing some of the limitations inherent to classical polynomials. These models can be easily fitted to seroprevalence data with R or, e.g., SAS. As usual, we focus on the use of R, with the functions *glm* and *mle*. SAS offers similar functionality with the *GENMOD* and *NLMIXED* procedure.

6.1 Modeling the Force of Infection: A Historical Perspective

In this section we briefly discuss the first (age-dependent) models for the force of infection as they appeared in literature from about 75 years ago, starting from basic parametric models to nonlinear models. We also refer to Hens et al. (2010a) for an overview of 75 years of estimating the force of infection from current status data.

6.1.1 Polynomial Models

The first references on the estimation of the force of infection go back to the early work of Muench, followed by Griffiths.

N. Hens et al., *Modeling Infectious Disease Parameters Based on Serological and Social Contact Data*, Statistics for Biology and Health 63, DOI 10.1007/978-1-4614-4072-7_6, © Springer Science+Business Media New York 2012

Muench (1934) and Griffiths (1974)

Muench (1934, 1959) suggested to model the infection process with a so-called "catalytic model," in which the distribution of the time spent in the susceptible class in the SIR model is exponential with rate β. More precisely, Muench (1934) proposed to model the prevalence by $\pi(a) = k\{1 - \exp(-\beta a)\}$ where $1 - k$ is the proportion of the population staying uninfected for lifetime. Under this catalytic model and assuming that $k = 1$, it follows from identity (5.4) that $\lambda(a) = \beta$. So in this case the force of infection is age-independent. This model fits into the GLM overview of Table 5.1 with log link and linear predictor $\eta(a) = \beta a$.

Using the R-function *glm* (Appendix B.2), Muench's model can be specified through the use of a log link function for binary data and the model specification -1+*Age* in order to specify a model without intercept, i.e., $\eta(a) = \beta a$. The model should be fitted to the number of seronegatives (*Tot-Pos*) in order to fit $1 - \pi(a)$ as $\exp(\beta a)$. Equivalently, Muench's model can also be estimated using the complementary log-log link function with linear predictor equal to $\eta(a) = \log(\beta) + \log(a)$. In this case the logarithm of the age (variable *log(Age)*) has to be specified as an offset variable using the option *offset = log(Age)*.

```
# R-code to fit Muench's model
model1=glm(cbind(Tot-Pos,Pos)~-1+Age,
                    family=binomial(link="log"))
summary(model1)

# Alternative R-code to fit Muench's model
model2=glm(cbind(Pos,Tot-Pos)~1,offset=log(Age),
                    family=binomial(link="cloglog"))
summary(model2)
exp(coef(model2))
```

Griffiths (1974) proposed a model for measles in which the force of infection increases linearly in the age range $(\tau, 10)$, $\tau \geq 0$:

$$\lambda(a) = \begin{cases} \beta_1(a + \beta_0) & a > \tau, \\ 0 & a \leq \tau. \end{cases}$$

He focused on the interval $(\tau, 10)$ as the interval $(0, \tau)$ represents the period of inherited immunity and since more than 95% of the measles cases occur before the age of 10 years. Note that since Griffiths (1974) specified τ as a parameter in the model, Griffiths' model should be interpreted as a changepoint model. Interestingly, Griffiths (1974) justified his choice of a linear force of infection by using a basic nonparametric estimate for the force of infection, $\lambda(a) = \Delta\pi/(1 - \pi(a))$, which he plotted against age and showed the linear trend of the force of infection. In coming chapters, we will discuss more advanced nonparametric models for the force of infection. Griffiths (1974) himself mentioned that his model for the prevalence corresponds to a model in which the linear predictor is a quadratic function of age.

Griffiths' model with linear force of infection $\lambda(a) = \beta_1 + 2\beta_2 a$ can be estimated using a GLM for which the linear predictor is a quadratic function of the age, i.e., $\eta(a) = \beta_1 a + \beta_2 a^2$. In the code below, the variables Age and Age^2 correspond to a and a^2, respectively.

```
# R-code to fit Griffiths' model
model3=glm(cbind(Tot-Pos,Pos)~-1+Age+I(Age^2),
                        family=binomial(link="log"))
summary(model3)
```

Grenfell and Anderson (1985)

Grenfell and Anderson (1985) extended the models of Muench and Griffiths further and used polynomial functions to model the force of infection. The advantage of higher-order polynomials is that they allow flexible curve shapes. Grenfell and Anderson (1985) did not restrict a priori the force of infection to be constant or linear but let the data determine the order of the polynomial. Their model assumes that $\pi(a) = 1 - e^{-\Sigma_i \beta_i a^i}$ which implies that, again using a GLM with log link (as in Table 5.1), the force of infection equals $\lambda(a) = \sum \beta_i i a^{i-1}$. For example, R-code for a possible model with quadratic force of infection such as $\lambda(a) = \eta'(a) = \beta_1 + 2\beta_2 a + 3\beta_3 a^2$ is given by

```
# R-code to fit Grenfell and Anderson's quadratic model
model4=glm(cbind(Tot-Pos,Pos)~-1+Age+I(Age^2)+I(Age^3),
                        family=binomial(link="log"))
summary(model4)
```

Application to Bulgarian Hepatitis A data

Here we illustrate and discuss selected R-output from running the above code for Muench's and Griffiths' model, to estimate the FOI of hepatitis A, based on the Bulgarian data (Chap. 4).

```
# R-output:  parameter estimates of Muench's model

> summary(model1)
```

(continued)

```
(continued)
Coefficients:
        Estimate Std. Error z value Pr(>|z|)
Age -0.050500    0.002457   -20.55   <2e-16 ***

AIC: 219.19

# R-output of alternative version of
# of Muench's model

> summary(model2)

Coefficients:
              Estimate Std. Error z value Pr(>|z|)
(Intercept) -2.98577     0.04866   -61.36   <2e-16 ***

AIC: 219.19

> exp(coef(model2))
(Intercept)
  0.0505004


# R-output:  parameter estimates of Griffiths' model

> summary(model3)

Coefficients:
            Estimate Std. Error z value Pr(>|z|)
Age       -0.0442616  0.0053697   -8.243   <2e-16 ***
I(Age^2)  -0.0001889  0.0001491   -1.266    0.205

AIC: 219.36

# R-output: parameter estimates Grenfell and
# Anderson's model

> summary(model4)

Coefficients:
            Estimate Std. Error z value Pr(>|z|)
Age       -5.326e-02  1.032e-02   -5.159 2.49e-07 ***
I(Age^2)   5.065e-04  6.508e-04    0.778    0.436
I(Age^3)  -1.019e-05  9.149e-06   -1.114    0.265

AIC: 219.72
```

The first fit of Muench's model produces an estimated force of infection equal to 0.0505. Using the alternative code, *Intercept* is the parameter estimate for $\log(\beta)$ and consequently the parameter estimate for the force of infection is again equal

Fig. 6.1 Estimated prevalence and force of infection for the Bulgarian Hepatitis A serological data. *Solid lines*: Muench's model with constant force of infection. *Long dashed lines*: Griffiths' model with linear force of infection. *Dotted lines*: Grenfell and Anderson's model with quadratic force of infection

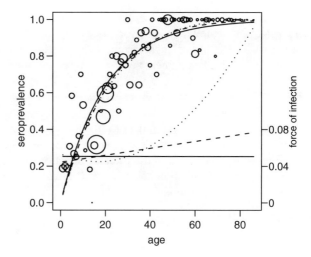

to $\exp(-2.9858) = 0.0505$. The R-code for Griffiths' model produces an estimate for a linear force of infection $-((-0.0443) + 2 \times (-0.0002)a)$. And finally the age-dependent force of infection estimated by Grenfell and Anderson's model equals $-((-0.0533) + 2 \times 0.0005a + 3 \times (-0.00001)a^2)$. The AIC values of all three models are very close with the one of Muench's model slightly smaller. Figure 6.1 shows the estimated prevalence and force of infection curves. Note that the prevalence curves are very close, whereas the FOI curves deviate more with increasing age.

Although polynomial models are quite flexible, they have some disadvantages: limited flexibility of polynomial type, unbounded and uncontrolled behavior at $\pm$infinity and intrinsic non-monotonicity. This is the motivation to turn to the more flexible family of fractional polynomials on the one hand and nonlinear models on the other hand. In the next section we discuss nonlinear models, some of which can be reformulated to fit within the framework of GLMs.

6.1.2 Nonlinear Models

One problem that arises when a higher-order polynomial model is fitted to the data is that the estimate for the force of infection can get negative. In fact, a force of infection estimate turns negative whenever the estimated probability to be infected before age a (i.e. the seroprevalence $\pi(a)$) is a non-monotone (increasing) function. In Chap. 9 we discuss this issue in more depth, for different types of models, including nonparametric models.

A possible solution to this problem is to define a nonnegative force of infection, $\lambda(a) \geq 0$ for all a, and to estimate $\pi(a)$ under these constraints. Farrington (1990), Edmunds et al. (2000a), and Farrington et al. (2001) applied this method for measles, mumps, and rubella, using a nonlinear model for $\pi(a)$. However, Farrington's method requires prior knowledge about the dependence of the force of infection on age. In particular, Farrington's model assumes that the force of infection increases to a peak in a linear fashion followed by an exponential decrease:

$$\lambda(a) = (\alpha a - \gamma)e^{-\beta a} + \gamma. \tag{6.1}$$

In order to ensure that the force of infection satisfies $\lambda(a) \geq 0$, Farrington (1990) constrained the parameter space to be nonnegative. The parameter γ is called the long-term residual value of the force of infection, as $a \to \infty$, $\lambda(a) \to \gamma$. If $\gamma = 0$, then the force of infection decreases to 0 as a tends to infinity. Integrating $\lambda(a)$ results in a nonlinear model:

$$\pi(a) = 1 - e^{-\int_0^a \lambda(s)ds} = 1 - \exp\left\{\frac{\alpha}{\beta}ae^{-\beta a} + \frac{1}{\beta}\left(\frac{\alpha}{\beta} - \gamma\right)\left(e^{-\beta a} - 1\right) - \gamma a\right\}. \tag{6.2}$$

The nonlinear model of Farrington (1990) can be fitted using the R-function *mle* (available in the *stats4* package), for instance for the rubella data, introduced in Chap. 4:

```
#R-code to fit Farrington's model
farrington=function(alpha,beta,gamma)
{
p=1-exp((alpha/beta)*Age*exp(-beta*Age)
        +(1/beta)*((alpha/beta)-gamma)*(exp(-beta*Age)-1)-gamma*Age)
ll=Pos*log(p)+(Tot-Pos)*log(1-p)
#alternative definition of the log-likelihood
#ll=sum(log(dbinom(Pos,Tot,prob=p)))
return(-sum(ll))
}

# R-package needed for mle function
library(stats4)
model5=mle(farrington,start=list(alpha=0.07,beta=0.1,gamma=0.03))
summary(model5)
AIC(model5)
```

The R-function *glm* cannot be used as it is limited to generalized linear models. Farrington's model is an example of a generalized nonlinear model. The above R-code is more generic as it allows to maximize a user-defined loglikelihood. The user-defined function *farrington* defines the (negative) loglikelihood (up to a constant) in our case, given the data. The user-defined function *ll* can be defined explicitly or alternatively using the R-function *dbinom* (binomial probabilities). The R-function *mle* computes the maximum likelihood estimates by minimizing minus

Fig. 6.2 Estimated prevalence and force of infection for the rubella data from the UK, using Farrington's model with three (*solid curves*) and two parameters (*dashed curves*), respectively

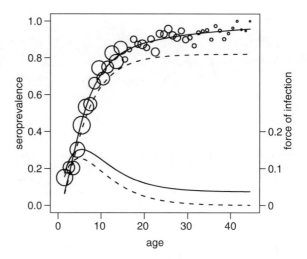

the loglikelihood. All previous models in this chapter could be modeled as well in this manner, essentially by modifying the definition of the age-dependent prevalence (the object p).

Parameter estimates are given in the output panel below.

```
Maximum likelihood estimation

Call:
mle(minuslogl = farrington, start = list(alpha = 0.07, beta
                                                       = 0.1,
    gamma = 0.03))

Coefficients:
          Estimate    Std. Error
alpha  0.07034904   0.005429317
beta   0.20243950   0.026093340
gamma  0.03665599   0.014751768

-2 log L: 3893.879

> AIC(model5)
[1] 3899.879
```

The estimated prevalence and force of infection of Farrington's model are shown in Fig. 6.2. The parameter estimate for the long-term residual value of the force of infection $(\hat{\gamma})$ is equal to 0.036 (95% C.I: 0.0077–0.0656). Note that a two-parameter model which assumes that $\gamma = 0$, with force of infection given by $\lambda(a) = \alpha a \exp(-\beta a)$ (decreasing to zero as age increases), can be fitted by the following mle-call (fixing $\gamma = 0$).

```
model6=mle(farrington,fixed=list(gamma=0),
                            start=list(alpha=0.07,beta=0.1))
summary(model6)
AIC(model6)
```

As can be seen in the output panel below, the AIC value of the two-parameter model (3902.393) is larger than the AIC of the three-parameter model (3899.879), indicating that the assumption that the force of infection decreases to zero as age increases is not reasonable for the rubella dataset. This is also confirmed by the fitted prevalence curve for the two-parameter model in Fig. 6.2, showing a severe negative bias in the prevalence curve.

```
> summary(model6)
Maximum likelihood estimation

Call:
mle(minuslogl = farrington, start = list(alpha = 0.07, beta = 0.1),
    fixed = list(gamma = 0))

Coefficients:
          Estimate   Std. Error
alpha  0.06744689  0.004074743
beta   0.15858061  0.007358578

-2 log L: 3898.393

> AIC(model6)
[1] 3902.393
```

Other parametric models fitted within the GLM-framework with binomial error were discussed by Becker (1989), Diamond and McDonald (1992), and Keiding et al. (1996), who used models with complementary log–log link function in order to parametrize the prevalence and the force of infection as a Weibull model. For the hepatitis C data from Belgium, introduced in Chap. 4, the time unit is the exposure time or duration d, which is defined as the difference between the age at first injection and the age at test. For a Weibull model, the prevalence is given by

$$\pi(d) = 1 - e^{-\beta_0 d^{\beta_1}} .$$

This at first sight nonlinear model can be reformulated as a GLM model with complementary log–log link and with linear predictor (using $\log(d)$) given by

$$\eta(d) = \log(\beta_0) + \beta_1 \log(d).$$

The Weibull model implies that the force of infection is a monotone function of the exposure time:

$$\lambda(d) = \beta_0 \beta_1 d^{\beta_1 - 1}.$$

In case that $\beta_1 > 1$, the force of infection is monotone increasing, while $\beta_1 < 1$ implies that the force of infection decreases with the exposure time. For the hepatitis C data, the Weibull model can be fitted by using the R-function *glm*, specifying the binomial distribution and complementary log–log link function.

```
log.d=log(d)
hcvfit=(glm(infected~log.d, family=binomial(link="cloglog")))
summary(hcvfit)
```

Parameter estimates for both prevalence and force of infection obtained from the Weibull model are shown in the output below. Note that $\hat{\beta}_1 = 0.3807 < 1$, and hence the FOI decreases as a function of exposure time. The *Residual deviance* equals 419.38 on 419 degrees of freedom, indicating that the Weibull model fit the data well.

```
> summary(hcvfit)

Call:
glm(formula=infected~log.d, family=binomial(link="cloglog"))

Deviance Residuals:
     Min        1Q    Median        3Q       Max
 -2.2378    0.4222    0.5527    0.7523    1.2040

Coefficients:
              Estimate Std. Error z value Pr(>|z|)
(Intercept)  -0.27596    0.14603   -1.890   0.0588 .
log.d         0.38074    0.07113    5.353 8.65e-08 ***
---
Signif. codes:  0 *** 0.001 ** 0.01 * 0.05 . 0.1   1

(Dispersion parameter for binomial family taken to be 1)

    Null deviance: 452.06  on 420  degrees of freedom
Residual deviance: 419.38  on 419  degrees of freedom
AIC: 423.38
```

The intercept estimate is the estimate for $\log(\beta_0)$. Hence, $\hat{\beta}_0 = \exp(-0.2760) = 0.758$. The estimated prevalence is given by $\hat{\pi}(d) = 1 - e^{-0.758 d^{0.3807}}$, while the force of infection is estimated as $\hat{\lambda}(d) = 0.758 \times 0.3807 d^{-0.6193}$. Estimated prevalence and FOI as a function of exposure time are shown in Fig. 6.3.

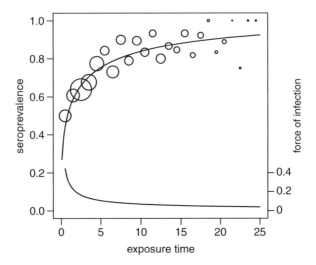

Fig. 6.3 Estimated prevalence and force of infection for the hepatitis C data from Belgium, using a Weibull model

Becker (1989) suggested to model a piecewise constant force of infection by fitting a model with log link. For the case that other covariates, in addition to age, are included in the model, Jewell and Van Der Laan (1995) proposed, in the context of current status data, a proportional hazards model with constant force of infection, which can be fitted as a GLM with complementary log–log link. Grummer-Strawn (1993) discussed two parametric models, the first being a Weibull proportional hazards model with complementary log–log link and the second being a log-logistic model with logit link function. For the latter, the proportionality in the model is interpreted as proportional odds.

6.1.3   Discussion

The estimation of the force of infection from a single cross-sectional serological sample is based on a series of landmark papers which established the modeling framework as we know it today. From the first paper of Muench (1934) who introduced the two scales of interest, the prevalence and the derivative, via the paper of Griffiths (1974), who introduced the GLM as the modeling framework and nonparametric methods as an exploratory tool, to the paper of Grenfell and Anderson (1985). Keiding (1991) presented in his paper the first appropriate nonparametric method, while Farrington (1990) introduced nonlinear models and addressed the issue of monotonicity of the prevalence. These five landmark papers established the framework which is still used today for the estimation of the force of infection. In recent years, using more up-to-date statistical models, the estimation procedures for the force of infection became much more advanced and consequently more computer intensive, as we will discuss in the remainder of this part of the book. But the basic ideas and issues, flexibility and monotonicity, remain crucial in the estimation process of the force of infection.

6.2   Fractional Polynomial Models

In this section we introduce fractional polynomials as a natural extension of polynomial models and their application to the estimation of the prevalence and the force of infection.

6.2.1   Motivating Example

For the Hepatitis A data from Belgium anno 1993–1994 (see Chap. 4), we consider two generalized linear models with logit and complementary log–log link functions. For the logit model the linear predictor is $\eta(a) = \beta_0 + \beta_1 a + \beta_2 a^3$. This model has a deviance of 82.74 on with 83 degrees of freedom. For the complementary log–log model $\eta(a) = \log(\beta_0) + \beta_1 a^2 + \beta_2 a^3$, the deviance is 81.41, also on with 83 degrees of freedom. The force of infection of these models can be derived from Table 5.1. Although both models fit the data well, Fig. 6.4 shows that both models predict negative forces of infection at the higher age groups. The motivation to model the force of infection with fractional polynomials is to extend the family of polynomial models, allowing for (1) more flexibility in combination with (2) improved behavior at the extremes of the observed age range. Low-order conventional polynomials

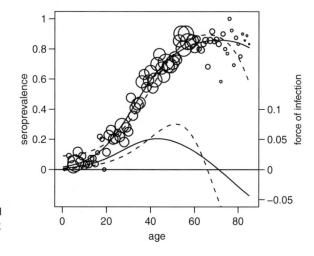

Fig. 6.4 Estimated prevalence and force of infection for the Belgian Hepatitis A data. *Solid line*: model with logit link function. *Dashed line*: model with complementary log–log link function

Table 6.1 Parametric models for the prevalence from literature, represented as fractional polynomials, and their corresponding force of infection

Publication	Fractional polynomial	Link function	Force of infection
Muench (1959), Farrington et al. (2001), Jewell and Van Der Laan (1995)	$\eta(m=1, p=0, \beta_1 = 1)$	cloglog	Constant
Griffiths (1974)	$\eta(m=1, p=0, \beta_1 = 2)$	cloglog	Linear
Grenfell and Anderson (1985)	$\eta(m=k, p_i = i)$	log	Polynomial
Keiding et al. (1996), Becker (1989), Diamond and McDonald (1992), Grummer-Strawn (1993)	$\eta(m=1, p=0, \beta_1 \neq 0)$	cloglog	Monotone
Grummer-Strawn (1993)	$\eta(m=1, p=0, \beta_1 \neq 0)$	logit	Flexible

have limited flexibility, do not have asymptotes, and tend to fit the data poorly whenever asymptotic behavior of the infection process is expected. Royston and Altman (1994) introduced the family of fractional polynomials as a generalization of the conventional polynomial class of functions. In the context of binary responses, a fractional polynomial (FP) of degree m for the linear predictor is defined as

$$\eta_m(a, \beta, p_1, p_2 \ldots p_m) = \sum_{i=0}^{m} \beta_i H_i(a), \qquad (6.3)$$

where m is an integer, $p_1 \leq p_2 \leq \cdots \leq p_m$ is a sequence of powers, and $H_i(a)$ is a transformation given by

$$H_i(a) = \begin{cases} a^{p_i} & \text{if } p_i \neq p_{i-1}, \\ H_{i-1}(a) \times \log(a) & \text{if } p_i = p_{i-1}, \end{cases} \qquad (6.4)$$

with $p_0 = 0$ and $H_0 \equiv 1$, and $a^{p_i} = \log(a)$ if $p_i = 0$. Royston and Altman (1994) argued that, in practice, fractional polynomials of degree higher than 2 are rarely needed and suggested to choose the value of the powers from the set $\{-2, -1, -0.5, 0, 0.5, 1, 2, \max(3, m)\}$. Note that the model with log link and with predictor function $\eta_1(a, \beta, p = 1)$ coincides with Muench's model, $\eta_2(a, \beta, p_1 = 1, p_2 = 2)$ corresponds to the model proposed by Griffiths (1974), and the models considered by Grenfell and Anderson (1985) have the general form of $\eta_m(a, \beta, p_1, p_2 \ldots, p_m)$ with $p_i = i$ for $i = 1, 2, \ldots, m$.

Table 6.1 shows a selection of parametric models discussed in the literature and their representation as fractional polynomials. For example, the model proposed by Keiding et al. (1996) is a first degree fractional polynomial with $p = 0$. The model with linear force of infection can be parameterized as a first degree fractional polynomial with complementary log–log link for which $p = 0$ with the constraint that $\beta_1 = 2$. In this case $\lambda(a) = 2\beta_0 a$ which implies that the force of infection is zero at birth and increases linearly thereafter. The models presented by Grummer-Strawn (1993) and Jewell and Van Der Laan (1995) include other covariates in addition to age. For these models $\eta(m, p, \beta)$ is the fractional polynomial used to model the dependency of prevalence on age. For the models discussed in Grummer-Strawn (1993), we do not include the adjusted parameter in our analysis since it is assumed that susceptibility is 100% at birth. The models discussed by Grummer-Strawn (1993) and Jewell and Van Der Laan (1995) were used in the context of current status data. When these models are implemented for infectious disease data, they result in constant, monotone, or/and flexible force of infection models.

6.2.2 Model Selection

Within the fractional polynomials framework the deviance of the model with $\eta_1(a,\beta,1)$ is taken to be the baseline deviance and improvement or gain by other models is measured by

$$G(m,p) = D(1,1) - D(m,p), \tag{6.5}$$

where $D(m,p)$ is the deviance of the model with fractional polynomial of degree m and sequence of powers $p = (p_1, p_2, \ldots p_m)$. Note that a large value of G indicates a better fit. Fitting models within the framework of fractional polynomials requires to start the modeling procedure from first degree fractional polynomials. To decide whether a model of first degree is adequate or a second degree model is needed, Royston and Altman (1994) recommend to use the criterion $D(1,\tilde{p}) - D(2,\tilde{p}) > \chi^2_{2,0.9}$ where $\tilde{p}$ is the power sequence for the model that has the best goodness of fit among models of the same degree.

6.2.3 Constrained Fractional Polynomials

Although fractional polynomials provide a wide range of flexible curve shapes, there is no guarantee that $\pi(a)$ will be a monotone function of age and therefore fractional polynomials can still result in a negative estimate for the force of infection at some range of age values. It is clear from Table 5.1 that the estimate for the force of infection is negative whenever $\eta'_m(a,\hat{\beta},p) < 0$ (since $\delta(\eta_m(a,\hat{\beta},p))$ is strictly positive). Therefore, one should fit model (6.3) subject to the constraint that $\eta'_m(a,\hat{\beta},p) \geq 0$, for all ages a in the predefined range. In the framework of fractional polynomials this cannot be done analytically. But in practice, one can fit a large number of fractional polynomials, over a grid of powers, and check for each fitted model whether $\eta'_m(a,\hat{\beta},p) \geq 0$, for all ages a. In case that a given sequence of powers leads to a negative derivative of the linear predictor, the model is not considered as an appropriate model. This means that we choose the model with the best goodness of fit among all fractional polynomials for which $\eta'_m(a,\hat{\beta},p) \geq 0$.

6.2.4 Selection of Powers and Back to Nonlinear Models

Although Royston and Altman (1994) suggested to choose the value of the powers from the set $\{-2, -1, -0.5, 0, 0.5, 1, 2, \max(3, m)\}$, one can extend the family of candidate models by refining the grid of possible powers, such as for instance an equidistant grid on the interval $[-2, \max(3, m)]$ with stepsize 0.1 or even 0.01. Selection of the best fractional polynomial can proceed in the same way. When refining the grid, one expects that the best fractional polynomial gets close to the genuinely nonlinear model (for the degree $m = 2$):

$$\eta_m(a, \boldsymbol{\beta}) = \beta_0 + \beta_1 a^{\tilde{\beta}_1} + \beta_2 a^{\tilde{\beta}_2}, \tag{6.6}$$

where now $\boldsymbol{\beta} = (\beta_0, \beta_1, \tilde{\beta}_1, \beta_2, \tilde{\beta}_2)$. Whereas the estimation of fractional polynomials is a two-step procedure, with in a first step the selection of the best powers and in a second step the estimation of intercept and slopes, both sets of unknown parameters are estimated in the nonlinear model in one step. Whereas inference based on the final fractional polynomials ignores that powers were also selected using the data, the nonlinear model fully recognizes the sample variability in the estimation of both sets of parameters. Another approach to account for the power-selection step is to compute the model averaged estimate and to apply multi-model inference (Burnham and Anderson 2002). This latter approach has been applied in, e.g., Faes et al. (2003) and will be explained in more detail when applied to the estimation of mixing patterns in Chap. 15.

6.2.5 Application to the Data

In this section, we apply our method to some datasets mentioned in Chap. 4. For each dataset, first and second degree fractional polynomials were fitted and the criterion proposed by Royston and Altman (1994) was used to decide whether the second degree model is needed or not. The optimal second degree FP is first selected without monotonicity constraint, and next the best monotone fractional polynomial is selected by excluding all non-monotone fits. The R-function and R-package *mpf* can be applied, but it does not examine the monotonicity constraint and it does not allow to change the grid of powers. Using own code (available on the web site) with the finer grid (stepsize 0.01 for first degree and 0.1 for second degree, in both dimensions) mentioned in Sect. 6.2.4, Table 6.2 presents the deviance for the best first and second degree fractional polynomials. For the second degree polynomials, the optimal powers are shown with and without monotonicity constraint. Clearly, for all datasets except the Bulgarian dataset, first degree fractional polynomials are not adequate and second degree fractional polynomials are required. For the first degree models, the gain values in Table 6.2 also indicate that, for all datasets except the Bulgarian dataset, the first degree fractional polynomials with $p = 1$ are not adequate and other powers are needed.

Table 6.2 Deviance and gain values for first and second degree fractional polynomials with logit link function

Dataset	First degree ($m = 1$)			Second degree ($m = 2$)		
	Deviance	p	$G(1,p)$	Monotone	Deviance	p_1, p_2
Hepatitis A (BE93)	114.25	0.42	35.31	No	79.58	+1.9,+2.0
				Yes	93.45	+1.0,+1.6
Hepatitis A (BG)	79.51	1	0	No	77.75	+1.9,+2.0
				Yes	77.89	+1.6,+2.1
Varicella	82.33	0.1	75.36	No	47.69	−1.2,−1.1
				Yes	71.81	−0.6,−0.2
Rubella	56.19	0.05	165.23	No	37.58	−0.9,−0.9
				Yes	42.34	−0.9,−0.4
Mumps	82.05	−0.17	75.36	No	44.60	−2.0,−0.8
				Yes	49.18	−1.0,−1.0

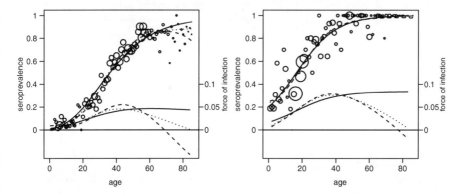

Fig. 6.5 Estimated prevalence and force of infection for Hepatitis A in Belgium (*left panel*) and in Bulgaria (*right panel*). *Solid lines*: first degree FP-model, *dashed lines*: unconstrained second degree FP-model, *dotted lines*: constrained second degree FP-model. Models were fitted with logit link function

Hepatitis A

The left panel in Fig. 6.5 shows the estimated models for the prevalence and the force of infection for hepatitis A in Belgium. The best unconstrained model with powers (1.9, 2.0) has deviance 79.58 with 83 degrees of freedom, whereas the deviance of the best constrained model with powers (1.0, 1.6) has a deviance value 93.45. The estimated force of infection of the constrained second degree fractional polynomial reaches a peak at age 41 ($\hat{\lambda}(41) = 0.046$) and drops down thereafter. Figure 6.6 shows the deviance surface for second degree fractional polynomials, as a function of both powers p_1 and p_2 (symmetrized for $p_2 < p_1$). The gray and black surface together correspond to all possible powers, regardless of any monotonicity constraint, whereas the black surface corresponds to only those powers for which the corresponding prevalence is monotone as a function of age. The optimal powers

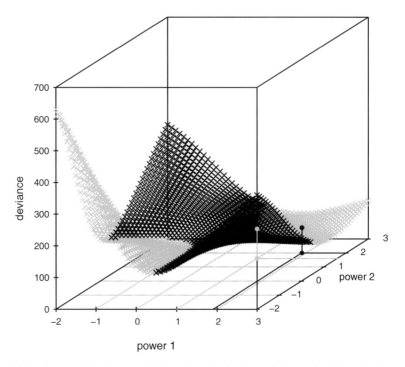

Fig. 6.6 Deviance surface for second degree fractional polynomials, as a function of both powers p_1 and p_2 (symmetrized for $p_2 < p_1$), for hepatitis A in Belgium. The *gray* and *black* surface together correspond to all possible powers, regardless of any monotonicity constraint; the *black* surface corresponds to those powers for which the corresponding prevalence is monotone as a function of age. Indicated are the optimal powers: in *black* for the overall, unconstrained *gray* surface: (1.9, 2) with deviance value 79.58; in *gray* for the constrained *black* surface: (1.0, 1.6) with deviance value 93.45

(1.9, 2) are indicated in black for the overall unconstrained gray surface with deviance value 79.58 and (1.0, 1.6) in gray for the constrained black surface with deviance value 93.45.

For the Bulgarian dataset, the second degree unconstrained fractional polynomial with powers (1.9, 2.0) has a deviance of 77.75 on with 80 degrees of freedom, whereas the constrained version with powers (1.6, 2.1) has a deviance of 77.89. This model suggests that the force of infection is maximal at age 37 ($\hat{\lambda}(37) = 0.076$). However, using statistical measures, the first degree fractional polynomial is to be preferred since $D(1,1) - D(2,(1.6,2.1)) = 1.63 < \chi^2_{2,0.9} = 4.605$. Using AIC, lower is better (see Appendix B.1), also leads to the simpler one degree polynomial, although borderline (AIC = 203.4 for the first degree polynomial, against AIC = 203.8 for the second degree polynomial). Interestingly, the first degree fractional polynomial with optimal power $p_1 = 1$ and logit link is just a simple linear logistic regression model. For this model $\lambda(a) = \beta_1 \pi(a)$ such that it predicts an upward

Fig. 6.7 Estimated prevalence and force of infection for varicella. *Solid lines*: first degree FP-model, *dashed lines*: unconstrained second degree FP-model, *dotted lines*: constrained second degree FP-model. Models were fitted with logit link function

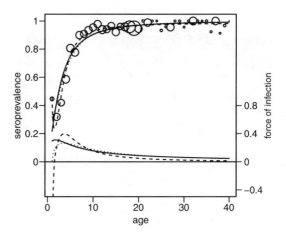

trend for the force of infection. This illustrates that estimated age-dependent force of infection curves can exhibit quite different qualitative characteristics, even if the estimated age-dependent prevalence curves are very similar (see right panel of Fig. 6.5).

Varicella, Rubella and Mumps

Figure 6.7 shows the estimated fractional polynomials for both prevalence and force of infection for the varicella data. Although observations for ages below 6 months were excluded, the unconstrained FP of degree 2 decreases up to about the age of 1.5 year and then increases rapidly, leading to a negative estimate for the force of infection. This example clearly shows the flexibility of FPs which is almost of a nonparametric nature. The constrained FP of degree 2 results in an estimated curve for the FOI that reaches a maximum at age 3.5 with value $\hat{\lambda}(3.5) = 0.27$ and drops down thereafter. At age 40 years the force of infection is estimated to be 0.045.

For rubella and mumps, we observe the same phenomenon at the lowest ages, but less pronounced. Although the selected powers for the unconstrained and constrained FP are quite different, the fitted curves are very close. Figure 6.8 (left panel) shows that for rubella the force of infection rises to a peak at age 6.3 with $(\hat{\lambda}(6.3) = 0.14)$. For mumps, the force of infection reaches a maximum value at age 4.6 with $\hat{\lambda}(4.6) = 0.32$.

6.2.6   Influence of the Link Function

In the previous section, all models were fitted with the logit link function. In this section, we illustrate the influence of using other link functions. In particular,

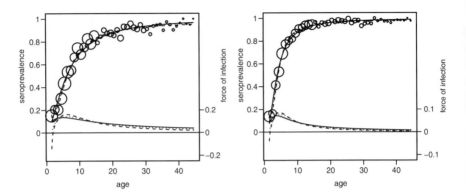

Fig. 6.8 Estimated prevalence and force of infection for rubella (*left panel*) and mumps (*right pane*). *Solid lines*: first degree FP-model, *dashed lines*: unconstrained second degree FP-model, *dotted lines*: constrained second degree FP-model. Models were fitted with logit link function

we focus on the use of the complementary log–log link function. More precisely, for the first degree fractional polynomials we specify the model for the prevalence as

$$\pi(a) = \begin{cases} 1 - \exp\left(-\beta_0 e^{\beta_1 H(a)}\right) & p \neq 0, \\ 1 - \exp\left(-\beta_0 a^{\beta_1}\right) & p = 0. \end{cases} \tag{6.7}$$

For the second degree fractional polynomials, we consider the following specification:

$$\pi(a) = 1 - \exp\left(-\beta_0 e^{\beta_1 H_1(a) + \beta_2 H_2(a)}\right), \tag{6.8}$$

with corresponding linear predictor

$$\begin{cases} \eta_2(a,\beta,p_1,p_2) = \log(\beta_0) + \beta_1 a^{p_1} + \beta_2 a^{p_2} & \text{if } p_1 \neq p_2, \\ \eta_2(a,\beta,p_1,p_2) = \log(\beta_0) + \beta_1 a^{p_1} + \beta_2 a^{p_1}\log(a) & \text{if } p_1 = p_2, \\ a^{p_1} = \log(a) & \text{if } p_1 = 0. \end{cases} \tag{6.9}$$

Note that indeed the models specified in (6.7) and (6.8) are GLM with a complementary log–log link function. The first degree model specified in (6.7) with $p = 0$ implies a Weibull distribution for the time spent in the susceptible class. Such a Weibull model was used by Keiding et al. (1996) to model the force of infection for rubella from an Austrian seroprevalence sample. A model with a constant force of infection is a special case of a first degree fractional polynomial with complementary log–log link function with β_1 fixed at value 1; in that case $\eta(a,\beta) = \log(\beta_0) + \log(a)$. Such a model was used by Farrington et al. (2001) to model the force of infection for hepatitis A in Bulgaria. Furthermore, a model with linear force of infection is a first degree fractional polynomial with $p = 0$ and $\beta_1 = 2$.

Table 6.3 Selected powers and deviance summaries of the fitted FP-models for the Belgian hepatitis A dataset

Model (link)	Monotone	Deviance	p	AIC
First degree (logit)	Yes	114.25	0.42	391.8
Second degree (logit)	No	79.58	1.9,2.0	359.2
Second degree (logit)	Yes	93.45	1.0,1.6	373.0
First degree (cloglog)	Yes	135.73	-0.04	413.3
First degree (cloglog)	Yes	136.00	$0\ (\beta_1 \neq 1)$	413.5
First degree (cloglog)	Yes	290.80	$0\ (\beta_1 = 1)$	566.4
Second degree (cloglog)	No	81.60	1.5,1.6	361.2
Second degree (cloglog)	Yes	106.00	0.5,1.1	385.5

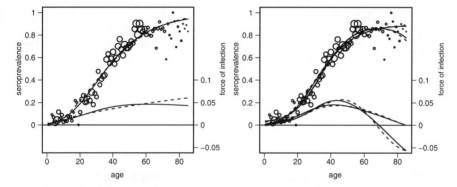

Fig. 6.9 Estimated prevalence and force of infection for the Belgian Hepatitis A data, based on models with logit and complementary log–log link function. *Left panel*: fits from first degree fractional polynomials with logit (*solid curves*) and complementary log–log link function (*dashed curves*); *right panel*: fits from second degree fractional polynomials with logit (*solid curves*) and complementary log–log link function (*dashed curves*), for unconstrained (non-monotone prevalence and negative FOI) and constrained models

Table 6.3 summarizes the characteristics of all fits to the Belgian hepatitis A data. One can observe that the logit models fit the data better, as compared to the cloglog counterparts. The Weibull model (FP of degree 1 with $p = 0$) does not fit well. The influence of the link function reduces as the model gets more flexible, going for FPs from degree one to degree two. This is confirmed in Fig. 6.9. For the first degree models, the fitted FOI curve based on the cloglog link deviates from the logit-based fit for ages above 60 years, as it does not reach a maximum. The unconstrained and constrained second degree FP fits though are remarkably close, even though the selected powers are quite different. This is in line with what is known also for nonparametric models: the more flexible the predictor models, the less the influence of the link function. Comparing all models, the best unconstrained model is the second degree logit-based FP model with powers 1.9 and 2.0 (deviance 79.58, AIC 359.2), closely followed by its cloglog-based counterpart with powers 1.5 and 1.6

Table 6.4 Belgian Hepatitis A data: estimates and standard errors for FPs of first and second degree, together with those of the equivalent nonlinear models

Model	β_0	β_1	$\tilde{\beta}_1$	β_2	$\tilde{\beta}_2$
FP1	−6.51(0.26)	1.44(0.06)	0.42(fixed)	–	–
NL1	−6.57(1.39)	1.47(0.81)	0.42(0.09)	–	–
FP2	−3.27(0.16)	0.03(0.002)	1.90(fixed)	−0.02(0.001)	2.00(fixed)
NL2	−3.30(0.24)	0.04(0.011)	1.88(0.11)	−0.02(0.008)	1.98(0.09)

(deviance 81.60, AIC 361.2). The best model that leads to a monotone prevalence and positive FOI fit is the second degree logit-based model with powers 1.0 and 1.6 (deviance 93.45, AIC 373.0), followed by again its cloglog counterpart with powers 0.5 and 1.1 (deviance 106.00, AIC 385.5).

6.2.7 From Fractional Polynomials Back to Nonlinear Models

The main advantage of an FP is its flexibility while remaining a parametric GLM and consequently fitting such a model is straightforward. As indicated in Sect. 6.2.4, a fractional polynomial with powers selected from a fine grid of powers gets close to the genuinely nonlinear model, but inference ignores that powers were also selected using the data. On the other hand treating the powers as parameters, we get nonlinear models with similar flexibility and correct inference, but convergence of nonlinear models may become problematic (no convergence, convergence to a local optimum, etc.). To get proper inference and to solve the computational difficulties of the nonlinear model, one could first select the FP over a fine grid of powers and use the resulting estimates and selected powers as starting values for the equivalent nonlinear model. The nonlinear equivalent of a fractional polynomial model of degree one is given by

$$\eta_m(a, \beta) = \beta_0 + \beta_1 a^{\tilde{\beta}_1}, \tag{6.10}$$

where now $\beta = (\beta_0, \beta_1, \tilde{\beta}_1)$, and for a second degree FP by

$$\eta_m(a, \beta) = \beta_0 + \beta_1 a^{\tilde{\beta}_1} + \beta_2 a^{\tilde{\beta}_2}, \tag{6.11}$$

with $\beta = (\beta_0, \beta_1, \tilde{\beta}_1, \beta_2, \tilde{\beta}_2)$.

Table 6.4 shows estimates and standard errors for FPs of first and second degree (rows FP1 and FP2), together with those of the equivalent nonlinear models (rows NL1 and NL2) as applied to the Belgian Hepatitis A data. The power of the FP of degree 1 was selected based on a grid with stepsize 0.01; the powers of the FP of degree 2 were selected based on a two-dimensional grid with stepsize 0.1 in each dimension. As expected the estimates (or selected powers) do not change much, but the standard errors are much larger for the nonlinear model. How does

Table 6.5 Belgian
Hepatitis A data: estimates,
standard errors, and 95%
confidence intervals for the
prevalence and force of
infection at age 40 years, for
FPs of first and second degree
and the equivalent nonlinear
models

Model	Parameter	Estimate(se)	95% CI
FP1	$\pi(40)$	0.57(0.011)	(0.548, 0.591)
NL1	$\pi(40)$	0.57(0.012)	(0.546, 0.594)
FP2	$\pi(40)$	0.59(0.013)	(0.564, 0.615)
NL2	$\pi(40)$	0.59(0.013)	(0.563, 0.616)
FP1	$\lambda(40)$	0.04(0.002)	(0.037, 0.044)
NL1	$\lambda(40)$	0.04(0.002)	(0.037, 0.044)
FP2	$\lambda(40)$	0.05(0.002)	(0.049, 0.058)
NL2	$\lambda(40)$	0.05(0.003)	(0.048, 0.059)

this affect the estimates for the prevalence and the force of infection? Table 6.5 shows the estimated prevalence and force of infection with standard errors and confidence intervals at the age 40 (age at which the FOI is close to its maximal value). With the increased standard errors of Table 6.4 in mind, it might be surprising to observe that standard errors and confidence intervals are very close. The reason is that in nonlinear models the estimated coefficients and corresponding estimated powers are highly correlated. For the first degree fractional polynomial the estimated correlation between $\hat{\beta}_1$ and $\widehat{\tilde{\beta}}_1$ equals -0.9975; for the second degree polynomial the estimated correlation between $\hat{\beta}_1$ and $\widehat{\tilde{\beta}}_1$ is equal to -0.5076, between $\hat{\beta}_2$ and $\widehat{\tilde{\beta}}_2$ 0.3379 (which seems rather moderate) but the correlation between $\hat{\beta}_1$ and $\hat{\beta}_2$ equals -0.8752 and that of $\widehat{\tilde{\beta}}_1$ and $\widehat{\tilde{\beta}}_2$ is equal to 0.9501. So, the main conclusion is that inference based on fractional polynomials seems acceptable, even when ignoring the sample variability in the power-selection step. The nonlinear models in this section were fitted using *PROC NLMIXED* in SAS.

6.3   Discussion

We have shown that modeling the prevalence and the force of infection with fractional polynomials is a very flexible method, allowing a variety of different types of relationships between the force of infection and age. The method can compete with nonparametric smoothers while keeping the attractive features of parametric models. Furthermore, we have shown that well-known parametric models can be expressed as special cases of fractional polynomials. Thus, by fitting a large number of fractional polynomials with logit and complementary log–log link function we account for the possibility of constant, linear, monotone, or flexible curve shapes for the force of infection. However, we do not require the force of infection to have a specific curve shape in advance, the choice is data-driven.

In case that other covariates, in addition to age, are included, the following semi-parametric additive model parameterizes the prevalence as

$$\text{link}(\pi(a)) = \phi(a) + Z\alpha, \tag{6.12}$$

where Z represents the additional categorical covariate(s). The nonparametric component of the model, $\phi(a)$, is used to model the dependency of $\pi(a)$ on age while $Z\alpha$, the parametric component of the model, is used to model the covariate effects. This modeling approach is further discussed in Chap. 8. In order to ensure a nonnegative estimate for the force of infection, one needs to estimate $\pi(a)$ with a nondecreasing function. This can be done by applying the pool adjacent violators algorithm to the data (Barlow et al. 1972; Robertson et al. 1988). This approach has been followed by Grummer-Strawn (1993) and Shiboski (1998). Within the framework of fractional polynomials, we can replace the nonparametric component of the model with a fractional polynomial

$$\mathrm{link}(\pi(a)) = \eta_m(a, p, \beta) + Z\alpha,$$

where $\eta_m(a, p, \beta)$ is the fractional polynomial modeling the dependence on age. Similar to the semiparametric model in (6.12), depending on the link function, this model implies proportionality. For example, suppose that Z is a binary variable, then for models with complementary log–log link we get $\lambda(a|Z = 1) = \exp(\alpha)\lambda(a|Z = 0)$ and for models with logit link we obtain $\lambda(a|Z = 1) = (\pi(a|Z = 1)/\pi(a|Z = 0))\lambda(a|Z = 0)$.

The problem of estimating a negative force of infection was addressed by fitting constrained fractional polynomials, excluding models that lead to negative force of infection as appropriate models. In our opinion, blind use of conventional linear predictors to model the force of infection can yield misleading results. Flexible models should be considered and the family of fractional polynomials offers an interesting choice. They can also be used as an exploratory tool or to perform a sensitivity analysis of a particular parametric model that, for instance, reflects prior information about the force of infection.

All models discussed in this chapter are generalized linear or nonlinear parametric models, which can be fit easily with standard software, such as the functions *glm()* or *mle()* in R, or *PROC GENMOD* or *PROC NLMIXED* in SAS.

Chapter 7
Nonparametric Approaches to Model the Prevalence and Force of Infection

7.1 Nonparametric Approaches

In the previous chapter, parametric models, including the flexible family of fractional polynomials, were fitted in the framework of generalized linear models. Such models, although quite flexible, are of a predetermined shape through their specific analytical form. They might not be able to capture unusual and unexpected features of the data. Nonparametric regression methods allow to accommodate flexible, highly nonlinear relationships for the age-dependent seroprevalence and consequently for the force of infection. Unlike parametric models, the shape of the functional relationship of the disease prevalence or the force of infection as a function of age is not predetermined. There are many nonparametric so-called "smoothing" methods, and there is a vast literature available (see e.g. Fan and Gijbels 1996; Efromovich 1999; Simonoff 1996; Ruppert et al. 2003; Bowman and Azzalini 1997).

Nonparametric methods are originating from different approximating principles, but roughly speaking one could classify them in "series" and "non-series" methods. Series methods (polynomial series, trigonometric series, wavelets, ...) originate from the mathematics of series approximation (Fourier series), whereas non-series methods are motivated through local approximations (kernel and local polynomial estimators, nearest neighbor methodology), interpolating theory (splines), models for the human brain (neural networks), separating hyperplanes (support vector machine), etc. The line between parametric and nonparametric models can be very thin, leading to "semiparametric" models. Penalized regression splines fitted as a mixed model is such an example. These types of models will be discussed and illustrated in the next chapter.

The focus in this chapter is on the local polynomial estimator. One reason for this choice is that we believe it is an appropriate smoothing approach for typical seroprevalence data. Another more technical argument is that this method allows

N. Hens et al., *Modeling Infectious Disease Parameters Based on Serological and Social Contact Data*, Statistics for Biology and Health 63, DOI 10.1007/978-1-4614-4072-7_7, © Springer Science+Business Media New York 2012

simultaneous estimation of a parameter, its derivatives, and functions thereof, such as the force of infection. But we start with a short historical tour on the first nonparametric approaches in the field of statistical models for infectious diseases.

7.1.1 The First Nonparametric Approaches

As mentioned in Chap. 6, Griffiths (1974) presented the first attempt to estimate the force of infection nonparametrically. The importance of Griffiths' method is the idea behind it. He justified his choice for a parametric model with linear force of infection using a nonparametric estimate for the same parameter. Farrington (1990) used a smoothed version of Griffiths' estimator. However, both can lead to a negative estimate for the force of infection. Although the discussion on the issue of constrained estimation of prevalence and FOI is postponed to Chap. 9, it is interesting to introduce Keiding's two-step approach (Keiding (1991)) already in this section. In the first step the prevalence is estimated by isotonic regression (Barlow et al. 1972; Robertson et al. 1988), and in the second step a kernel smoother is used in order to estimate the force of infection.

The isotonic regression estimator of the observed prevalence is the nonparametric maximum likelihood estimator (NPMLE) for (5.2). It is a step function with respect to age. Barlow et al. (1972) and Robertson et al. (1988) discussed the NPMLE for the general case of the binomial likelihood and Keiding (1991), Greenhalgh and Dietz (1994), and Keiding et al. (1996) discussed it in the context of infectious diseases (using the form of the likelihood in (5.2)). In the second step the force of infection, assumed to be a smooth function of age, is estimated by

$$\hat{\lambda}(a) = \frac{1}{h} \int_{a-h}^{a+h} K\left(\frac{x-a}{h}\right) \frac{d\hat{\pi}(x)}{1 - \hat{\pi}(x^-)}, \qquad (7.1)$$

where K is a kernel function, h is the bandwidth, and $\hat{\pi}(\cdot)$ is the isotonic regression estimator of the observed prevalence. Note that $\hat{\pi}(x^-)$ is the shorthand notation for the left limit of $\hat{\pi}$ with respect to x. As discussed in Greenhalgh and Dietz (1994), in case that $\hat{\pi}$ has discontinuities at the points $x_1, x_2, \ldots, x_n$, then

$$\hat{\lambda}(a) = \frac{1}{h} \sum_{x_i \in [a-h, a+h]} K\left(\frac{x_i - a}{h}\right) \frac{\hat{\pi}(x_i) - \hat{\pi}(x_{i-1})}{1 - \hat{\pi}(x_{i-1})}. \qquad (7.2)$$

Keiding's method requires the crucial choice of an optimal bandwidth h. This issue was not addressed by Keiding, who chose the smoothing parameter by visual inspection. Later on, Keiding et al. (1996) proposed to replace the kernel estimate in the second step with a smoothing spline. However, This method also requires the selection of a smoothing parameter as well. Figure 7.1 shows the hepatitis A

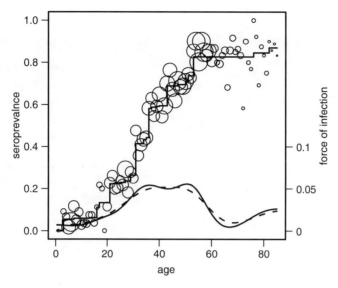

Fig. 7.1 Estimated prevalence and force of infection for Hepatitis A in Belgium using Keiding's method: isotonic regression to estimate the prevalence and a kernel smoother for the force of infection, based on a standard normal density K and bandwidths $h = 15$ (*solid curve*) and $h = 20$ (*dashed curve*)

data from Belgium with the prevalence estimated using isotonic regression and a kernel smoother to estimate the force of infection (with K the standard normal density and with two choices $h = 15$ and $h = 20$ for the bandwidth parameter). As mentioned before, the estimation of the prevalence and the force of infection from a serological sample is closely related to the problem of estimation from current status data (Keiding et al. 1996). While in the literature related to the estimation of parameters from current status data attention is placed on estimating the prevalence, in the context of infectious diseases one focuses on the estimation of the force of infection (as well as other disease-related parameters). In the context of current status data, Shiboski (1998) proposed a semiparametric model, based on generalized additive models (Hastie and Tibshirani 1990), in which the dependency of the force of infection on age is modeled nonparametrically and the covariate effect is the parametric component of the model. Depending on the link function, the model proposed by Shiboski (1998) assumes proportionality; proportional hazards (complementary log–log link) or proportional odds (logit and probit links). Other semi–parametric models, assuming a logit link, were proposed by Rossini and Tsiatis (1996).

The use of a kernel function to smooth out neighboring data information, as illustrated in formulas (7.1) and (7.2), is also the key idea in local polynomial estimation, as discussed in the next section.

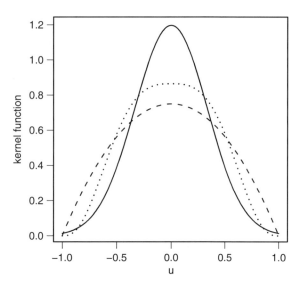

Fig. 7.2 Kernel functions: tricube (*dotted line*), Epanechnikov (*dashed line*), and Gaussian (*solid line*)

7.1.2 Local Estimation by Polynomials

Within the local polynomial framework, the linear predictor $\eta(a)$ is approximated locally, at one particular value a_0 for age, by a line (local linear, degree $p = 1$), or a parabola (local quadratic, degree $p = 2$), etc. The appropriate degree p is a first choice to be made. For a general degree, it holds that the (Taylor) approximation

$$\eta(a_i) \approx \eta(a_0) + \eta^{(1)}(a_0)(a_i - a_0) + \frac{\eta^{(2)}(a_0)}{2}(a_i - a_0)^2 + \ldots + \frac{\eta^{(p)}(a_0)}{p!}(a_i - a_0)^p,$$

(7.3)

is quite accurate, under the condition that a_i is close enough to a_0, and that the curve $\eta(\cdot)$ is sufficiently smooth at the age a_0 (smoothness is mathematically translated into the existence of the derivatives $\eta^{(1)}(a_0), \ldots, \eta^{(p)}(a_0)$). This mathematical fact naturally inspires the idea to fit a polynomial locally, only for observations with a_i close to a_0. This "closeness" is governed by the so-called kernel function K_h, assigning high weights to data points with age values close to a_0 and low or zero weights to data points further or far away. The kernel function K_h is typically a density function (such as the bell-shaped gaussian density), having mean 0 and variance h. This variance parameter h is the so-called smoothing parameter. Figure 7.2 graphs three popular kernels: the Gaussian kernel, the tricube kernel ($70/81 \times (1 - (|u|)^3)^3$ ($|u| \leq 1$)), and the Epanechnikov kernel ($3/4 \times (1 - u^2)(|u| \leq 1)$).

This idea to use a variance parameter to control and optimize the level of smoothness is a recurrent concept in smoothing (see the next chapter and the use of a variance component in mixed models as a smoothing parameter). The kernel

K_h and the value h are two other choices to be made. In general, one can say that a degree p higher than two is seldom required, that the choice of the form of the kernel K_h is relatively unimportant compared to the most crucial parameter in the game, the smoothing parameter h, also called the "window width." There are several options to select an appropriate value for h. We will illustrate some of these criteria in Sect. 7.2 and refer to the statistical literature for more details.

Instead of maximizing (5.2), the local polynomial approach is based on the maximization of

$$\sum_{i=1}^{N} \ell_i \left\{ Y_i, g^{-1} \left(\beta_0 + \beta_1(a_i - a_0) + \beta_2(a_i - a_0)^2 + \ldots + \beta_p(a_i - a_0)^p \right) \right\} K_h(a_i - a_0),$$

(7.4)

where

$$\ell_i \{ Y_i, \pi \} = Y_i \log\{\pi\} + (1 - Y_i) \log\{1 - \pi\}$$

are the individual binomial type contributions to the likelihood (as in expression (5.2)). Identification of the polynomial expressions in (7.3) and (7.4) leads to the following estimator for the k-th derivative of $\eta(a_0)$, for $k = 0, 1, \ldots, p$:

$$\hat{\eta}^{(k)}(a_0) = k! \hat{\beta}_k(a_0).$$

(7.5)

The estimator for the seroprevalence at age a_0 is then given by

$$\hat{\pi}(a_0) = g^{-1} \left\{ \hat{\beta}_0(a_0) \right\},$$

(7.6)

and for the force of infection at age a_0 by assuming $p \geq 1$ and using identity (5.5):

$$\hat{\lambda}(a_0) = \hat{\beta}_1(a_0) \delta \{ \hat{\beta}_0(a_0) \},$$

(7.7)

where $\delta\{\hat{\beta}_0(a_0)\} = dg^{-1}\{\hat{\beta}_0(a_0)\}/d\hat{\beta}_0(a_0)$ (see Chap. 6). Fitting a local polynomial model is straightforward and can be done by standard software for (logistic) regression. Indeed, as likelihood expression (7.4) indicates, the local fit at a particular value a_0 is the result of a simple weighted logistic regression with weights $w(a) = K_h(a - a_0)$. Figure 7.3 shows two such local fits at the age $a_0 = 5.5$ and $a_0 = 20.5$ for the UK Mumps data (Chap. 4). It concerns a local quadratic fit with tricube kernel.

Local polynomials are one of the most mathematically studied nonparametric methods (see aforementioned literature). For the specific application to the force of infection, Shkedy et al. (2003) derived some theoretical properties, such as asymptotic normality and formulas for the optimal choice of h, based on the asymptotic expression for the mean squared error.

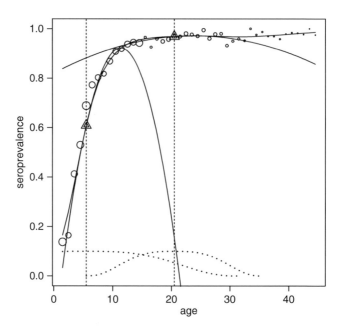

Fig. 7.3 UK Mumps data. Local quadratic fit with tricube kernel. Local quadratic polynomials (*solid curves*) are shown at ages 5.5 and 20.5, as well as the tricube kernels (*dotted curves*) which are used for locally weighting the observations

In R local polynomials can be fit through the *locfit* package as follows:

```
# R-code to fit a local polynomial
library(locfit)

# For binary response data y and age a
lpfit=locfit(y~a,family="binomial")

# For binomial response data with number of positives
# and total number
lpfit=locfit(pos/tot~a,family="binomial",alpha=0.7,deg=2,
kernel="tcub")

# local fit force of infection based on the derivative
# on the logit scale
lpfitd1=locfit(y~a,deriv=1,family="binomial",alpha=0.7,deg=2,
kernel="tcub")
lpfoi=fitted(lpfitd1)*fitted(lpfit)
```

Most of this code is self-explanatory, but the last line might need some explanation. The function *fitted* returns the fitted values on the probability π-scale for the probability function, but on the predictor η-scale for the derivative function. Since the default link is the logit link, Table 5.1 shows that the two factors in the rhs of $\lambda(a) = \eta'(a)\pi(a)$ are exactly the two scales provided by *fitted*. The option *family = "binomial"* has to be specified for seroprevalence data, as the default option is *"gaussian."* The other options *alpha = 0.7, deg = 2, kernel = "tcub"* are the default options. Full details on the use of *locfit* can be found in Loader (1999) and in the R-help files.

In the next section some details on the use of these options of *locfit* are illustrated on the UK Mumps data (see Chap. 4).

7.2   Application to UK Mumps Data

In this section we go briefly into the different *locfit*-options when fitting a local polynomial: the degree of the polynomial, the kernel, and most importantly, the smoothing parameter. The upper panel of Fig. 7.4 shows the data with size

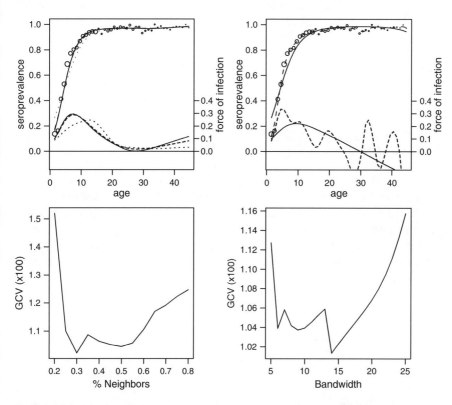

Fig. 7.4 UK Mumps data. *Upper panels*: proportion positive, as function of the corresponding half-year age categories, overlaid with different local polynomial fits for the seroprevalence and the force of infection; *left*: default options (*solid lines*), Epanechnikov kernel (*dashed line*), degree 1 (*dotted line*); *right*: default options but with local constant bandwidths 100 (*solid*) and 5 (*dashed*). *Lower panels*: GCV curves for the nearest neighbor method (*left*) and constant bandwidth (*right*). Note that the models for the prevalence are not constrained to be monotone and therefore $\lambda(a)$ is not always positive. Monotonicity constraints will be discussed in details in Chap. 9

proportional to the number of observations in the half-year age group, overlaid with different local polynomials. The solid curves in the upper left panel show the fitted seroprevalence (upper curve) and the fitted force of infection (lower curve) using the default options $alpha = 0.7$, $deg = 2$, $kernel = $ "tcub."

The option $alpha = 0.7$ refers to a local fit only incorporating 70% of the data, namely the 70% closest neighbors, when fitting the curve at a particular age a_0 (as in 7.3 and 7.4). This way of local fitting implies a varying value of $h = h(a_0)$ in formula (7.4), as neighbors are more spread out in sparse data areas. More precisely, specifying $alpha = \alpha$, the nearest neighbor bandwidth $h(a_0)$ is computed as follows: (1) compute all distances $|a_0 - a_i|$, $i = 1, \ldots, N$; (2) take $h(a_0)$ to be the kth smallest distance, where $k = \lfloor n\alpha \rfloor$. In general, this is preferred above a constant bandwidth h, which does not adapt to the data density. In *locfit*, a constant bandwidth of, e.g., $h = 5$ can be specified as $alpha = c(0,5)$.

The second option $deg = 2$ specifies the degree of the local polynomial, in this case a local quadratic fit ($p = 2$ in formula 7.4). Shkedy et al. (2003) showed that this is the optimal degree when estimating the force of infection. Finally the last option $kernel = $ "tcub" specifies the use of the tricube kernel. The dashed curves show the fitted curves with the same options using the Epanechnikov kernel. As expected, for this application, the differences are very minor and the curves are almost identical. The dotted curve corresponds to the fit where the only change was the degree to be equal to one. This has a bit more impact as it changes the location and the value of the maximal force of infection.

Of course all curves in this panel are nonoptimal since they are not based on the optimal smoothing parameter, and the optimal value of the smoothing parameters depends on the degree of the polynomial. The effect of the smoothing parameter is illustrated in the right upper panel, showing the constant bandwidth fits for two extreme cases: (1) a very high value $h = 10^6$ implying that all data are equally weighted, leading to a parametric polynomial fit of degree 2; (2) a very low value $h = 5$ leading to a too wiggly curve. Clearly both fits are bad, showing that the smoothing parameter has to be selected with caution.

There are different criteria to select the optimal value for the smoothing parameter, based on the data. Plug-in estimators are based on asymptotic expressions for bias and variance, combined into an asymptotic mean (integrated) squared error (MSE) expression. This approach however replaces the problem to the estimation of some unknown quantities in the asymptotic expression, which are even more complicated to estimate (such as a higher-order derivative of the function of interest). This approach was taken by Shkedy et al. (2003) and they used fractional polynomials as an initial estimate for the unknown quantities in the MSE expression. Other approaches to bandwidth selection are extensions of model selection methods for parametric models, such as AIC, Mallows C_p, and cross-validation. In what follows we illustrate the cross-validation and the generalized cross-validation (GCV) method. For more information on bandwidth selection, see Ruppert et al. (2003) and Simonoff (1996).

The cross-validation bandwidth minimizes the cross-validation criterion

$$CV(h) = \sum_{i=1}^{N} \ell_i\{Y_i, \hat{\pi}_i^h(a_i)\},$$

where $\hat{\pi}_i^h(a_i)$ is defined as the local estimator at a_i leaving out the ith observation and using bandwidth h. The CV-criterion is minimized as a function of h for a constant bandwidth or as a function of the percentage of neighbors α for a nearest neighbor bandwidth. GCV provides an approximation to cross-validation based on the so-called fitted or effective degrees of freedom and does not require the possibly expensive calculation of the N leave-i-out estimates $\hat{\pi}_i^h(a_i)$ (see e.g. Ruppert et al. 2003). The lower panels of Fig. 7.4 show the GCV curves for the nearest neighbor (left) and constant bandwidth (right) approaches. The R code to produce these GCV plots is as follows.

```
# R-code to compute the cross-validation criterion on a grid
# "lowgp" to "uppergp" with resolution "gridres"
lowgp=0.2; uppergp=0.8; gridres=0.05

alpha=seq(lowgp,uppergp, by=gridres)
plot(gcvplot(y~a,family="binomial",alpha=alpha,type="l"))

# plot with horizontal axis given by alpha
cvres=cbind(alpha,summary(gcvplot(y~a,family="binomial",
            alpha=alpha)))
plot(cvres[,1],cvres[,3],type="n",main="Nearest Neighbor GCV",
     xlab="\% Neighbors",ylab="GCV")
lines(cvres[,1],cvres[,3])
```

The left GCV-curve in Fig. 7.4 shows two minimums, at percentages 30% and 50%. Since a flat curvature at the minimum is typical and since a more parsimonious model is to be preferred, we opted for $\alpha = 0.50$ as a final choice. For a constant bandwidth, the right GCV-curve suggests an optimal bandwidth $h = 14$. The seroprevalence and force of infection fit well for both optimal bandwidth choices as shown in Fig. 7.5. Both fits are very similar, except for the fact that above the age of 40 years, the fit based on the local constant bandwidth suffers more from boundary effects as a result of data sparseness.

7.3 Concluding Remarks

We have shown how nonparametric models such as local polynomials can be used to fit seroprevalence data and to estimate the force of infection. Such models can also be extended to encompass a setting with multiple covariates. In case the additional

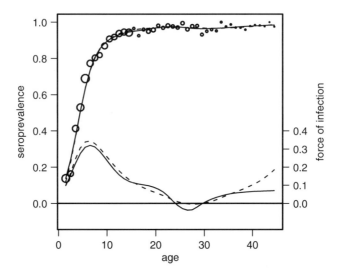

Fig. 7.5 UK Mumps data. proportion positive, as function of the corresponding half-year age categories, overlaid with two local polynomial fits for the seroprevalence and the force of infection: with GCV optimal nearest neighbor percentage 0.5 (*solid line*) and with GCV optimal constant bandwidth 14 (*dashed line*)

covariate is categorical (such as gender), the local nature of this nonparametric approach boils down to separate fits for all categories. In case other covariates are continuous, the concept of local fitting can be readily extended to higher dimensional neighborhoods and windows. Of course, selecting the optimal bandwidth can become cumbersome and the curse of dimensionality will complicate the estimation in case of several covariates. In the latter case additive and semiparametric models are typically better choices and will be discussed in the next chapter.

Chapter 8
Semiparametric Approaches to Model the Prevalence and Force of Infection

8.1 Semiparametric Approaches

While Chap. 6 presented an overview of different parametric models, imposing a specific structure on the age-specific seroprevalence and FOI, Chap. 7 showed how nonparametric methods allow to capture unusual or unexpected features of the data. Although, these two frameworks are often considered to be mutually exclusive, nonparametric methods can be looked upon as an extension of parametric methods. This combination is often referred to as semiparametric regression (Ruppert et al. 2003).

The idea of semiparametric regression is best illustrated by means of an example. Figure 8.1 shows the proportion of B19 seropositives as a function of age for the Belgian B19 data (Chap. 4). To capture the systematic trend in these data, one could opt to carry out a generalized linear regression analysis with a linear, quadratic, or higher-order polynomial in age. While such an analysis will be able to capture the overall trend, it is not straightforward to adapt the function to capture systematic deviations from the overall trend such as the decrease in B19 seroprevalence around 25 years of age.

In semiparametric regression, the parametric analysis is extended by including segment-wise parametric functions that are able to follow deviations from the overall trend in the data. One typically imposes continuity and differentiability up to a certain order by constraining these segment-wise functions in the knots, i.e., the points where two adjacent segments join. This approach is known as spline smoothing (de Boor 1978). To overcome overfitting, penalized spline smoothing has been introduced by O'Sullivan (1986), while Eilers and Marx (1996) actually gave it the name "P-spline smoothing." The idea of penalized spline smoothing has led to a series of approaches including the work of Eilers and Marx (1996), Eilers et al. (2006), Ruppert et al. (2003), and Wood (2006).

In this chapter, an overview of different semiparametric approaches will be presented. The primary aim is to model the seroprevalence in a flexible way, ignoring constraints as monotonicity (steady-state assumption), distortions in the

N. Hens et al., *Modeling Infectious Disease Parameters Based on Serological and Social Contact Data*, Statistics for Biology and Health 63, DOI 10.1007/978-1-4614-4072-7_8, © Springer Science+Business Media New York 2012

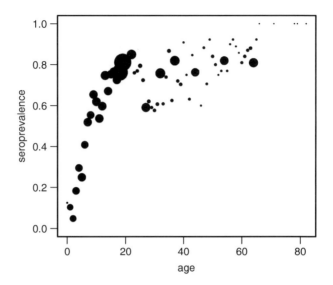

Fig. 8.1 Age-specific proportion of B19 seropositives for the Belgian B19 data

seroprofile due to, e.g., the presence of maternal antibodies, waning immunity- and test-uncertainty. Using the general form of the hazard function in the current status data framework, the estimate for the FOI is easily obtained from the estimated seroprevalence using $\hat{\lambda}(a) = \hat{\pi}'(a)/(1 - \hat{\pi}(a))$ (see (5.4)). The inclusion of monotonicity constraints will be discussed in Chap. 9.

We start by introducing penalized splines in a more formal way in Sect. 8.2 where we distinguish between the penalized likelihood framework and the generalized linear mixed model alternative. In Sect. 8.3, we address taking other predictors such as gender into account. While the methods discussed up to that moment use a common smoothing parameter for the whole range of the predictor variable, an extension towards adaptive smoothing methods is provided in Sect. 8.4. We end by contrasting the aforementioned semiparametric methods to the parametric and nonparametric methods as introduced in Chaps. 6 and 7 using a case study on rubella in the UK (Chap. 4).

8.2 Penalized Splines

As before let y_i indicate whether individual i has experienced the infection before age a_i, $i = 1, \ldots, N$. A general model relating the prevalence to age can be written as a GLM:

$$g(P(Y_i = 1|a_i)) = g(\pi(a_i)) = \eta(a_i), \tag{8.1}$$

where g is the link function and η is the linear predictor. The linear predictor $\eta(a_i)$ can be estimated semiparametrically using penalized splines. A popular approach is the penalized spline with truncated power basis functions of degree p and fixed knots $\kappa_1, \ldots, \kappa_K$ where (see e.g. Friedman and Silverman 1989; Ruppert et al. 2003):

$$\eta(a_i) = \beta_0 + \beta_1 a_i + \cdots + \beta_p a_i^p + \sum_{k=1}^{K} u_k (a_i - \kappa_k)_+^p , \qquad (8.2)$$

with

$$(a_i - \kappa_k)_+^p = \begin{cases} 0, & a_i \leq \kappa_k \\ (a_i - \kappa_k)^p, & a_i > \kappa_k. \end{cases} \qquad (8.3)$$

In matrix notation, the mean structure model for $\eta(a_i)$ becomes

$$\eta = \mathbf{X}\beta + \mathbf{Z}\mathbf{u}, \qquad (8.4)$$

where $\eta = [\eta(a_1) \cdots \eta(a_N)]^T$, $\beta = [\beta_0 \ \beta_1 \ \cdots \ \beta_p]^T$, and $\mathbf{u} = [u_1 \ u_2 \ \cdots \ u_K]^T$ are the regression coefficients with corresponding design matrices:

$$\mathbf{X} = \begin{bmatrix} 1 & a_1 & a_1^2 & \cdots & a_1^p \\ 1 & a_2 & a_2^2 & \cdots & a_2^p \\ \vdots & \vdots & \vdots & \cdots & \vdots \\ 1 & a_N & a_N^2 & \cdots & a_N^p \end{bmatrix}, \ \mathbf{Z} = \begin{bmatrix} (a_1 - \kappa_1)_+^p & (a_1 - \kappa_2)_+^p & \cdots & (a_1 - \kappa_K)_+^p \\ (a_2 - \kappa_1)_+^p & (a_2 - \kappa_2)_+^p & \cdots & (a_2 - \kappa_K)_+^p \\ \vdots & \vdots & \cdots & \vdots \\ (a_N - \kappa_1)_+^p & (a_N - \kappa_2)_+^p & \cdots & (a_N - \kappa_K)_+^p \end{bmatrix}.$$

Within the parametric regression framework, η can be estimated by maximizing the likelihood. However, it is always possible to choose η sufficiently complicated that it interpolates the data in the sense that the fitted values agree with the observed responses. In the semiparametric framework, following Ruppert et al. (2003), we consider a number of knots that is large enough (typically 5–20) to ensure the desired flexibility. But, to overcome the problem of overfitting we restrict the influence of $\mathbf{Z}$ by constraining the corresponding vector of coefficients. How this is typically done is described in Sect. 8.2.1. Once $(\beta, \mathbf{u})$ has been estimated, the FOI can easily be derived as

$$\hat{\lambda}(a_i) = \left[\hat{\beta}_1 + 2\hat{\beta}_2 a_i + \cdots + p\hat{\beta}_p a_i^{p-1} + \sum_{k=1}^{K} p\hat{u}_k (a_i - \kappa_k)_+^{p-1} \right] \delta(\hat{\eta}(a_i)),$$

where $\delta()$ is determined by the link function used in the model (See $\delta(\cdot)$ and Chap. 5).

Before going into the different methods to control the smoothness of the semiparametric regression, we graphically present the semiparametric procedure as outlined above. We use the Belgian B19 data and without loss of generality, we restrict attention to those individuals aged 0–40 years. We use the penalized splines with truncated power basis functions of degree 2 and use three knots for illustrative purposes. The selected knots were located at ages 8.07, 14.04, and 19.38 years, i.e., the 25%, 50% and 75% percentiles of the age distribution.

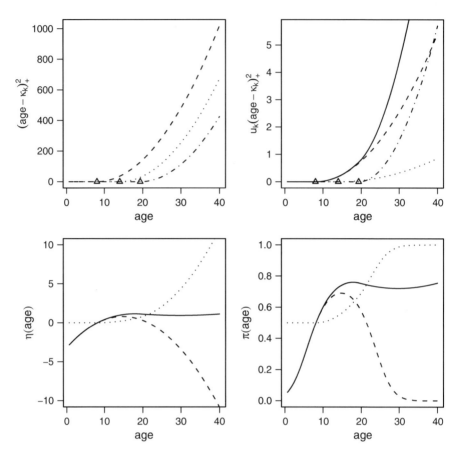

Fig. 8.2 Illustration of penalized splines with truncated polynomial basis functions of degree 2 and three knots (*triangles*; *upper left panel*: *dashed, dotted, dashed–dotted lines*) with their respective contributions (*upper right panel*: *dashed, dotted, dashed–dotted lines*) to the semiparametric part of the linear predictor (*solid line*). In the *lower left panel*, the parametric part (*dashed line*) and the semiparametric part (*dotted line*) add up to the linear predictor (*solid line*). The *lower right panel* shows this addition on the scale of the prevalence

In the upper left panel of Fig. 8.2, the basis functions, i.e., the truncated poly-nomials of degree 2, as defined by (8.3), are shown at the respective knots. Using the estimated values for (β, u), we show the contributions of each of those basis functions to the semiparametric part of the linear predictor (8.2): $\sum_{k=1}^{3} \hat{u}_k (a - \kappa_k)_+^2$, in the upper right panel of Fig. 8.2. In the lower left panel of Fig. 8.2 (solid line), $\hat{\eta}(a_i)$ as defined by (8.2) is shown together with its decomposition into the parametric part ($\hat{\beta}_0 + \hat{\beta}_1 a + \hat{\beta}_2 a^2$, dashed line) and the semiparametric part (dotted line). In the lower right panel of Fig. 8.2 the same decomposition is shown on the prevalence scale (logit-link). Note that the latter decomposition doesn't add up directly whereas the decomposition on the scale of the linear predictor does.

While the underlying function (here: the quadratic function of age) is able to capture the trend in the data, the three semiparametric components jointly allow for a more local adaptation of the function to the data. Note that the $\hat{u}_k, k = 1, 2, 3$ are estimated at 5.3×10^{-3}, 1.2×10^{-3}, and 13.4×10^{-3}, respectively. These values are all positive which in general is not necessarily so.

Note that the semiparametric approaches in this book all allow for a similar graphical representation as outlined here. We however do not pursue these and advise the reader, when interested, to the references mentioned throughout this chapter.

8.2.1 Penalized Likelihood Framework

A first approach to control the influence of $\mathbf{Z}$ is obtained by maximizing the penalized likelihood:

$$\phi^{-1} \left[y^T (\mathbf{X}\beta + \mathbf{Z}\mathbf{u}) - \mathbf{1}^T c(\mathbf{X}\beta + \mathbf{Z}\mathbf{u}) \right] - \frac{1}{2} \lambda^2 \begin{bmatrix} \beta \\ \mathbf{u} \end{bmatrix}^T D \begin{bmatrix} \beta \\ \mathbf{u} \end{bmatrix}, \tag{8.5}$$

with D a known positive semi-definite penalty matrix (Wahba 1978; Green and Silverman 1994), y the response vector, $\mathbf{1}$ the unit vector and where $c(\cdot)$ is determined by the link function used in the GLM. The first term in (8.5) measures the goodness-of-fit while the second term is the roughness penalty. λ is the smoothing parameter for which large values produce smoother curves while smaller values produce more wiggly curves. The parameter ϕ is the overdispersion parameter and equals 1 if there is no overdispersion.

In general, the smoothness of a P-spline is determined by the choice of basis function, selection of knots, and the way penalization is done. Next to the truncated power basis functions, a variety of other spline basis functions are used in literature. Most commonly used basis functions include the polynomial, truncated polynomial, and B-spline basis function. The knot selection is mostly either equidistant over the range of the covariate space or based on the quantiles of the covariate distribution (Ruppert et al. 2003). However, user-defined criteria can be used too. Finally, penalization can be done in a variety of ways such as penalizing for large finite differences of adjacent coefficients or for large curvatures. The trade-off between smoothness and closely matching the data is governed by the smoothing parameter. The choice of the smoothing parameter is crucial in the practical use of splines. Several smoothing parameter selection methods as Akaike's information criterion (AIC), its corrected version (AIC$_c$), the Bayesian information criterion (BIC), unbiased risk estimation (UBRE), and generalized cross-validation (GCV) have proven to be effective.

The degree of the basis function and continuity constraints on the function and its derivatives in the knots, the placement of the knots, the choice of penalty, and smoothing parameter selection are very important for a spline. Basic references in this field are: de Boor (1978), Eilers and Marx (1996), Ruppert et al. (2003), and Wood (2006). In what follows, several methods for which code is readily available will be presented.

8.2.1.1 Smoothing Splines

Smoothing splines (Hastie and Tibshirani 1990) avoid knot selection problems by using the maximal set of knots, i.e., all unique age values. Regularization is then done by penalizing the curvature of the function. The resulting spline is a natural spline, i.e., a cubic spline where the function is linear beyond the endpoints of the data (Chambers and Hastie 1992).

The implementation of smoothing splines in R is given through the *gam*-library (Chambers and Hastie 1992). The following code fits a smoothing spline with logit- and cloglog-link, respectively.

```
# R-code Smoothing Splines
library(gam)
gam(y~s(a,df=dfopt1),family=binomial(link="logit"))
gam(y~s(a,df=dfopt2),family=binomial(link="cloglog"))
```

The amount of smoothing is fixed by *df*, the effective degrees of freedom or equivalently *spar*, the smoothing parameter. Given a grid of *df* (or *spar*)-values, the optimal amount of smoothing is chosen, e.g., by minimizing the BIC criterion. Note that different link functions could result in different optimal smoothing parameters, here denoted by *dfopt1* and *dfopt2*, respectively.

Applying the above procedure to the Belgian B19 data resulted in *dfopt1 = 3.5* and *dfopt2 = 4.5* for logit- and cloglog-link, respectively. The resulting seroprevalence curves and the thereof derived FOI curves are given in the left upper panel of Fig. 8.3. There is little difference in seroprevalence and FOI when comparing logit (solid line) and cloglog (dashed line) curves. Note that of both models the model with logit-link is the preferred one according to the BIC criterion (Table 8.1).

8.2.1.2 B-Splines

Eilers and Marx (1996) used B-splines of which the basis functions are defined as differences of truncated polynomials of degree p (de Boor 1978). They proposed to use m-order difference penalties on the coefficients of adjacent B-spline basis functions to control the smoothness of the curve and consequently used the term "P-splines" (penalized splines). Throughout the remainder of the book we will mostly use the term B-spline even when using its penalized version. The degree p,

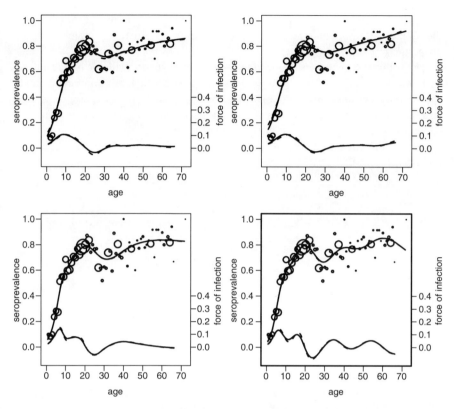

Fig. 8.3 Fitted seroprevalence and FOI curves for the Belgian B19 data using smoothing splines (*left upper panel*), B-splines (*right upper panel*), cubic regression splines (*left lower panel*), and thin plate regression splines (*right lower panel*) for both logit-link (*solid line*) and cloglog-link (*dashed line*). In each graph, the *lower curves* represent the FOI curves derived from the corresponding seroprevalence curves. The *dots* are the observed seroprevalence per integer age value with size proportional to the number of samples taken

Table 8.1 Overview of BIC values for the different P-spline methods in the penalized likelihood framework

Method	Smoothing parameter selection	Link	BIC
Smoothing splines	BIC	logit	3,480.80
		cloglog	3,488.43
B-splines	BIC	logit	3,472.70
		cloglog	3,481.32
Cubic regression splines	UBRE	logit	3,481.38
		cloglog	3,485.31
Thin-plate regression splines	UBRE	logit	3,489.90
		cloglog	3,491.57

the order m, and the number of (equidistant) knots determine the flexibility of the spline. The popularity of B-splines is mainly due to their stable numerical properties (Eilers et al. 2006).

The following code uses the *pspline.fit*-function as made available by the authors of Eilers and Marx (1996). It is often advised to use a large number of knots, specified by *ps.intervals*, while a B-spline basis function of degree $p = 3$ or larger ensures a differentiable FOI. We choose order $m = 2$ but higher-order difference penalties resulting in smoother curves can be chosen too. Similar to the smoothing splines setting, the optimal smoothness parameter *lambda* is selected using the BIC criterion.

```
# R-code B-splines
# Function Code Eilers and Marx (see book's website)
pspline.fit(response=y,x.var=a,ps.intervals=20,degree=3,
            order=2,link="logit",family="binomial",
            lambda=lambdaopt1,x.predicted=a)
pspline.fit(response=y,x.var=a,ps.intervals=20,degree=3,
            order=2,link="cloglog",family="binomial",
            lambda=lambdaopt2,x.predicted=a)
```

Applying the procedure to the Belgian B19 data with logit- and cloglog-link resulted in optimal smoothing parameters *lambdaopt1 = 80* and *lambdaopt2 = 200*. The fitted seroprevalence and FOI curves are shown in the upper right panel of Fig. 8.3. Note the similarity with the results of the smoothing spline, although in terms of BIC, this method is the preferred one (Table 8.1).

8.2.1.3 Cubic Regression Splines

Cubic regression splines fall into the more general class of regression splines, joining (cubic) polynomials at the knots of the spline to ensure continuity and differentiability up to degree two. In contrast to smoothing splines, the number of knots is smaller than the unique number of data points and the placement of knots is user-defined. The cubic regression spline is available in the R-library *mgcv*-package (Wood 2006), where the default knot location is governed by the quantiles of the covariate distribution. An additional advantage of the *mgcv*-package is the automated selection of the smoothness parameter by either GCV or UBRE (Wood 2006).

The code hereunder shows the implementation of the cubic regression spline approach using logit- and cloglog-link, respectively. The resulting seroprevalence fits are shown in the left lower panel of Fig. 8.3. Although the BIC values are close to those for the smoothing splines (Table 8.1), the seroprevalence fit is not so smooth. This is also reflected by the shape of the FOI.

```
# R-code Cubic Regression Spline
library(mgcv)
gam(y~s(a,bs="cr"),family=binomial(link="logit"))
gam(y~s(a,bs="cr"),family=binomial(link="cloglog"))
```

8.2.1.4 Thin Plate Regression Splines

Another regression spline, available in the *mgcv*-package in R, is the thin plate regression spline. Changing the option *bs* in the previous code to *tp* allows these thin plate regression splines to be fitted.

```
# R-code Thin Plate Regression Spline
library(mgcv)
gam(y~s(a,bs="tp"),family=binomial(link="logit"))
gam(y~s(a,bs="tp"),family=binomial(link="cloglog"))
```

Thin plate regression splines (Wood 2006) do not use knots, are computationally harder but provide nested models which for model building is in line with general linear modeling methods. Thin plate splines use less parameters and posses optimality properties in the use of generalized additive models. The resulting seroprevalence curves are the most non-smooth curves of all methods (Fig. 8.3). The BIC values are the largest ones for both "cloglog" and "logit" link function (Table 8.1).

Applying the four aforementioned methods resulted mainly in differences regarding smoothness. This is not surprisingly so since the different methods use different basis functions, different penalties, and different knot selection. In Table 8.2, an overview of the different components for each smoothing method is shown.

Let us now turn to the generalized linear mixed model framework to facilitate an integrated smoothing parameter selection method.

8.2.2 Generalized Linear Mixed Model Framework

Generalized linear mixed models (GLMM) are commonly used to handle correlations in the data (e.g., longitudinal data, clustered data). In addition, they are a standard tool for smoothing discrete data. Several authors have made an explicit connection between semiparametric regression and mixed models (Speed 1991; Wang et al. 1998; Zhang et al. 1998; Verbyla et al. 1999). This connection allows penalized splines to be fitted as a GLMM, possibly combined with complex

Table 8.2 Overview of the different smoothing methods and their basis function, knot selection, penalty and smoothing parameter selection method

Method	Basis function	Knots	Penalty	Smoothing parameter selection
Smoothing splines (*gam-library*)	Cubic	All grid points	Second order derivative	Manual
B-splines (*pspline.fit*)	Differences of truncated polynomials	User-defined (ps.intervals)	Difference penalty	Manual
Cubic regression splines (*mgcv-library*)	Cubic	User-defined (mgcv-default)	Second order derivative	Automated
Thin-plate regression splines (*mgcv-library*)	Thin plate	None	Eigenvalue decomposition	Automated

correlation structures in the data. Since then, using smoothing splines within the mixed model framework has become more and more appreciated and the number of applications in literature is growing.

Starting from the penalized likelihood framework and truncated basis functions as in (8.5), an obvious constraint on the parameters $\mathbf{u}$ would be $\sum_k u_k^2 < C$, for some positive value C. This is equivalent to choosing $(\beta, \mathbf{u})$ to maximize the penalized loglikelihood (8.5) with $D = diag(\mathbf{0}, \mathbf{1})$ where $\mathbf{0}$ denotes the zero vector of length $p + 1$ and $\mathbf{1}$ denotes the unit vector of length K. For a fixed value of λ, this is equivalent to fitting the generalized linear mixed model (Ruppert et al. 2003; Wand 2003; Ngo and Wand 2004):

$$f(y|\mathbf{u}) = \exp\left\{\phi^{-1}\left[y^T(\mathbf{X}\beta + \mathbf{Z}\mathbf{u}) - c(\mathbf{X}\beta + \mathbf{Z}\mathbf{u})\right] + \mathbf{1}^T c(y)\right\},$$

$$\mathbf{u} \sim N(0, \mathbf{G}), \tag{8.6}$$

with similar notation as before and where $\mathbf{G} = \sigma_u^2 \mathbf{I}_{K \times K}$. Thus, the nonlinear part of the spline $\mathbf{Z}$ is penalized by assuming that the corresponding coefficients $\mathbf{u}$ are random effects with $\mathbf{u} \sim N(0, \sigma_u^2 \mathbf{I})$.

Given this equivalence, the penalized spline model can be fitted using standard statistical software for GLMM where the amount of smoothing $\lambda = 1/\sigma_u$ is automatically selected via the estimation routine, being an important asset of the GLMM framework. The smaller the variance σ_u of the random effects distribution, the smoother the resulting curve. As in the penalized likelihood framework, a generalization towards different basis functions and different choices of knots can be used (Ruppert et al. 2003; Wood 2006). Next to the simple and often used truncated line basis, also penalized splines with a higher-order truncated polynomial basis, a radial basis, and a B-spline basis have a mixed model representation with corresponding basis (Currie and Durban 2002; Ruppert et al. 2003).

A challenge of this method is the model estimation because of the nonlinear nature of the GLMM. Maximum likelihood estimation requires the marginal likelihood of Y, which is obtained by integrating over the random effects. In general, this integration cannot be solved analytically, and maximum likelihood estimation is hindered by the presence of this integral. Several alternative methods to estimate parameters in a random effects model are available (Molenberghs and Verbeke 2005). A possible approach is to compute the integration numerically. Different integral approximations are available, the principal one being (adaptive) Gaussian quadrature (Anderson and Aitkin 1985). Alternatively, the generalized linear random effects model can be cast into a Bayesian framework, avoiding the need for numerical integration by taking repeated samples from the posterior distributions using Gibbs sampling techniques (Zeger and Karim 1991) as discussed in Chap. 10. Other methods use approximations of the likelihood to circumvent the computational burden caused by numerical integration. A possible method involves Laplace approximation of integrals (Breslow and Clayton 1993; Wolfinger and O'Connell 1993), which is commonly referred to as penalized quasi-likelihood (PQL). However, the latter approach, although the simplest method among the presented alternatives, can be seriously biased for binary response data.

The connection between the penalized spline smoother and the optimal predictor in a GLMM framework, assuming normality for the parameters u_k, presents an opportunity for using standard mixed model software, such as, e.g., the "nlme" library in R or the "nlmixed" procedure in SAS. The penalized spline model, using the PQL estimation method, is also routinely implemented in the SAS procedure "glimmix." Also the "mcgv"-library in R (Wood 2006) and the "SemiPar"-library in R (Ruppert et al. 2003) contain a function to fit a penalized spline in the GLMM framework, using PQL estimation. In "mgcv," the code is very similar to the R-code for a thin plate regression spline or a cubic regression spline.

```
# R-code to fit Penalized Spline in GLMM framework
library(mgcv)
gamm(y~s(a,bs="tp"),family=binomial(link="logit"))
gamm(y~s(a,bs="cr"),family=binomial(link="logit"))
```

The resulting seroprevalence and force of infection curves are shown in Fig. 8.4.

Note that no formal likelihood-based comparison of different basis functions is possible because of the PQL-estimation method. As such there is no formal way to compare the method with those proposed in Sect. 8.2.1. Based on a visual inspection, the results of the different GLMM-based methods are similar to those of the penalized likelihood methods.

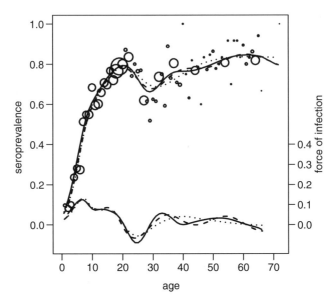

Fig. 8.4 Fitted seroprevalence and FOI curves for the Belgian B19 data using penalized splines fitted in the GLMM framework, using a radial basis (*solid line*), a thin plate basis (*dashed line*), and cubic basis (*dotted line*). The *dots* are the observed seroprevalence per integer age value with size proportional to the number of samples taken

8.3   Covariate Effects

So far, focus was on the specification of a spline describing the prevalence and the force of infection as a function of age. Often, it is also of interest to compare the prevalence and force of infection curves among different populations such as comparisons among males and females or among different countries. This is naturally embedded in the generalized additive model framework (see e.g. Hastie and Tibshirani 1990; Wood 2006) and its mixed model variant (Lin and Zhang 1999). For illustrative purposes, we focus on a comparison among the Belgian and Italian B19 data.

The semiparametric model discussed in Sect. 8.2.2 implies that the overall trend for each group can be represented by an additive model of two components, a linear component $X\beta$ and a smooth component Zu. Figure 8.5 illustrates, with hypothetical examples, several possible scenarios related to the evolution of the prevalence as a function of age in two groups.

In the top left panel, the two groups have a similar trend, the linear components of the splines in the two groups differ only by a constant. The top right panel shows the prevalence curves when the groups are different in the linear part (different intercept and slope) but the smooth component of the mean is identical. The bottom panels reveal patterns in which the prevalence for the two groups has a different evolution over age and the groups are different in both the linear and smooth part.

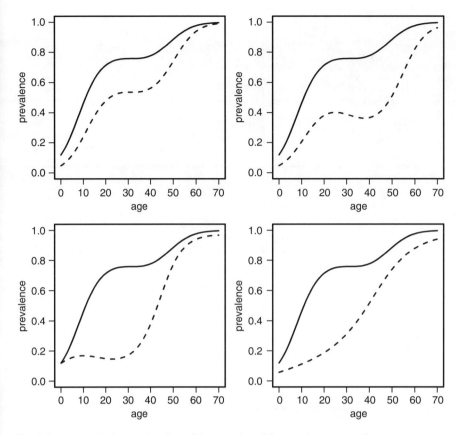

Fig. 8.5 Hypothetical examples of possible scenarios of the prevalence curves in two groups

In the left panel, both groups have the same smoothing parameter; in the right panel, the smoothing parameter for the two groups is different. In what follows, we formulate possible penalized splines in the generalized linear mixed model framework, following each of the scenarios illustrated in Fig. 8.5.

First, we assume that the underlying linear trend in both groups differs by a shift only. The model can be represented as

$$\eta(a_i) = (\beta_0 + \gamma_0 G_i) + \beta_1 a_i + \cdots + \beta_p a_i^p + \sum_{k=1}^{K} u_k (a_i - \kappa_k)_+^p, \qquad (8.7)$$

where the coefficients u_k are common to all groups, with $\mathrm{Var}(u_k) = \sigma_u^2$ and G_i is a group indicator. Note that the same nonparametric part is fitted to both groups. This model thus assumes that the difference amongst the groups, if present, does not depend on age.

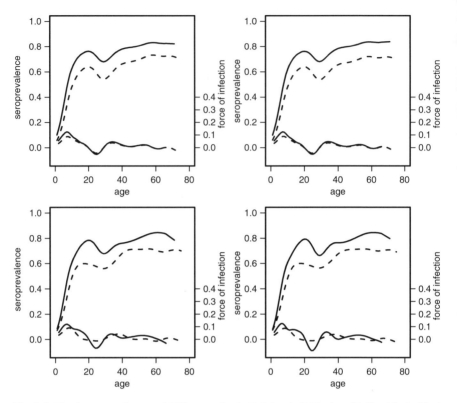

Fig. 8.6 Fitted seroprevalence and FOI curves for the Belgian (*solid line*) and Italian (*dashed line*) B19 data using penalized splines fitted in the GLMM framework using a radial basis

All models discussed in this section were fitted in SAS. We use the Belgian and Italian B19 data for illustration. This resulted in the seroprevalence and force of infection curves as given in the upper left panel of Fig. 8.6. There seems to be a higher prevalence for Belgium as compared to Italy, which is slightly reflected by an increased force of infection at 0–10 years of age for the Belgian B19 data.

Second, assume that the linear parts of the models differ while the same smooth part is considered for both groups (model 2). In this case, the group effect is no longer constant over age. A representation of such a model is

$$\eta(a_i) = (\beta_0 + \gamma_0 G_i) + (\beta_1 + \gamma_1 G_i)a_i + \cdots + (\beta_p + \gamma_p G_i)a_i^p + \sum_{k=1}^{K} u_k (a_i - \kappa_k)_+^p, \quad (8.8)$$

with $\text{Var}(u_k) = \sigma_u^2$. The top right panel of Fig. 8.5 graphically illustrates such a scenario. The SAS program to be used to fit this model is very similar to the one of the previous model. The resulting seroprevalence and force of infection curves for the Belgian and Italian B19 data are given in the upper right panel of Fig. 8.6 and are found to be similar to the previous model.

All models considered so far assume that the same smooth component is fitted to both groups. It is possible to go one step further and fit a model with different nonparametric parts for Belgium and Italy, although the same smoothing parameter is used. The linear part of the model is assumed to be different and, although the random effects are assumed to be independent from Belgium to Italy, a single smoothing parameter is used for both groups (model 3). A representation of such a model is

$$\eta(a_i) = (\beta_0 + \gamma_0 G_i) + (\beta_1 + \gamma_1 G_i)a_i + \cdots + (\beta_p + \gamma_p G_i)a_i^p + \sum_{k=1}^{K} (u_{kg})(a_i - \kappa_k)_+^p.$$

(8.9)

Note that the part of the design matrix corresponding to smoothing Z_i is now block-diagonal with each diagonal entry corresponding to a particular group and the coefficients for the truncated lines basis, u_{kg}, are now group-specific with $\mathrm{Var}(u_{kg}) = \sigma_u^2$. This situation is similar to the illustration in the left lower panel of Fig. 8.5. The resulting prevalence and force of infection curves for the Belgian and Italian B19 data are given in the lower left panel of Fig. 8.6. There is a considerable difference in the estimated seroprevalence and force of infection when compared to those estimated based on the previous two models.

A final extension is to relax the assumption of a constant smoothing parameter across the groups and thereby to assume that the groups can be smoothed separately with different smoothing parameters (model 4). Hence, both the fixed effects part and the nonparametric part differ by group. The penalized spline representation of this model and the Z matrix are the same as in previous model, but with the variance components $\mathrm{Var}(u_{kg}) = \sigma_{ug}^2$ being group-specific. The bottom right panel of Fig. 8.6 shows the resulting prevalence and force of infection curves when applied to the Belgian and Italian B19 data.

Again, as in Sect. 8.2.2, no formal likelihood-based comparison of the different models can be made due to the PQL estimation procedure as used in "glimmix."

However, when turning to the penalized likelihood framework, one can use for instance AIC or BIC to select the most appropriate model from the candidate set of fitted models. This is done for models 1, 2, and 4 using the *gam*-function in R (library "mgcv").

```
# R code to fit the interaction of a spline of age with country
# Model 1
gam(y~country+s(a,bs="tp"),family=binomial(link="logit"))
# Model 2
gam(y~country+country*a+s(a,bs="tp"),
    family=binomial(link="logit"))
# Model 4
gam(y~s(a,bs="tp",by=country1)+s(a,bs="tp",by=country2),
    family=binomial(link="logit"))
```

In the code *country1* and *country2* denote the dummy variables associated with Belgium and Italy, respectively. Based on the corresponding BIC values (6,565.31, 6,573.14, 6,700.05), one can decide that there is only a shift when comparing the B19 seroprofile for Belgium and Italy (p-value < 0.0001 when compared to identical seroprofiles). Note that model 3, although possibly formulated in a penalized likelihood framework, is not implemented as such in the using the *gam*-function in R.

8.4   Adaptive Spline Smoothing

In the preceding section, smoothing methods were either embedded in the penalized likelihood framework or in the generalized linear mixed model framework. Both approaches differ in the way the smoothing parameter is selected/estimated. Recall the GLMM-approach (8.6):

$$f(y|\mathbf{u}) = \exp\left\{\phi^{-1}\left[y^T(\mathbf{X}\beta + \mathbf{Z}\mathbf{u}) - c(\mathbf{X}\beta + \mathbf{Z}\mathbf{u})\right] + \mathbf{1}^T c(y)\right\},$$

$$\mathbf{u} \sim N(0, \sigma_u^2 I),$$

where $1/\sigma_u$ is the smoothing parameter that is determined by the behavior of the penalized spline fit on the entire age range and as such it does not allow for locally adaptive smoothing.

One way to allow for a locally adaptive smoothing parameter in the GLMM framework is to, in its turn, model the variance σ_u^2 as a smooth function of age. This can be done by modeling σ_u^2 as a penalized spline as well in a hierarchical mixed model framework. To surpass the associated computational burden of integrating the random effects distribution, a Laplace approximation can be used (Krivobokova et al. 2008). The following code presents the library "AdaptFit" in R which employs the Laplace approximation to fit an adaptive penalized spline in the GLMM framework:

```
# R code for the (non-)adaptive penalized spline
library(AdaptFit)
kn.mean=knots.default(a,20)
kn.var=knots.default(a,5)
asp(y~f(a,knots=kn.mean),adap=F,
    family="binomial",spar.method="ML")
asp(y~f(a,knots=kn.mean,var.knot=kn.var),adap=T,
    family="binomial",spar.method="ML")
```

The *asp*-function allows to fit both adaptive and nonadaptive penalized spline smoothing by changing the *adap* option. Because of the additional computational burden of fitting adaptive splines rather than nonadaptive, the number of knots

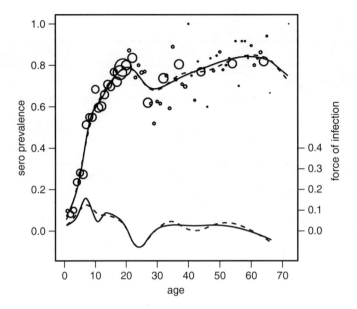

Fig. 8.7 Adaptive (*solid line*) and nonadaptive (*dashed line*) penalized spline applied to the Belgian B19 data. The *dots* are the observed seroprevalence per integer age value with size proportional to the number of samples taken

used in the mean and mixed model variance estimation was limited to 20 and 5, respectively. The function *knots.default* generates knots based on the quantiles of the covariate distribution. Figure 8.7 shows the nonadaptive and adaptive penalized spline for the Belgian B19 data.

There is a moderate difference between both adaptive and nonadaptive penalized spline fit. The adaptive penalized spline fit results in a less smooth curve for lower age values and a smoother curve for higher age values, reflecting the lower and higher uncertainty in those specific regions, respectively. Note that a formal comparison is again not possible because of the PQL estimation procedure.

8.5 Synthesis

In summary, Table 8.3 presents the different approaches as described in this chapter. We focused on R-code throughout this chapter whereas we did not explicitly present SAS code. Note that other packages to model P-splines exist (e.g., "nlmixed" in SAS, the library "SemiPar" in R), that in addition B-splines have also been

Table 8.3 Overview of the different smoothing approaches together with the libraries in SAS and R as presented in this chapter

Method	Framework	Library	Estimation method	Adaptive
Smoothing splines	Pen Lik	R:"gam"	ML	No
B-splines	Pen Lik	R:"psplinefit"	ML	No
Cubic regression splines	Pen Lik	R:"mgcv"	ML	No
Thin plate regression splines	Pen Lik	R:"mgcv"	ML	No
Radial P-spline	GLMM	SAS:"glimmix"	PQL	No
Cubic regression splines	GLMM	R:"mgcv"	PQL	No
Thin plate regression splines	GLMM	R:"mgcv"	PQL	No
Adaptive splines	GLMM	R:"AdaptFit"	PQL	Yes

implemented in the GLMM framework (Currie and Durban 2002) and that code for certain penalized splines is available in other software packages as, e.g., STATA and Matlab too.

8.6 Non-, Semi- and Parametric Methods to Estimate the Prevalence and Force of Infection: A Case Study

Using the UK data on rubella we present an overview of the methods as described in Chaps. 5–8. More specifically, we compare Farrington's model (see (6.1) with $\gamma = 0$, i.e., yielding the best fit) with the best fractional polynomial fit, the best local polynomial fit, and the best spline among the set of spline approaches in the penalized likelihood framework (Sect. 8.2.1). The best second degree fractional polynomial for the UK data on rubella was obtained for the powers $(-0.9, -0.9)$. Based on GCV, the best local polynomial fit was obtained when using 0.8% of its nearest neighbors. Finally, in the penalized likelihood framework the best spline was a B-spline with smoothing parameter chosen using BIC. Note that, whenever choices needed to be made for other parameters like the degree of the local polynomials or spline basis functions and number of knots, the default option was used.

Figure 8.8 shows the fitted seroprevalence and FOI curves for the four different models. While there is only a moderate difference in the fitted seroprevalence, the FOI curves exhibit considerable differences for ages 4–14 years with respect to the age of maximal FOI and its value, while the estimated FOI using the B-spline approach yields a higher FOI at 30 years of age and older as compared to the fractional and local polynomial as well as Farrington's model. Since these approaches are ML-based, the optimal model can be chosen using, e.g., BIC.

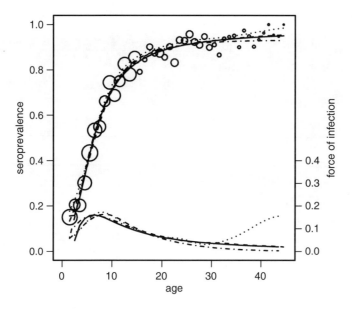

Fig. 8.8 Fitted seroprevalence and FOI curves for rubella in the UK based on the best fractional polynomial fit (*solid line*), the best local polynomial fit (*dashed line*), the best spline fit (*dotted line*), and Farrington's model (*dashed–dotted line*). The *dots* are the observed seroprevalence per integer age value with size proportional to the number of samples taken

While the BIC value for Farrington's model equals 3,915.09, the local polynomial and the B-spline have BIC values of 3,917.42 and 3,911.47, respectively, the fractional polynomial fit seems to be the most parsimonious model with a BIC value of 3,898.31. However, one can argue that for a fractional polynomial, one needs to penalize for the selection of the most optimal set of powers too. By doing so, the BIC value of the FP amounts to 3,915.01, making it comparable to the local polynomial fit in terms of BIC and favoring the B-spline to be the most appropriate model to use.

A similar exercise for the Belgian B19 data showed that the best fractional polynomial model, having powers $(-1.3, -1.3)$, has a BIC value of 3,480.54 (without penalization for the powers). This now turns out to be the worst fit in terms of BIC when compared to the best local polynomial (0.3% nearest neighbors, BIC value: 3,451.07), the best penalized spline model (B-spline, BIC value: 3,472.70), and the nonlinear model of Farrington ($\gamma = 0$; BIC value: 3,472.26). The local polynomial fit turns out to be the best fit in terms of BIC. This is not surprisingly so when realizing that the B19 seroprofile shows more local changes. This is also reflected in several local maxima for the FOI, unable to be captured by the fractional polynomial model and the nonlinear model.

Chapter 9
The Constraint of Monotonicity

9.1 Introduction

In Chaps. 6–8, (flexible) parametric, nonlinear, nonparametric, and semi-parametric models to estimate the force of infection from seroprevalence data have been introduced. All these methods rely on the steady-state assumption of which the plausibility is untestable in case of one cross-sectional sample (Keiding 1991; Nagelkerke et al. 1999).

When the observed prevalence increases monotonically with age, the problem of estimating the force of infection is straightforward. However, unless samples at each age are very large and the steady-state assumption is fulfilled, a monotone increase of the observed prevalence with age only rarely occurs. As the survival function, one minus the prevalence, is a monotonically decreasing function, one typically estimates the prevalence function under order restrictions.

In Sect. 6.1, we already mentioned how the problem of non-monotonicity is dealt with using particular nonnegative functions for the force of infection (Farrington 1990; Farrington et al. 2001; Edmunds et al. 2000b). However, these methods rely on prior knowledge about the dependence of the force of infection on age and are as such limited in their flexibility. One way around this is to use a rich candidate set of unconstrained flexible models and then select the best monotonic model using model selection criteria as AIC. This is the approach used in Chap. 6 when using fractional polynomials. A drawback of this approach is that these models are parametric and potentially all candidate models could be non-monotone at, e.g., the tails of the age range. It is therefore useful to consider non- and semiparametric models that are monotonized in some way.

In this chapter, we introduce the most commonly used methods to obtain a monotone seroprevalence curve and thus a positive FOI. We first show how piecewise constant forces of infection can be adapted to provide monotonic seroprevalence curves by altering the age categories, a rather ad hoc way of monotonizing a curve. We then introduce the general concept of isotonic regression and proceed by describing the pool adjacent violator algorithm (PAVA), a simple monotonization

N. Hens et al., *Modeling Infectious Disease Parameters Based on Serological and Social Contact Data*, Statistics for Biology and Health 63, DOI 10.1007/978-1-4614-4072-7_9, © Springer Science+Business Media New York 2012

algorithm often used in this context. We show how using the PAVA, Keiding (1991) adapted a monotone nonparametric kernel-based estimation procedure and illustrate the refinements proposed by Shkedy et al. (2003) with respect to the local polynomials, described in Chap. 7, to incorporate monotonicity. We further show how a straightforward extension of the P-spline approach introduced by Eilers and Marx (1996) can be used to obtain monotone seroprevalence curves (Bollaerts et al. 2006). We illustrate these methods using the Bulgarian Hepatitis A data and the Belgian Parvovirus B19 data (Chap. 4).

Note that there exist other ways to estimate monotone curves, mostly relying on constrained optimization. We however will not cover these methods in this chapter and advise the reader to textbooks like Silvapulle and Sen (2005) and articles such as Leitenstorfer and Tutz (2007).

9.2 Piecewise Constant Forces of Infection

Using a piecewise constant force of infection, monotonicity is often achieved by redefining the age categories over which a constant force of infection is assumed. We illustrate this using the Bulgarian Hepatitis A data and the Belgian Parvovirus B19 data. We choose two different sets of five half-closed half-open age categories for both datasets. While one is a rather ad hoc choice, $S1 = \{0, 10, 20, 40, 60, 100\}$; the second one is based on school enrollment ages, $S2^{BE} = \{0, 6, 12, 18, 60, 100\}$ and $S2^{BG} = \{0, 5, 11, 18, 60, 100\}$ for Belgium and Bulgaria, respectively. Table 9.1 and Fig. 9.1 present the estimated FOI for both sets of age categories and both infections. Depending on the choice of the set of age categories, the estimated FOIs are all positive or not. Together with the although possibly well motivated but rather ad hoc choice of the set of age-categories, this illustrates the need for more objective methods to estimate the prevalence and FOI under monotonicity constraints. Note that in this case, when comparing both piecewise constant FOIs, the lowest deviances were observed for the non-monotone fits.

Table 9.1 Overview of estimated piecewise constant forces of infection according to two different choices for the age categories for both the Bulgarian Hepatitis A data (HAV) and the Belgian Parvovirus B19 (B19) data

HAV	Cat 1	Cat 2	Cat 3	Cat 4	Cat 5	dev
S1	0.06	0.01	0.08	0.04	0.11	790.9
$S2^{BG}$	0.11	−0.02	0.03	0.07	0.07	781.3
B19	Cat 1	Cat 2	Cat 3	Cat 4	Cat 5	dev
S1	0.08	0.07	−0.02	0.04	−0.03	3485.8
$S2^{BE}$	0.07	0.12	0.04	4e−3	0.06	3486.8

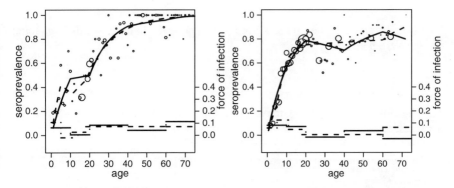

Fig. 9.1 Piecewise constant forces of infection according to two different choices of age categories (*solid* and *dashed line*) for the Bulgarian Hepatitis A data (*left panel*) and the Belgian B19 data (*right panel*). The *dots* are the observed seroprevalence per integer age value with size proportional to the number of samples taken

9.3 Isotonic Regression

Barlow et al. (1972) defines isotonic regression as the statistical theory that deals with problems in which conditional expectations are subject to order restrictions.

Let us introduce the concept of isotonic regression in a simple linear regression setting. Let $X = \{x_1, x_2, \ldots, x_n\}$, where $x_1 \leq x_2 \leq \ldots \leq x_n$ denote the finite set of n ordered observed values for the independent variable and $y_1, y_2, \ldots, y_n$ denote the corresponding observed values for the dependent variable. Let $\mu(x) = \mathrm{E}(Y|X = x)$ denote the mean of the conditional distribution $Y|X = x$. Estimating $\mu(x)$ is typically done minimizing the least-squares criterion in the class of arbitrary functions f on X. However, it might be assumed or known that $\mu(x)$ is nondecreasing in x; i.e., isotonic with respect to the simple order on X. In that situation isotonic regression refers to minimizing the least-squares criterion in the class of isotonic functions f on X, i.e., f is isotonic, if $x_i \leq x_j, i \neq j$ implies that $f(x_i) \leq f(x_j), i, j = 1, \ldots, n$. To this respect Barlow et al. (1972) introduced the PAVA, where successive approximation is used to isotonize the minimizer of the least-squares criterion. Note that Barlow et al. (1972) showed that the PAVA is optimal for the least-squares criterion with equal weights and that currently no such result exists in case of a binomial likelihood.

9.3.1 The Pool Adjacent Violator Algorithm

Let us focus again on modeling seroprevalence data. Assume we have estimated the seroprevalence function π using seroprevalence data $\{(a_i, y_i)\}, i = 1, \ldots, n$. Without loss of generality we assume $a_1 \leq a_2 \leq \ldots \leq a_n$. Denote the maximum likelihood estimate of $\pi(a_i)$ by $\hat{\pi}(a_i)$. Suppose i^* is the first index for which $\hat{\pi}(a_{i^*}) < \hat{\pi}(a_{i^*-1})$, i.e., the first index for which a "violation" of monotone behavior is observed. The PAVA now states that these values need to be "pooled." In other words $\hat{\pi}(a_{i^*})$ and $\hat{\pi}(a_{i^*-1})$ are both replaced by

$$\frac{\hat{\pi}(a_{i^*}) + \hat{\pi}(a_{i^*-1})}{2}.$$

The algorithm proceeds by recursively checking monotone behavior and by pooling if necessary and finally stops if monotonicity is achieved.

The R code for the PAVA algorithm, where the number of positives *pos* out of a total of *tot* trials ordered by increasing age are the input variables, is specified below.

```
# The pool adjacent violator algorithm in R
# 'pos' represents the successes out of 'tot' trials
# 'pos' and 'tot' should be ordered by age
pavit= function(pos=pos,tot=rep(1,length(pos)))
{
pai1 = pai2 = pos/tot
N = length(pai1)
ni=tot
for(i in 1:(N - 1)) {
if(pai2[i] > pai2[i + 1]) {
pool = (ni[i]*pai1[i] + ni[i+1]*pai1[i + 1])/(ni[i]+ni[i+1])
pai2[i:(i + 1)] = pool
k = i + 1
for(j in (k - 1):1) {
if(pai2[j] > pai2[k]) {
   pool.2 = sum(ni[j:k]*pai1[j:k])/(sum(ni[j:k]))
   pai2[j:k] = pool.2
                                                 }
                                      }
                           }
                 }
return(list(pai1=pai1,pai2=pai2))
}
```

The PAVA algorithm gained popularity because it is straightforward to apply. For an elaborate overview of different R functions for isotonic/monotonic regression we refer to De Leeuw et al. (2009). We will show how the PAVA algorithm was used before to estimate the FOI (Keiding 1991; Shkedy et al. 2003; Hens et al. 2008b).

Following Friedman and Tibshirani (1984) and Mammen et al. (2001), Shkedy et al. (2003) suggested to estimate $\pi(a)$ and $\lambda(a)$ using local polynomials and smoothing splines and, if necessary, a posteriori apply the PAVA to isotonize the resulting estimate. This is in line with the finding of Mammen et al. (2001), who showed that constrained smoothing leads to estimates of the form "smooth then constrain." One could also opt to estimate $\pi(a)$ and $\lambda(a)$ based on the idea "constrain then smooth" as proposed by Keiding (1991).

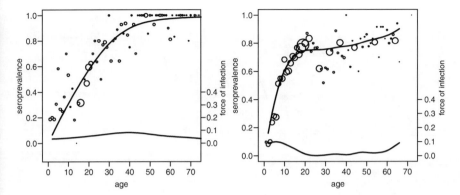

Fig. 9.2 The fitted seroprevalence and FOI according to Keiding (1991) for the Bulgarian Hepatitis A data (*left panel*) and the Belgian B19 data (*right panel*). The *dots* are the observed seroprevalence per integer age- value with size proportional to the number of samples taken

9.3.2 Keiding (1991)

To estimate the FOI under monotonicity constraints, Keiding (1991) first applied the PAVA to the empirical prevalence. The monotonized prevalence was then used to estimate the FOI using the kernel smoothing as described in Sect. 7.1.1.

The R code hereunder shows how to obtain the monotonized kernel-based FOI-estimate according to Keiding (1991). *foi.num* calculates the FOI from seroprevalence data using formula (7.1), while *ksmooth* calculates the kernel-based estimate with normal kernel (*kernel = "normal"*) and bandwidth chosen by visual inspection (*bandwidth = bw*). The last line in the code is used to calculate the prevalence from the estimated FOI.

```
# Keiding 1991
xx=pavit(pos=pos,tot=tot)
foi.k=foi.num(grid,xx$pai2)$foi
age.k=foi.num(grid,xx$pai2)$grid
fit.k=ksmooth(age.k,foi.k,kernel="normal",
bandwidth=bw,n.points=length(age))
pihat=1-exp(-cumsum(c(age.k[1],diff(age.k))*fit.k$y)
```

Figure 9.2 shows the resulting seroprevalence- and FOI curves based on Keiding (1991)'s method. Bandwidths were chosen by visual inspection (*bw = 10* for Hepatitis A, *bw = 30* for B19).

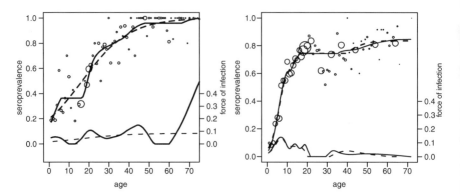

Fig. 9.3 The fitted seroprevalence and FOI according to Shkedy et al. (2003) (*solid line,* bandwidths 0.35 (left) and 0.30 (right)) and Namata et al. (2007) (*dashed line*) for the Bulgarian Hepatitis A data (*left panel*) and the Belgian B19 data (*right panel*). The *dots* are the observed seroprevalence per integer age value with size proportional to the number of samples taken

9.3.3   *"Smooth Then Constrain"*

The local polynomial approach used by Shkedy et al. (2003) to estimate the FOI as described in Chap. 7 is easily adapted to achieve an isotonic estimate of the prevalence by a posteriori applying the PAVA algorithm. Following this approach, Namata et al. (2007), Mossong et al. (2008a), and Hens et al. (2008b) have used the same idea with different smoothing techniques. In Fig. 9.3, the fitted seroprevalence and FOI according to Shkedy et al. (2003) and Namata et al. (2007) for the Bulgarian Hepatitis A data and the Belgian B19 data are shown. Note that the estimated local polynomial clearly leads to undersmoothing in the case of the Bulgarian Hepatitis A data. This is somewhat reflected in the estimated FOI for the Belgian B19 data as well. Recall that determining the optimal smoothing parameter is done using GCV which indeed has a tendency to undersmooth (Burnham and Anderson 2002).

9.4   P-spline Regression with Shape Constraints

In Sect. 8.2.1, the penalized spline approach based on B-spline basis functions was introduced (Eilers and Marx 1996). These authors used an extensive amount of B-spline basis functions:

$$B_1(a,q),\ldots,B_r(a,q), \tag{9.1}$$

where $B_j(a,q)$ denotes a B-spline of degree q with left most knot j evaluated at age a. Typically $q = 3$ and although unequally spaced knots exist, Eilers and Marx (1996) argue that using equally spaced knots from which the boundaries are located outside the covariate range shows good performance in terms of estimation and avoids boundary problems.

Using the B-spline basis functions, the linear predictor $\eta(a)$ is expressed as

$$\eta(a) = \sum_{j=1}^{r} \beta_j B_j(a,q). \tag{9.2}$$

To overcome overfitting, one penalizes on the coefficients of the adjacent B-splines using second (or higher) order differences. This corresponds to maximizing

$$\ell(\beta;y,a) - \frac{1}{2}\alpha\beta' D^{2'} D^2 \beta, \tag{9.3}$$

where $\ell(\beta;y,a)$ denotes the binomial loglikelihood corresponding to (9.2) and D^2 is the matrix representation of the difference operator Δ^2, $\Delta^2\beta_j = \Delta^1(\Delta^1\beta_j) = \beta_j - 2\beta_{j-1} + \beta_{j-2}$. The smoothing parameter α regulates the smoothness of the predictor function and is often chosen by minimizing an information criterion as AIC or BIC (see Sect. 8.2.1).

Using B-splines, it is straightforward to ensure monotonicity by adding large penalties on the negative first-order differences of the coefficients β in (9.3) (Bollaerts et al. 2006). Equation (9.3) now becomes

$$\ell(\beta;y,a) - \frac{1}{2}\alpha\beta' D^{2'} D^2 \beta - \frac{1}{2}\kappa\beta' D^{1'} V W D^1 \beta, \tag{9.4}$$

where V denotes a diagonal matrix with elements v_{ij} indicating whether ($v_{ij} = 1$) or not ($v_{ij} = 0$) the constraint should hold on at least part of the support of B_j, $j = 1,\ldots,r$ and W is the diagonal matrix with elements $w_{ij}(\beta_i) = 0$ if $\Delta^1(\beta_{ij}) \geq 0$ and 1 otherwise. Note that $V = I$ yields monotonicity over the entire age range. The more general approach could prove useful when considering maternal antibodies. We however do not consider this situation here.

While the value of κ is typically chosen to be large (since it imposes to what extent non-monotone behavior is penalized), the choice of α concerns the usual smoothing parameter selection.

The following code uses the *mpspline.fit*-function, an adjusted version of the original *pspline.fit*-function introduced in Sect. 8.2.1. Similar to the non-monotone version, the optimal smoothness parameter *alpha* is selected using the BIC criterion.

```
# R-code B-splines with monotonicity constraint
# Function Code Eilers and Marx (see book's website)
mpspline.fit(response=y,x.var=a,ps.intervals=20,degree=3,
            order=2,link="logit",family="binomial",
            alpha=alphaopt)
```

Figure 9.4 shows the fitted seroprevalence and FOI using the P-spline with monotonicity constraints, the PAVA applied to the unconstrained P-spline and the

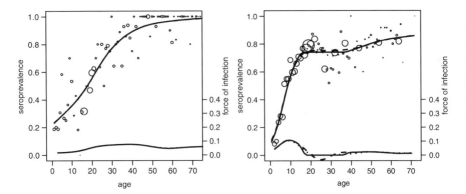

Fig. 9.4 The fitted seroprevalence and FOI using the P-spline with monotonicity constraints (*solid line*), the PAVA applied to the unconstrained P-spline (*dashed line*), and the unconstrained P-spline (*dotted line*) for the Bulgarian Hepatitis A data (*left panel*) and the Belgian B19 data (*right panel*). The *dots* are the observed seroprevalence per integer age value with size proportional to the number of samples taken

unconstrained P-spline for the Bulgarian Hepatitis A data and the Belgian B19 data. While there is no difference between the methods for the Bulgarian Hepatitis A, the initial unconstrained fit is monotone; there is a minor difference between the PAVA applied to the unconstrained fit and the P-spline with monotonicity constraints for the Belgian B19 data. Note that different smoothing parameters were found for the unconstrained and constrained P-splines for the Belgian B19 data.

The advantage of using a method such as the P-spline approach with monotonicity constraints lies in simultaneously acquiring the estimated seroprevalence and FOI together with pointwise confidence intervals. This is not straightforward to do in case of a posteriori applying the PAVA for which the bootstrap can serve as a way out (Shkedy et al. 2003; Mossong et al. 2008a; Hens et al. 2008b). We refer to Bollaerts et al. (2006) for the exact calculations for the P-splines with shape constraints.

9.5   Concluding Remarks

Although several methods to estimate the prevalence under monotonicity constraints have been proposed, one has to realize that monotonicity is likely to be violated due to departures from the steady-state assumption. Unless multiple serological samples are available there is no way to tell whether the estimated parameters are truly valid.

In this chapter, several approaches to estimate the seroprevalence (and consequently the FOI) under monotonicity constraints have been introduced. In the light of the previous comment, we strongly advise the reader to verify, to the extent possible, whether distortions in the seroprofile can be identified. We refer to Nagelkerke et al. (1999) and a more recent paper by Hens et al. (2010a) for a more elaborate discussion on this matter.

Chapter 10
Hierarchical Bayesian Models for the Force of Infection

10.1 Introduction

So far the prevalence and the FOI were estimated within the frequentist framework. In this chapter we estimate the prevalence and the FOI within the Bayesian framework. We refer to Sect. B.5 of Appendix B for an introduction to Bayesian inference.

In the frequentist framework, Farrington (1990) and Farrington et al. (2001) proposed nonlinear models for the FOI based on prior knowledge about the relationship between the FOI and the host age. In Farrington (1990) the FOI is defined as

$$\lambda(a) = (\alpha_1 a - \alpha_3)e^{-\alpha_2 a} + \alpha_3. \tag{10.1}$$

To ensure that the FOI is positive, $\lambda(a) \geq 0$, Farrington (1990) constrained the parameter space to be nonnegative ($\alpha_j \geq 0$, $j = 1,2,3$).

In a parametric Bayesian framework the prevalence has a parametric form, $\pi(a_i, \alpha)$, where α is a parameter vector. In this case $\pi = (\pi_1, \ldots, \pi_m)$ has a deterministic relationship with the predictor a and one can constrain the parameter space of the prior distribution $P(\alpha)$ in order to achieve the desired monotonicity of the posterior distribution $P(\pi_1, \pi_2, \ldots, \pi_m | y, n)$, where $y = (y_1, y_2, \ldots, y_m)$, $n = (n_1, n_2, \ldots, n_m)$, and y_i is the number of infected individuals from the n_i sampled subjects at age a_i. Hierarchical nonlinear and generalized linear models for the prevalence and the FOI are discussed in Sect. 10.3.

In Sect. 10.4 we return to the nonparametric framework. Within the framework of nonparametric Bayesian modeling, the problem is estimating $\pi_1, \pi_2, \ldots, \pi_m$ under the order restriction $\pi_{(1)} \leq \pi_{(2)} \leq \cdots \leq \pi_{(m)}$, where $\pi_{(k)}$ denotes the prevalence with kth rank according to (the) age(-group). For ease of notation we assume $\pi_i = \pi_{(i)}, i = 1, \ldots, m$. The prevalence is assumed to be an isotonic nonparametric function satisfying $0 \leq \pi_i \leq 1$. Likewise, in the hierarchical parametric Bayesian models we focus on the posterior distribution of the prevalence $P(\pi | y, n)$. The m dimensional parameter vector is constrained to lie in a subset of $\mathbb{R}^m$. The constrained

N. Hens et al., *Modeling Infectious Disease Parameters Based on Serological and Social Contact Data*, Statistics for Biology and Health 63, DOI 10.1007/978-1-4614-4072-7_10, © Springer Science+Business Media New York 2012

set is determined by the order restrictions among the components of π. In this case it is natural to incorporate the constraints into the specification of the prior distribution, $P(\pi)$. In the context of bioassay modeling, Gelfand and Kuo (1991) showed that the constrained posterior distribution has the same form as the unconstrained posterior distribution restricted to the constrained set. This implies that if $P(\pi)$ is a product-beta distribution, and the likelihood $P(y|n,\pi)$ is binomial, then the posterior distribution $P(\pi_i|y,n,\pi_{-i})$, $\pi_{-i} = (\pi_1,\dots,\pi_{i-1},\pi_{i+1},\dots,\pi_m)$, is a beta distribution restricted to the interval $[\pi_{i-1},\pi_{i+1}]$. The hierarchical nonparametric approach will be discussed in Sect. 10.4. The methods are illustrated on the rubella and mumps datasets (see Chap. 4) for which an exploratory data analysis is briefly presented in Sect. 10.2.

10.2   Exploratory Data Analysis

Although local polynomial models and isotonic regression were discussed in Chaps. 7 and 9, respectively, we briefly discuss the results for rubella and mumps in this section as well. Figure 10.1 shows both local polynomials and isotonic regression estimates for $\pi(a)$ and $\lambda(a)$. For rubella, the estimated FOI based on the local quadratic model rises steeply to a peak at age 7–8 years, followed by a steady decrease. The two methods result in somewhat different patterns. The FOI estimated by the kernel estimate predicts a secondary peak at age 24 years and a third peak at age 40 years. The same pattern is revealed for mumps. We note that the second peak at age 10 years estimated by the local polynomial is smoothed by the kernel smoother which also predicts peaks at 20 and 33 years of age.

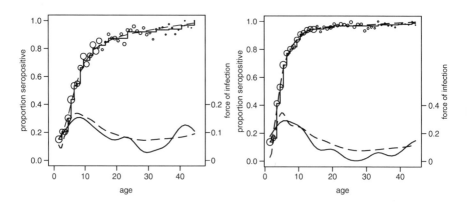

Fig. 10.1 Nonparametric estimate for the prevalence and the FOI. *Solid line*: isotonic regression for the prevalence and kernel smoother for the FOI. *Dashed line*: local quadratic model. *Left panel*: rubella in the UK. *Right panel*: mumps in the UK

10.3   Hierarchical Bayesian Models for the Force of Infection

In this section, we present the hierarchical Bayesian models for the FOI. We first discuss the nonlinear hierarchical and log-logistic model and its application in Winbugs whereas we then discuss model selection and its application to the data.

10.3.1   Nonlinear Hierarchical Model

The model in (10.1) assumes that the FOI is zero at birth ($\lambda(0) = 0$) and then rises to a peak in a linear fashion followed by an exponential decrease. The peak is reached at an age corresponding to the maximum transmission rate between susceptible and infectious individuals. The parameter α_3 is called the long-term residual value of the FOI. If $\alpha_3 = 0$, then the FOI decreases to 0 as a tends to infinity. Integrating $\lambda(a)$ results in the following nonlinear model:

$$\pi(a) = 1 - \exp\left\{ \frac{\alpha_1}{\alpha_2}ae^{-\alpha_2 a} + \frac{1}{\alpha_2}\left[\frac{\alpha_1}{\alpha_2} - \alpha_3\right]\left[e^{-\alpha_2 a} - 1\right] - \alpha_3 a \right\}. \qquad (10.2)$$

In what follows we refer to (10.2) as the exponentially damped linear model. The average age at infection, the mean of the distribution of the age of infection, is given by $A = \int_0^L (1 - \pi(x))dx$, where L is the life expectancy. Following Farrington (1990), we assume that $L = 75$ years. In case that the data are observed up to a certain age U, $U \leq L$, the average age at infection is given by

$$A = \int_0^U (1 - \pi(x))dx + f \times (L - U). \qquad (10.3)$$

Here, f is the fraction of individuals that remains uninfected, which can be estimated from the data by $f = 1 - \pi(U)$. Farrington (1990) estimated unrestricted models for measles, mumps, and rubella based on (10.2) and performed a sensitivity analysis for f by estimating the model in (10.2) conditional on several values for f. In these analyses, the parameter α_1 is no longer a free parameter but can be calculated conditional on the values of α_2, α_3, and f.

In the present chapter we use hierarchical nonlinear models to estimate the parameters in the exponentially damped linear model (10.2). Independent binomial distributions are assumed for the number of infected individuals at age a_i:

$$y_i \sim \text{Bin}(n_i, \pi_i), \text{ for } i = 1, 2, \dots, m, \qquad (10.4)$$

where n_i is the sample size at age a_i. The constraints on the parameter space can be incorporated in the hierarchical model by assuming truncated normal distributions for the components of $\boldsymbol{\alpha}$, $\boldsymbol{\alpha} = (\alpha_1, \alpha_2, \alpha_3)$, in $\pi_i = \pi(a_i, \boldsymbol{\alpha})$,

$$\alpha_j \sim \text{truncated } N(\mu_j, \tau_j) \quad j = 1, 2, 3.$$

Here, the normal prior distributions are left truncated at 0 to ensure that $\lambda(a) \geq 0$. The joint posterior distribution for α can be derived by combining the likelihood and the prior model as

$$P(\alpha|y) \propto \prod_{i=1}^{m} \text{Bin}(y_i|n_i, \pi(a_i, \alpha)) \prod_{i=1}^{3} -\frac{1}{\tau_j} \exp\left(\frac{1}{2\tau_j^2}(\alpha_j - \mu_j)^2\right). \tag{10.5}$$

The full conditional distribution of α_i, derived from (10.5), is given by

$$P(\alpha_i|\alpha_j, \alpha_k, k, j \neq i) \propto -\frac{1}{\tau_i} \exp\left(\frac{1}{2\tau_i^2}(\alpha_i - \mu_i)^2\right) \prod_{i=1}^{m} \text{Bin}(y_i|n_i, \pi(a_i, \alpha)), \tag{10.6}$$

which cannot be simplified any further. To complete the specification of the probability model we assume flat hyperprior distributions at the third level of the model, i.e., $\mu_j \sim N(0, 10000)$ and $\tau_j^{-2} \sim \Gamma(100, 100)$.

10.3.2 Fitting Farrington's Model in Winbugs

In Winbugs 1.4, the data can be entered as a list with *posi* and *ni* the number of infected individuals and the sample size at each age group, respectively. *Nage* is the number of age groups.

```
list(
age=c(1.5,2.5,3.5,4.5,5.5,6.5,7.5,8.5,9.5,10.5,11.5,12.5,13.5,
      14.5,15.5,16.5,17.5,18.5,19.5,20.5,21.5,22.5,23.5,24.5,
      25.5,26.5,27.5,28.5,29.5,30.5,31.5,32.5,33.5,34.5,35.5,
      36.5,37.5,38.5,39.5,40.5,41.5,42.5,43.5,44.5),
posi=c(31,30,34,57,95,104,90,96,134,110,111,147,138,141,53,49,
       73,69,97,65,74,84,82,79,90,84,81,72,71,51,45,45,35,39,
       36,37,37,37,28,26,25,21,18,18),
ni=c(206,146,168,189,219,195,164,145,180,160,148,178,177,165,
     67,58,81,79,111,76,82,101,88,85,94,91,89,76,79,56,52,48,
     37,41,40,38,39,41,30,27,25,22,19,18),
Nage=44)
```

The likelihood of the three-parameter model, in the first stage of the hierarchical model, can be defined using the following code:

```
for(i in 1:Nage) {
posi[i]  ~ dbin(theta[i],ni[i])
theta[i] <- 1-exp((alpha1/alpha2)*age[i]*exp(-alpha2*age[i]))
             +(1/alpha2)*((alpha1/alpha2)-alpha3)*
             (exp(-alpha2*age[i])-1)-alpha3*age[i])
foi[i] <- (alpha1*age[i]-alpha3)*exp(-alpha2*age[i])+alpha3
}
```

where *theta[i]* and *foi[i]* denote the prevalence and the FOI, respectively. The constraint on the parameter space of α_1, α_2, and α_3 can be imposed using the function *I()*:

```
alpha1 ~ dnorm(mu.alpha1,tau.alpha1)I(0.00001,)
alpha2 ~ dnorm(mu.alpha2,tau.alpha2)I(0.00001,)
alpha3 ~ dnorm(mu.alpha3,tau.alpha3)I(0.00001,)
```

Finally, we need to specify the hyperprior distributions:

```
tau.alpha1 ~ dgamma(0.01,0.01)
tau.alpha2 ~ dgamma(0.01,0.01)
tau.alpha3 ~ dgamma(0.01,0.01)
mu.alpha1 ~ dnorm(0,0.0001)
mu.alpha2 ~ dnorm(0,0.0001)
mu.alpha3 ~ dnorm(0,0.0001)
```

The complete code for the three-parameter model is as follows:

```
model
{
for(i in 1:Nage) {
posi[i] ~ dbin(theta[i],ni[i])
theta[i] <- 1-exp((alpha1/alpha2)*age[i]*exp(-alpha2*age[i])
            +(1/alpha2)*((alpha1/alpha2)-alpha3)*
            (exp(-alpha2*age[i])-1)-alpha3*age[i])
foi[i] <- (alpha1*age[i]-alpha3)*exp(-alpha2*age[i])+alpha3
ai[i]<- 1-theta[i]
}
ef<- 1-theta[Nage]
avei2<-sum(ai[])+ef*(75-age[Nage])
Pi<- 1-avei2/75
alpha1 ~dnorm(mu.alpha1,tau.alpha1)I(0.00001,)
alpha2 ~dnorm(mu.alpha2,tau.alpha2)I(0.00001,)
alpha3 ~dnorm(mu.alpha3,tau.alpha3)I(0.00001,)
tau.alpha1 ~dgamma(0.01,0.01)
tau.alpha2 ~dgamma(0.01,0.01)
tau.alpha3 ~dgamma(0.01,0.01)
mu.alpha1 ~dnorm(0,0.0001)
mu.alpha2 ~dnorm(0,0.0001)
mu.alpha3 ~dnorm(0,0.0001)
sig.alpha1<-1/tau.alpha1
sig.alpha2<-1/tau.alpha2
sig.alpha3<-1/tau.alpha3
}
```

The two-parameter model can be fitted by changing the parametric structure of the prevalence, i.e.,

```
for( i in 1 : Nage) {
posi[i]  ~ dbin(theta[i],ni[i])
theta[i]  <- 1-exp((alpha1/alpha2)*age[i]*exp(-alpha2*age[i])
                +(1/alpha2)*((alpha1/alpha2))*
                (exp(-alpha2*age[i])-1))
foi[i]  <- (alpha1*age[i])*exp(-alpha2*age[i])
ai[i]<- 1-theta[i]
}
```

10.3.3   Hierarchical Log-Logistic Model

The exploratory data analysis in Sect. 10.2 indicates that the FOI rises to a peak and drops down thereafter. Therefore we can conclude that the time spent in the susceptible class is not an outcome of neither an exponential nor a Weibull distribution since these distributions have a constant and a monotone FOI, respectively. In contrast, the log-logistic distribution offers a wide range of shapes for the hazard function, which is better able to capture the common pattern revealed in Fig. 10.1 (although, similar to model (10.2), the secondary peaks will be smoothed). Under the assumption that the time spent in the susceptible class follows a log-logistic distribution, the probability to become infected before age a is given by

$$\pi(a) = \frac{\beta a^{\alpha}}{1 + \beta a^{\alpha}}, \quad \alpha, \beta > 0, \tag{10.7}$$

and the FOI by

$$\lambda(a) = \frac{\alpha \beta a^{\alpha-1}}{1 + \beta a^{\alpha}}. \tag{10.8}$$

The log-logistic model can be fitted as a GLM with $\log(a)$ as a predictor and a logit link function. This leads to a Bayesian logistic regression model (Gilks et al. 1996; Gelman 1996) of y with covariate $\log(a)$. We specify the same likelihood as in (10.4) with linear predictor given by

$$\mathrm{logit}(\pi(a)) = \alpha_2 + \alpha_1 \log(a),$$

where $\alpha_2 = \log(\beta)$. For the prior model of α_1, we specify $\alpha_1 \sim$ truncated $N(\mu_1, \tau_1)$. We constrain β to be positive by specifying $\alpha_2 \sim N(\mu_2, \tau_2)$. The full conditional distribution of α_1 equals

$$P(\alpha_1 | \alpha_2) \propto -\frac{1}{\tau_1} \exp\left(\frac{1}{2\tau_1^2} (\alpha_1 - \mu_1)^2 \right) \prod_{i=1}^{m} \mathrm{Bin}(y_i | n_i, \pi(a_i, \alpha_1, \alpha_2)). \tag{10.9}$$

The full conditional distribution for α_2 can be derived in the same way. The same flat hyperprior distributions as in the previous section are assumed for the hyperparameters.

10.3.4 Fitting the Log-Logistic Model in Winbugs

The log-logistic model is a GLM and as such it can be fitted using the *logit( )* function in Winbugs as a link function, i.e., the parametric structure for the prevalence is given by

```
logit(theta[i]) <- alpha2+alpha1*log(age[i])
```

The code for the log-logistic model is given below.

```
model
{
for( i in 1 : Nage) {
posi[i] ~ dbin(theta[i],ni[i])
logit(theta[i]) <- alpha2+alpha1*log(age[i])
ai[i]<- 1-theta[i]
loglike[i] <- posi[i]*log(theta[i])
             +(ni[i]-posi[i])*log(1-theta[i])
foi[i]<-alpha1*exp(alpha2)*pow(age[i],(alpha1-1))*(1-theta[i])
}
}
```

10.3.5 Model Selection

Within the Bayesian framework, the unknown parameters are estimated by means of the posterior mean. However, since the full conditional distributions in (10.6) and (10.9) do not have a closed analytical form, we cannot evaluate it directly. We can approximate it using Markov Chain Monte Carlo (MCMC) methods (Gilks et al. 1996) and generate samples form the full conditional distributions using the Gibbs sampler. The sample averages are taken as the posterior means of the parameters of interest.

A model selection procedure is needed in order to compare the models mentioned above and to select the best model. Goodness of fit and complexity of the models were assessed using the deviance information criterion (DIC) as proposed by Spiegelhalter et al. (1998, 2002) who suggested to measure the effective number of parameters (the complexity) in the model by the difference between the posterior expectation of the deviance and the deviance evaluated at the posterior expectation of π, i.e.,

$$P_D = E_{\pi|y,n}(D) - D(E_{\pi|y,n}(\pi)) = \bar{D} - D(\bar{\pi}), \tag{10.10}$$

with the deviance given by $D(\pi) = -2\log(P(y|n,\pi)) + 2\log(f(y|n))$. The second term in the deviance is a standardizing factor which does not depend on π; we use -2 times the loglikelihood value of the saturated model. Hence, for the models discussed above the binomial deviance is given by

$$D(\pi) = 2\sum_{i=1}^{m}\left(y_i\log\frac{y_i}{n_i\pi_i} + (y_i - n_i)\log\frac{1 - \frac{y_i}{n_i}}{1 - \pi_i}\right). \tag{10.11}$$

In practice, $D(\pi)$ and π can be monitored during the MCMC run, $\bar{D}$ is the sample mean of $D(\pi)$ while $D(\bar{\pi})$ is the deviance evaluated at the posterior mean. For model selection, Spiegelhalter et al. (1998, 2002) defined the *Deviance Information Criterion*, DIC, as

$$\text{DIC} = \bar{D} + P_D = D(\bar{\pi}) + 2P_D. \tag{10.12}$$

Smaller values of DIC indicate a better fitting model.

10.3.6 Application to the Data

The panel below presents the deviance summaries obtained from Winbugs for the three models, Fig. 10.2 shows the fitted models for both the prevalence and the FOI and Table 10.1 presents the posterior means for the parameters.

```
RUBELLA

           Dbar       Dhat       pD      DIC
EXP(2)     231.190    229.229    1.961   233.151
EXP(3)     227.644    225.137    2.508   230.152
LL         225.244    223.273    1.971   227.215


MUMPS
           Dbar       Dhat       pD      DIC
EXP(2)     224.349    222.372    1.977   226.326
EXP(3)     225.912    223.791    2.121   228.033
```

Starting with rubella, the first model that was fitted assumes that $\alpha_3 = 0$ in the exponentially damped linear model in (10.2). For this model the posterior deviance

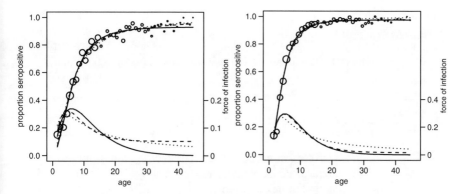

Fig. 10.2 Posterior means for the prevalence and the FOI for rubella (*left panel*) and mumps (*right panel*). *Solid line*: exponentially damped linear model with $\alpha_3 = 0$; *dashed line*: exponentially damped linear model with $\alpha_3 > 0$; *dotted line*: log-logistic model

Table 10.1 Posterior means for the parameters

	Rubella			Mumps		
	Exponential $\alpha_3 = 0$	Exponential $\alpha_3 > 0$	Log-logistic	Exponential $\alpha_3 = 0$	Exponential $\alpha_3 > 0$	Log-logistic
α_1	0.067	0.070	1.645	0.139	0.139	2.063
α_2	0.158	0.201	−2.964	0.192	0.198	−2.865
α_3		0.034			0.008	
f	0.07	0.044	0.036	0.023	0.021	0.007
A	11.11	10.16	9.86	5.72	5.61	5.05

Note that the α parameters of the log-logistic model and the exponentially damped linear model are not comparable

The exponentially damped linear model with $\alpha_3 = 0$ is the model proposed by Farrington (1990) with the assumption that $\lambda(a) = \alpha_1 a \exp(-\alpha_2 a)$

is 231.19 and $P_D = 1.96$, slightly lower than the "true" number of parameters. For the exponentially damped linear model with $\alpha_3 > 0$, $\bar{D} = 227.64$ and $P_D = 2.5$. The DIC of this model is 230.15, smaller than the DIC of the first model (233.15) indicating that among the exponentially damped linear models the second one is to be preferred. However, the log-logistic model with DIC $= 227.21$ has the best goodness-to-fit. For mumps, the model with the lowest DIC value is the exponentially damped linear model with $\alpha_3 = 0$ (226.32). Figure 10.2 shows that there is a substantial difference between the models at the age for which the FOI reaches its peak and in the level of the FOI at older age groups. Furthermore, for rubella, the posterior mean of the average age at infection for the exponentially damped linear model with $\alpha_3 > 0$ is 10.16 years and the posterior mean for f is 0.04. When α_3 is not included in the model, the average age of infection increases to 11.11 years and f increases to 0.07. The posterior mean of the average age at infection obtained from the log-logistic model is 9.86 years. For mumps, the effect of α_3 on f is less substantial, the reason for that is the small value of α_3 that was estimated in the second model (0.008). The smallest value of f is obtained for the log-logistic model (0.007) with average age at infection equal to 5.05 years.

10.4 Hierarchical Nonparametric Model

Whereas in the previous section we considered parametric models, in this section focus goes to a hierarchical nonparametric model in which we do not specify a parametric mean structure but define a probabilistic model for the order restricted prevalence.

10.4.1 Hierarchical Beta/Binomial Model

In the previous section the prevalence was assumed to have a parametric form $\pi(a, \alpha)$, and monotonicity was achieved by constraining the parameter space of α. In this section, we assume that π is a right-continuous nondecreasing function defined on $[0, \delta]$, $\pi_m \leq \delta \leq 1$, $\delta = 1 - f$. We do not assume any deterministic relationship between π_i and a_i but instead we specify a probabilistic model for π_i at each distinct level of a_i. Since the data are binomial, it is natural to use the product-beta prior (Gelfand and Kuo 1991) for π, since it is a conjugate prior for the binomial likelihood and ensures that the posterior distribution of $\pi | y, n$ is also a beta distribution. A product-beta prior has the form

$$P_B(\pi | \alpha, \beta) \propto \prod_{i=1}^{m} (\pi_i)^{\alpha_i - 1} (1 - \pi_i)^{\beta_i - 1} \quad (\alpha_i > 0, \beta_i > 0), \tag{10.13}$$

where $\alpha = (\alpha_1, \alpha_2, \ldots, \alpha_m)$ and $\beta = (\beta_1, \beta_2, \ldots, \beta_m)$. For the unconstrained case, combining the binomial likelihood and the product-beta prior leads to the posterior distribution:

$$P(\pi | y, \alpha, \beta) \propto \prod_{i=1}^{m} \pi_i^{y_i} (1 - \pi_i)^{n_i - y_i} \prod_{i=1}^{m} \pi_i^{\alpha_i - 1} (1 - \pi_i)^{\beta_i - 1}$$

$$\propto \prod_{i=1}^{m} \pi_i^{y_i + \alpha_i - 1} (1 - \pi_i)^{n_i - y_i + \beta_i - 1}, \tag{10.14}$$

which is $\text{Beta}(y_i + \alpha_i, n_i - y_i + \beta_i)$. The problem is to estimate π under the order restrictions, $\pi_1 \leq \pi_2 \leq \cdots \leq \pi_m$. Thus, the m dimensional parameter vector is constrained to lie in a subset S^m of $\mathbb{R}^m$. The constrained set S^m is determined by the order among the components of π. In this case it is natural to incorporate the constraints into the specification of the prior distribution. Gelfand et al. (1992) show that the posterior distribution of π given the constraints is the unconstrained posterior distribution normalized such that

$$P(\pi|y) \propto \frac{P(y|\pi)P(\pi|\alpha,\beta)}{\int_{S^m} P(y|\pi)P(\pi|\alpha,\beta)d\pi}, \quad \pi \in S^m. \tag{10.15}$$

Let $S_j^m(\pi_j, j \neq i)$ be a cross section of S^m defined by the constraints for the component π_i at a specified set of π_j, $j \neq i$. In our setting, $S_j^m(\pi_j, j \neq i)$ is the interval $[\pi_{i-1}, \pi_{i+1}]$. It follows from (10.15) that the posterior distribution for π_i is given by

$$\begin{cases} P(\pi_i|y,\alpha,\beta,\pi_{-i}) \propto P(y|\pi)P(\pi|\alpha,\beta) \;\; \pi_i \in S_j^m(\pi_j, j \neq i), \\ 0, \;\; \pi_i \notin S_j^m(\pi_j, j \neq i). \end{cases} \tag{10.16}$$

Here, $\pi_{-i} = (\pi_1, \ldots, \pi_{i-1}, \pi_{i+1}, \ldots, \pi_m)$. Hence, when the likelihood and the prior distribution are combined, the posterior conditional distribution of $\pi_i|y,\alpha,\beta,\pi_{-i}$ is the standard posterior distribution restricted to $S_j^m(\pi_j, j \neq i)$, i.e., $\text{Beta}(y_i + \alpha_i, n_i - y_i + \beta_i)$ restricted to the interval $[\pi_{i-1}, \pi_{i+1}]$ (Gelfand and Kuo 1991). This means that during the MCMC simulation the sampling from the full conditional distribution can be reduced to interval restricted sampling from the standard posterior distribution (Gelfand et al. 1992).

The hierarchical model we consider is given by

$$\begin{aligned} y_i &\sim \text{Bin}(n_i, \pi_i) & \text{likelihood,} \\ \pi_i &\sim \text{Beta}(\alpha_i, \beta_i)I(\pi_{i-1}, \pi_{i+1}) & \text{prior,} \end{aligned} \tag{10.17}$$

where $I(\pi_{i-1}, \pi_{i+1})$ is an indicator variable which takes the value of 1 if $\pi_{i-1} \leq \pi_i \leq \pi_{i+1}$ and zero elsewhere. In order to complete the specification of the hierarchical model in (10.17) we need to specify hyperprior distributions for α and β. Note that the special case $\alpha_i = \beta_i = 1$ for $i = 1, \ldots, m$ implies that the prior distribution of the prevalence in the ith age group, conditional on π_{i-1} and π_{i+1}, is a uniform distribution over the interval $[\pi_{i-1}, \pi_{i+1}]$, $\pi_i|\pi_{i-1}, \pi_{i+1} \sim \text{Uniform}(\pi_{i-1}, \pi_{i+1})$. Although, there is no reason to fix α and β to be equal to 1 albeit there is no clear way how to choose the hyperprior distribution for the components in α and β either. For the analysis presented below we specify noninformative distributions for the hyperparameters by specifying a left truncated (at zero) normal distribution with variance equal to 1,000 for each of the components in α and β at the third stage of the hierarchical model.

Once the prevalence values are obtained, the problem of estimating the FOI becomes straightforward. Let $\pi^{(k)}$ be the constrained value of π, obtained in the kth iteration of the MCMC simulation. The FOI $\lambda^{(k)}(a)$ can be estimated by $\hat{\lambda}^{(k)}(a) = \hat{\pi}'^{(k)}(a)/(1 - \hat{\pi}^{(k)}(a))$. However, since we assume that the FOI is a smooth function, we smooth $\lambda^{(k)}(a)$ with a twice successively third-order moving average

(Diggle 1990), i.e., $\lambda_S^{(k)}(a) = S\lambda^{(k)}(a)$ where $\lambda_S(a)$ is the smoothed FOI and S is the smoothing matrix. The posterior mean of $\lambda_S(a)$ is simply $\sum_{k=1}^{K} \lambda_S^{(k)}(a)/K$ where K is the number of MCMC iterations.

The fraction of uninfected individuals can be used in this model to specify the distribution of $\pi(U)$. If $f = 0$ is our prior assumption, then $\pi(U) \sim \text{Beta}(\alpha_m, \beta_m) \times I(\pi_{m-1}, 1)$, where $I(\pi_{m-1}, 1)$ is an indicator that takes the value of 1 if $\pi_{m-1} \leq \pi_m \leq 1$ and 0 otherwise. In case that we use the prior knowledge that $f > 0$, say $f = f^*$, then we can truncate the distribution of $\pi(U)$ at the right side with $1 - f^*$, $\pi(U) \sim \text{Beta}(\alpha_m, \beta_m) I(\pi_{U-1}, 1 - f^*)$.

10.4.2 Fitting the Model in Winbugs

As we mentioned above, for $\alpha = \beta = 1$, the prior distribution of the prevalence at the ith age group, conditional on π_{i-1} and π_{i+1}, is a uniform distribution over the interval $[\pi_{i-1}, \pi_{i+1}]$ which implies that $\pi_i | \pi_{i-1}, \pi_{i+1} \sim \text{Uniform}(\pi_{i-1}, \pi_{i+1})$. For the first age group, $\pi_1 \sim \text{Uniform}(0, \pi_2)$ this constraint can be implemented in Winbugs by

```
pi[1] ~ dunif(0,pi[2])
```

The constrained priors for π_i, $i = 2, \ldots, n-1$ are implemented using the following code:

```
for(k in 2:(Nage-1))
{
pi[k] ~dunif(pi[k-1],pi[k+1])
}
```

Finally, for the last age group $\pi_m \sim \text{Uniform}(\pi_{m-1}, f)$. For $f = 0.98$ this constraint is implemented by

```
pi[Nage] ~ dunif(pi[Nage-1],0.98)
```

The prevalence in the above model is a stochastic node. The FOI, on the other hand, is a deterministic node and can be estimated at each MCMC iteration by $\hat{\lambda}^{(k)}(a) = \hat{\pi}'^{(k)}(a)/(1 - \hat{\pi}^{(k)}(a))$ (assuming age groups of one year). In Winbugs we need to specify the following deterministic relationship:

```
model
foi[1]<-(pi[1]/(1-pi[1]))/1.5
for(k in 2:(Nage-1))
{
foi[k]<-  (pi[k]-pi[k-1])/(1-pi[k])
}
foi[Nage]<-(pi[Nage]-pi[Nage-1])/(1-pi[Nage])
```

Note that *foi[k]* is the rough FOI, and similar to the approach of Keiding (1991), it needs to be smoothed. In our example we use a twice successively third-order moving average (Diggle 1990), i.e., $\lambda_S^{(k)}(a) = S\lambda^{(k)}(a)$ where $\lambda_S(a)$ is the smoothed FOI and S is the smoothing, matrix. In the panel below *fois[h]* is the smoothed FOI.

```
fois[1]  <-  (foi[1]+foi[2]+foi[3])/6
fois[2]  <-  (foi[1]+3*foi[2]+foi[3])/5
for(h in 3:(Nage-2))
{
fois[h]  <-  (foi[h-2]+2*foi[h-1]+3*foi[h]+2*foi[h+1]+foi[h+2])/9
}
fois[Nage-1] <-  (foi[Nage-2]+3*foi[Nage-1]+foi[Nage])/5
fois[Nage]  <-  (foi[Nage-2]+2*foi[Nage-1]+3*foi[Nage])/6
}
```

The truncated beta prior model specified in (10.17) can be implemented in Winbugs by replacing the uniform prior with a Beta prior,

```
pi[1]  ~ dbeta(alpha[1],beta[1])I(,pi[2])
for(k in 2:(Nage-1))
{
pi[k]  ~dbeta(alpha[k],beta[k])I(pi[k-1],pi[k+1])
}
pi[Nage]  ~ dbeta(alpha[Nage],beta[Nage])I(pi[Nage-1],0.96)
```

Note that for this model we need to specify hyperprior distributions for α and β. In our example we used independent flat hyperpriors:

```
for(i in 1:Nage)
{
alpha[i]~dnorm(0,0.001)I(0,)
beta[i]~dnorm(0,0.00001)I(0,)}
}
```

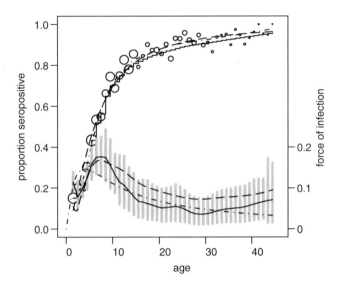

Fig. 10.3 Posterior means for the prevalence and the FOI (rubella). The gray area represents the 95% credible intervals for the FOI. *Solid lines*: the beta-binomial model; *dashed lines*: the nonparametric local polynomials. The parametric model is the log-logistic model (*dashed-dotted lines*) which, among the parametric models, has the smallest DIC value

10.4.3 Application to the Data

The posterior means for the prevalence and FOI are shown in Fig. 10.3 (rubella) and Fig. 10.4 (mumps). For rubella, the nonparametric models indicate essentially the same patterns, although the secondary peak at age 23 is less substantial in the beta-binomial model. In addition, from age 30 onwards, the beta-binomial model predicts a higher FOI. For mumps, the secondary peak at age 20 was smoothed by the beta-binomial model. Similar to rubella, the beta-binomial model predicts higher values for the FOI at the first peak, compared to the parametric model. This can be seen in Fig. 10.5 which presents the density estimates for the posterior distribution of the FOI between age 3.5 and 6.5. Note that the exponential and the beta-binomial models for the FOI reach a peak at age 4.5 and 5.5, respectively. The beta-binomial model predicts higher values for the FOI : 0.36 and 0.29 for the beta-binomial and the exponentially damped linear model, respectively.

The value of f has a substantial influence on the posterior mean of the average age at infection. We fitted the beta-binomial model with several values of f. That is, we truncated the distribution of $\pi(U)$ at the right-hand side with $1 - f$, $\pi(U) \sim \text{Beta}(\alpha_n, \beta_n) I(\pi_{U-1}, 1 - f)$. Table 10.2 presents the results and shows that the posterior mean of A increases with f. This can be seen in Fig. 10.7 which shows the 95% credible intervals for the average age at infection. This pattern was observed by Farrington (1990) for the estimated conditional models (see Farrington 1990,

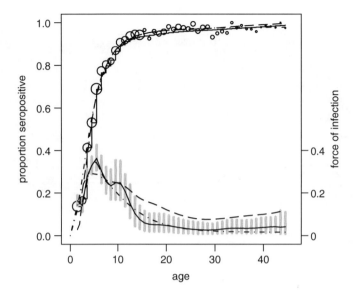

Fig. 10.4 Posterior means for the prevalence and the FOI (mumps). The gray area represents the 95% credible intervals for the FOI. *Solid lines*: the beta-binomial model; *dashed lines*: the nonparametric local polynomials. The parametric model is the exponentially damped linear model with $\alpha = 0$ (dashed-dotted lines) which, among the parametric models, has the smallest DIC value

Table 3). Note that in the first column in Table 10.2, $\bar{f} = 1 - \bar{\pi}(U)$ is the posterior mean for f. Figure 10.6 shows the estimated forces of infection for several values of f. Note that substantial differences are observed from age 30 and onwards. The FOI increases with higher values of f.

10.5 Discussion

As pointed out in several places in this book, the (age-dependent) FOI is a basic concept in any epidemiological model for an infectious disease. Furthermore, the average age at infection and the basic reproduction number, R_0, depend on the model for the FOI (Chaps. 14 and 15). In this chapter we modeled the prevalence within the framework of hierarchical Bayesian models in order to investigate the posterior distribution of $\lambda(a)$ and A. The parametric models are restrictive since they can estimate only a single peak model for the FOI. However, the beta-binomial model suggests secondary peaks which may be important from an epidemiological point of view. Furthermore, we have shown that compared to the parametric models, the beta-binomial models predict higher values for the FOI at its maximum.

The problem of estimation under order restrictions was addressed by choosing constrained priors for the hierarchical models in Sect. 10.3 or a truncated

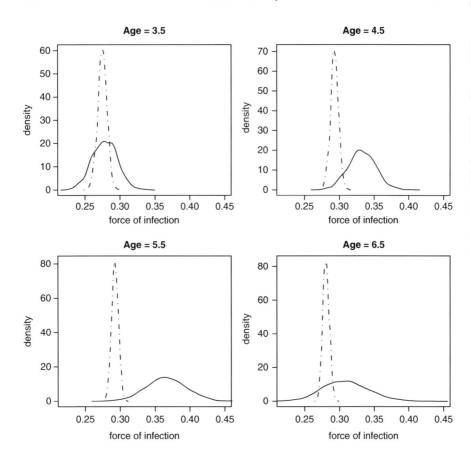

Fig. 10.5 Kernel estimates for the posterior distribution of the FOI for mumps at ages 3.5 (*top left*), 4.5 (*top right*), 5.5 (*lower left*) and 6.5 (*lower right*). The *dashed–dotted line* corresponds with the exponential model; the *solid line* with the nonparametric Bayesian model

Table 10.2 Posterior mean for the average age at infection and f obtained from the beta-binomial models

Rubella	$\bar{f}$	$\bar{A}$
	0.007	9.27
	0.016	9.58
	0.025	9.85
	0.033	10.24
	0.043	10.63
	0.053	11.08
	0.063	11.55
Mumps	0.004	5.29
	0.012	5.58
	0.021	5.99

Fig. 10.6 The 95% credible intervals for the average age at infection (rubella). *Solid lines*: beta-binomial models; *dotted line*: log-logistic model; *long dashed line*: the exponentially damped linear model. The numbers to the *left* of the credible intervals are the posterior means for f, $1 - \bar{\pi}(U)$

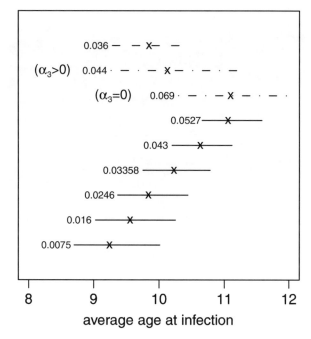

Fig. 10.7 Posterior mean for the FOI for several values of f. *Left Panel*: rubella; *right panel*: mumps. The *solid line* is the FOI estimated by local quadratic model. The numbers to the *right* are the values of f that were used to right truncate the prior distribution of $\pi(U)$

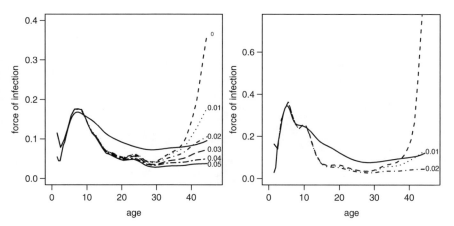

product-Beta for the prior model in the hierarchical beta-binomial model. Both models estimate a nondecreasing prevalence and therefore lead to a nonnegative FOI, as required. The beta-binomial model is highly sensitive for the values of f. It is necessary to fit the model with several values of f in order to investigate its influence on the posterior mean of A and $\lambda(a)$.

Chapter 11
Modeling the Prevalence and the Force of Infection Directly from Antibody Levels

11.1 Serological and Current Status Data

As discussed in previous chapters and illustrated by different methods, prevalence and force of infection (FOI) (and, as we will show in Chaps. 14 and 15, indirectly other parameters such as the basic reproduction number) are estimated from so-called seroprevalence data. Seroprevalence data are obtained by dichotomizing or trichotomizing disease-specific antibody levels using one or two threshold values, often provided by the test manufacturer. In particular, individuals are diagnosed as infected (left-censored age at infection, its value somewhere before the age at the time of the test) if their test result exceeds a certain threshold value τ_u and as being susceptible (right-censored age at infection) if their result falls below a possibly different threshold $\tau_\ell \leq \tau_u$. In case two different threshold values are used ($\tau_\ell < \tau_u$), individuals having test results in between are labeled *inconclusive* or *equivocal*. Individuals labeled inconclusive are either advised to have their sample retested, considered diseased (conservative approach) or non-diseased (liberal approach) or discarded from analysis. Figure 5.1 in Sect. 5.1 showed Belgian Parvovirus B19 antibody activity levels together with two thresholds. This is a situation where both groups can be nicely separated and one can expect a very limited number of misclassified subjects. Figure 11.1 shows a similar plot for data on varicella zoster Virus (VZV, see Chap. 4). This plot of the $\log((\text{antibody level in U/ml}) + 1)$ as a function of age shows more overlap between the infected and the susceptible populations and consequently more inconclusive cases (105 values between $\tau_l = \log(51)$ and $\tau_u = \log(101)$).

For a serological sample, the current status of the disease depends on the antibody level Z_i of the ith subject, $i = 1\ldots,N$ and, say, one manufacturer cutoff point (i.e., the threshold value) τ. In case τ is known, the current status of the disease Y_i is determined by

$$Y_i = \begin{cases} 1 \text{ if } Z_i > \tau, \\ 0 \text{ if } Z_i < \tau. \end{cases} \tag{11.1}$$

N. Hens et al., *Modeling Infectious Disease Parameters Based on Serological and Social Contact Data*, Statistics for Biology and Health 63, DOI 10.1007/978-1-4614-4072-7_11, © Springer Science+Business Media New York 2012

Fig. 11.1 Belgian VZV data. Logarithm of antibody activity levels in U/ml (+1) as a function of the individual's age, with threshold values represented by *solid horizontal lines. Upper dashed horizontal line*: estimated mean for the infected subpopulation. *Lower dashed horizontal line*: estimated mean for the susceptible subpopulation. *Solid smooth curve*: monotone least-squares fit using P-splines

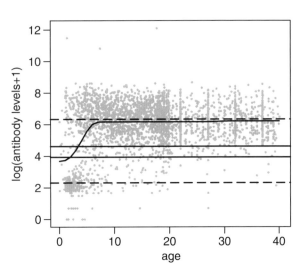

Several authors (see e.g. Gay et al. 2003; Vyse et al. 2004; Vyse et al. 2006; Nielsen et al. 2007; Hardelid et al. 2008) pointed out on the difficulty to interpret serological data based on predefined manufacturer cutoff points or thresholds. In particular, Hardelid et al. (2008) argued that due to the difficulty of applying a meaningful cutoff point value to the continuous distribution of antibody levels, cut-off point based methods are likely to set a high cutoff point level in order to avoid false-negative results. Furthermore, if cutoff point τ is unknown the true current status of the individual is unknown or subject to measurement error when one chooses the cutoff point arbitrarily. As a consequence, the use of threshold value(s) in order to diagnose individual subjects is virtually always prone to test misclassification, encompassing both false-negative (infected/diseased subjects testing negative) and false-positive results (susceptible/undiseased subjects testing positive), yielding biased estimates when not corrected for. Furthermore, in case two thresholds are used, discarded inconclusive classifications will add to the bias and over and above might result in information loss.

In this chapter we investigate the effect of test misclassification on the estimation of the prevalence and the FOI and show that the optimal threshold is different for both parameters. This complicates the application of thresholds and to avoid its use we discuss alternative methods using mixture models in Sects. 11.3 and 11.5. This method combines two concepts: the fact that all information is available on the original continuous scale of antibody activity levels, and the very natural idea to represent the antibody levels, collapsed over age, as coming from a mixture of two distributions (representing the *infected* and the *susceptible* subpopulations). Figure 11.2 shows a hypothetical example of a mixture of two normal distributions which represent the distribution of antibody levels according to the disease status. The first component of the mixture is the distribution of the (log) antibody level of

Fig. 11.2 A two-component mixture for the serological data

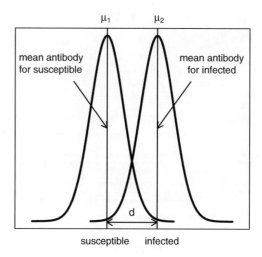

Fig. 11.3 Belgian VZV data, collapsed over the age dimension. Histogram overlaid with the fitted mixture of two Gaussian distributions on the logarithm of antibody activity levels in U/ml. *Triangles* on the horizontal axes represent the two estimated means

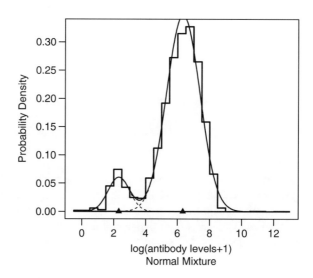

the susceptible individuals and the second component is the distribution of the (log) antibody level of the infected individuals.

Figure 11.3 shows such a mixture fitted to the VZV data. The triangles on the horizontal axes represent the two estimated means, also shown by the two horizontal lines in Fig. 11.1.

11.2   The Threshold Approach

We restrict our discussion to the one-threshold case and briefly summarize the main conclusions of the two-threshold case as studied by Bollaerts et al. (2012).

As in Sect. 11.1, consider a serological sample of N subjects, let Z_i be the test result for subject $i = 1, 2, \ldots, N$ and let τ be a single predefined threshold value. Then Z_i is dichotomized according to (11.1) and the current status of the disease for the ith subject Y_i is a binary variable for which 0 denotes test negative and 1 denotes test positive. To quantify the performance of a test, two test characteristics are typically used, namely the test sensitivity SE_τ (the probability of a positive test result given the individual has been infected) and the test specificity SP_τ (the probability of a negative test result given the individual is still susceptible). In case $SE_\tau = SP_\tau = 1$, the test is perfect (no misclassifications). Furthermore, for a test to be valid, it is required that $SE_\tau > 1 - SP_\tau$ (or equivalently, the probability of a test-positive result should be larger for an infected individual).

The mean of the binary data $\hat{\pi}_\tau = (\sum_{i=1}^{N} Y_i)/N$ is an unbiased estimate of the proportion π_τ of test positives. However, $\hat{\pi}_\tau$ is a biased estimate of the true prevalence π_{TRUE} unless the test is perfect. Starting from the deterministic relation between π_τ and π_{TRUE}:

$$\pi_\tau = \pi_{\text{TRUE}} SE_\tau + (1 - \pi_{\text{TRUE}})(1 - SP_\tau), \qquad (11.2)$$

simple calculus leads to the (asymptotic) bias expression

$$\pi_\tau - \pi_{\text{TRUE}} = (1 - \pi_{\text{TRUE}})F_\tau^+ - \pi_{\text{TRUE}}F_\tau^-, \qquad (11.3)$$

where $F_\tau^+ = 1 - SP_\tau$ is the false-positive probability and $F_\tau^- = 1 - SE_\tau$ is the false-negative probability. The bias depends on the choice of threshold τ and on the true prevalence π_{TRUE} and can be positive as well as negative. Note that only for a perfect test the bias disappears.

Using (11.2), an asymptotically unbiased estimator for π_{TRUE} can easily be derived (Rogan and Gladen 1978):

$$\hat{\pi}_{RG} = \frac{\hat{\pi}_\tau + \widehat{SP}_\tau - 1}{\widehat{SE}_\tau + \widehat{SP}_\tau - 1}, \qquad (11.4)$$

provided that $\widehat{SE}_\tau$ and $\widehat{SP}_\tau$ are asymptotically unbiased estimators for SE_τ and SP_τ, respectively.

Using one of the estimators $\hat{\pi}_\tau(a)$ from earlier chapters, all expressions (11.2)–(11.4) can be made age-dependent, and an age-dependent *sero-FOI* can be defined as

$$\lambda_\tau(a) = \frac{\pi_\tau'(a)}{1 - \pi_\tau(a)}, \qquad (11.5)$$

and a natural asymptotically unbiased estimator $\hat{\lambda}_\tau(a)$ follows from plugging in the estimator $\hat{\pi}_\tau(a)$ in definition (11.5).

Bollaerts et al. (2012) show that $\hat{\lambda}_\tau(a)$ is a biased estimate of the true FOI, $\lambda_{\text{TRUE}}(a) = \pi'_{\text{TRUE}}(a)/(1 - \pi_{\text{TRUE}}(a))$, and that the asymptotic bias can be expressed as

$$\lambda_\tau(a) - \lambda_{\text{TRUE}}(a) = - \left(\frac{F_\tau^-}{(1 - \pi_{\text{TRUE}}(a))(1 - F_\tau^+) + \pi_{\text{TRUE}}(a)F_\tau^-} \right) \lambda_{\text{TRUE}}(a). \quad (11.6)$$

It turns out that this bias is always negative and, for a valid test, it equals zero in case the false-negative rate F_τ^- is zero (or $SE_\tau = 1$). Bollaerts et al. (2012) show that the biases (11.3) and (11.6) are minimized for different values of the threshold τ. For the prevalence, the optimal choice is the *to be expected value* discriminating both infected and susceptible groups in a maximal way, the optimal choice for the FOI however can be substantially smaller (leading to fewer false negatives).

Plugging an age-dependent version of the Rogan–Gladen estimator $\hat{\pi}_{RG}(a)$ as an estimator for π_{TRUE} in the expression of $\lambda_{\text{TRUE}}(a)$, Bollaerts et al. (2012) derive the following estimator for $\lambda_{\text{TRUE}}(a)$, corrected for misclassification (asymptotically unbiased):

$$\hat{\lambda}_{RG}(a) = \frac{\hat{\pi}'_\tau(a)}{\widehat{SE}_\tau - \hat{\pi}_\tau(a)}, \quad (11.7)$$

provided that $\widehat{SE}_\tau$ is an asymptotically unbiased estimator for SE_τ. Note that only in case $\widehat{SE}_\tau = 1$, this estimator $\hat{\lambda}_{RG}(a)$ equals the threshold-based version $\hat{\lambda}_\tau(a)$.

For the two-threshold situation with equivocal/inconclusive cases discarded, the situation gets more complicated. The expressions for the bias include the probabilities that infected and susceptible individuals are inconclusive and hence deleted. Again RG-types of corrected estimators can be derived, but as estimators for the probabilities to be inconclusive are generally unavailable or hard to estimate, these estimators have very limited practical use. Figure 11.4 shows a plot of the estimated seroprevalence and sero-FOI (as discussed in previous chapters), using monotone P-splines, and using the dichotomized data excluding the inconclusive observations. As we are in a setting of two thresholds, it is not straightforward to correct this estimator for misclassifications and deletions. For more details, we refer to Bollaerts et al. (2012).

From this discussion it is clear that the use of threshold-based estimators is not without problems. In the next section we therefore introduce a direct approach to estimate $\pi_{\text{TRUE}}(a)$ and $\lambda_{\text{TRUE}}(a)$ without using any thresholds.

11.3   A Direct Approach

The true prevalence, $\pi_{\text{TRUE}}(a)$, and FOI, $\lambda_{\text{TRUE}}(a)$, can be derived directly by using a two-component mixture model for the antibody activity levels. The group of infected individuals and the group of susceptible individuals form the two

Fig. 11.4 Belgian VZV data. Proportion positive, as a function of the corresponding half-year age categories, overlaid with the monotone P-spline fit (using logit link and binomial likelihood) and the FOI: with BIC optimal smoothing parameter

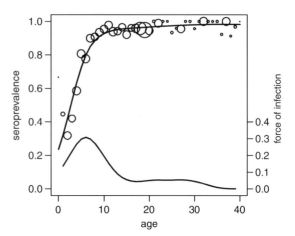

components with the true prevalence $\pi_{\text{TRUE}}(a)$ as age-dependent mixing probability. In general, it can be (equally well) assumed that π_{TRUE} depends on other covariate information or that π_{TRUE} does not depend on covariate information at all.

Formally, the two-component mixture model for non-dichotomized test results Z with Z_j ($j = \{I,S\}$) being the latent mixing component having density $f_j(z_j|\theta_j)$ and with $\pi_{\text{TRUE}}(a)$ being the age-dependent mixing probability can be represented as

$$f(z|z_1, z_S, a) = (1 - \pi_{\text{TRUE}}(a))f_S(z_S|\theta_S) + \pi_{\text{TRUE}}(a)f_I(z_I|\theta_I), \qquad (11.8)$$

based on which it is readily seen that the mean $E(Z|a)$ equals

$$\mu(a) = (1 - \pi_{\text{TRUE}}(a))\mu_S + \pi_{\text{TRUE}}(a)\mu_I, \qquad (11.9)$$

with μ_S and μ_I being the mean of $f_S(y_S|\theta_S)$ and $f_I(y_I|\theta_I)$, respectively, and with, for reasons of identifiability, the convention made that $\mu_I > \mu_S$.

From (11.9), it is straightforward to derive the identity

$$\pi_{\text{TRUE}}(a) = \frac{\mu(a) - \mu_S}{\mu_I - \mu_S}, \qquad (11.10)$$

which shows that $\pi_{\text{TRUE}}(a)$ is the excess of the mixture mean $\mu(a)$ to the mean of the susceptible population μ_S relative to the difference in means of both subpopulations. A natural estimator for the true prevalence is given by

$$\hat{\pi}_{\text{DIRECT}}(a) = \frac{\hat{\mu}(a) - \hat{\mu}_S}{\hat{\mu}_I - \hat{\mu}_S}. \qquad (11.11)$$

It is standard to estimate the mixture mean $\mu(a)$ using least-squares regression techniques, parametrically or nonparametrically depending on the application and research interests. The subpopulation means μ_s and μ_i can be estimated by density estimation methods for two-component mixture models, using Bayesian sampling algorithms (Gilks et al. 1996) or EM-algorithms, either parametric (e.g. Peel and McLachlan 2000) or semiparametric (e.g. Cruz-Medina et al. 2004; Bordes et al. 2007). Alternatively, classification methods can be used as well. If $\hat{\mu}_s$ and $\hat{\mu}_i$ are (asymptotically) unbiased estimates, so is the estimator $\hat{\pi}_{\text{DIRECT}}(a)$.

Differentiating both sides of identity (11.9), some straightforward calculus shows that

$$\lambda_{\text{TRUE}}(a) = \frac{\mu'(a)}{\mu_i - \mu(a)}, \tag{11.12}$$

which leads to the natural estimator

$$\hat{\lambda}_{\text{DIRECT}}(a) = \frac{\hat{\mu}'(a)}{\hat{\mu}_i - \hat{\mu}(a)}. \tag{11.13}$$

Note that these expressions do not depend on the mean μ_s of the susceptible subpopulation. Again, the estimator (11.13) is asymptotically unbiased.

Bollaerts et al. (2012) show that there is an explicit connection between the direct and corrected threshold approach. More precisely they show mathematically that both approaches are exactly identical using a particular transformation. This identity however concerns the population parameters, and in a simulation study, covering a variety of settings, they show that both methods do differ when applying them on data. Their main conclusions can be formulated as follows. On the true prevalence scale, the direct and corrected threshold approach behave very similar (in terms of MSE). On the true FOI scale however the results are more mixed. There is no clear overall winner, but for many settings the direct method performs more accurate (in terms of MSE) and more robust or stable (less variable over different settings).

In the next section we apply the direct approach to the VZV data, illustrate R code, and compare the results with those obtained from the dichotomized data.

11.4 Application to VZV Data

We start with illustrating how to fit a mixture model to the VZV data (collapsed over age), next how to fit a monotone least-squares P-spline, and finally how to combine both concepts to derive the estimates for the true prevalence and the true FOI.

11.4.1 Fitting a Mixture

There are several packages available in R to fit mixture models. The following code illustrates the use of the *mixdist* R-package. The estimates for the fitted mixture and Fig. 11.3 are produced by the following R-code:

```
# R-code to fit a Gaussian mixture
library(mixdist)
zmixdat=mixgroup(z,breaks=40)
zstartpar=mixparam(pi=c(0.2,0.8),mu=c(2,6),sigma=c(0.5,1))
mixfit=mix(zmixdat,zstartpar,dist="norm")
summary(mixfit)
plot(mixfit,cex.lab=2,cex.axis=2)
coef(mixfit)
```

resulting in the following estimates, based on the data pooled over age (variable z in the code above):

```
> coef(mixfit)
         pi        mu      sigma
1 0.1012956 2.316357 0.6660275
2 0.8987044 6.338433 1.0318659
```

The fit indicates that (as suggested by Figs. 11.1 and 11.3) a large majority (almost 90%) of the cases belongs to the infected group.

11.4.2   Fitting the Mean Antibody Levels as a Function of Age

The monotonicity of the true prevalence $\pi_{\mathrm{TRUE}}(a)$ implies, through identity (11.9), that also $\mu(a)$ is a nondecreasing function of age. As explained in Chap. 9, a monotone P-spline is an interesting option and the same R-code can be used, but now specifying the identity link and the gaussian family (resulting in a least-squares fit). The optimal smoothness parameter was selected using the BIC criterion.

11.4.3   Combining the Mixture with the Least Squares Regression Fit

Direct application of formula's (11.11) and (11.13) leads to the fits as shown in Fig. 11.5. The fits based on the direct method are shown as solid curves, those of the threshold method by dashed curves. The solid prevalence curve seems to fit the observed proportions not very well in the age range 5–10 as most of the bubbles are below the estimated curve. Remember however that this estimate is

Fig. 11.5 Belgian VZV data. Proportion positive, as a function of the corresponding half-year age categories, overlaid with the monotone P-spline fit and the FOI: estimated using the direct method (*solid curves*) and the threshold method (*dashed curves*)

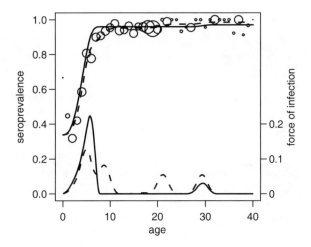

based on more data, as the 105 inconclusive cases are not excluded by the direct method. Moreover, the dashed curve should still be corrected for misclassifications, which might appear more frequently in this age range. As a consequence the directly estimated FOI reaches a much higher first peak at about the age of seven. The second peak at the age of about 30 is also much more pronounced. This is in line with the theoretical finding that the FOI based on the threshold method has a negative bias. Finally note that the fitted curves are less bumpy as the ones shown in Bollaerts et al. (2012), a consequence of choosing the smoothness parameter based on the BIC criterion rather than using (generalized) cross-validation.

11.5   Modeling the Force of Infection Directly from Antibody Titers Using Hierarchical Mixture Models

In Sect. 11.3 the estimated means of the two mixture components and the estimated mean antibody level were used in order to estimate $\pi_{\text{DIRECT}}(a)$ in (11.11). In this section we take a slightly different approach. In contrast with the previous section we do not focus on $E(Z|a)$ but rather on the prevalence itself. We use hierarchical mixture models and we show that the mixture probability $\pi(a)$ (the probability that a subject belongs to the infected component of the mixture) can be interpreted as the true prevalence, $\pi(a) = \pi_{\text{TRUE}}(a)$. Similar to the previous section we do not assume that the current infection status of the subject is known in advance but rather classify the subjects in the sample as seronegative (susceptible) or seropositive (infected) based on a hierarchical mixture model.

11.5.1 Model Formulation

Let $f(Z)$ be the density function of the antibody level Z. We assume that $f(Z)$ is a finite mixture distribution of the form

$$f(Z) = \sum_{j=1}^{k} \pi_j f(Z|\theta_j), \qquad (11.14)$$

where $f(Z|\theta_j)$, $j = 1,\ldots,k$, are called the mixture components, $\pi_j \geq 0$ with $\sum_{j=1}^{k} \pi_j = 1$ are the mixture probabilities, and θ_j are the parameters to be estimated (Gelman et al. 1995; Gilks et al. 1996; Congdon 2003). In what follows we focus on a mixture of two normal populations with possibly different mean and variance parameters. As discussed in Sect. 11.1 the first component of the mixture is the distribution of (log) antibody levels of the susceptible individuals and the second component is the distribution of the (log) antibody levels of the infected individuals (see also Figs. 11.2 and 11.3).

Finite mixture models for estimation of the prevalence have also been discussed by Gay et al. (2003) and Vyse et al. (2004, 2006). These authors focused on the estimation of the prevalence and fitted the mixture model for each age group. Hardelid et al. (2008) proposed a similar approach to model the distribution of rubella antibody levels using the EM algorithm implemented in the R packages *flexmix* and *gamlss.mx*. Hardelid et al. (2008) assigned each individual to one of the mixture components based on the maximum estimated mixture probability. Nielsen et al. (2007) proposed a two-component hierarchical mixture model for the estimation of within-herd prevalence of bovine paratuberculosis. The components' means and the mixture probability in Nielsen's model were formulated as a function of several covariates in order to model the dependence of both the means and the mixture probabilities upon these covariates.

Following the approach of Congdon (2003) and Nielsen et al. (2007), we formulate the mixture model in terms of a hierarchical model using a latent indicator variable. In this model, the latent variable Y_i represents the unknown true disease status. Hence, the likelihood in the first stage of the hierarchical model is given by

$$Z_i \sim N(Y_i\mu_1 + (1 - Y_i)\mu_2, Y_i\sigma_1^2 + (1 - Y_i)\sigma_2^2). \qquad (11.15)$$

Here, $\mu = (\mu_1, \mu_2)$, and $\sigma^2 = (\sigma_1^2, \sigma_2^2)$ are the mean and variance vectors for the susceptible and infected components, respectively. The variable Y_i can be seen as a latent classification random variable which represents the true (but latent) current status of the disease for which we assume a Bernoulli distribution:

$$Y_i = \begin{cases} 1 & \pi, \\ 0 & 1 - \pi. \end{cases} \qquad (11.16)$$

The mixture probability in (11.16) is the probability that an individual in the population belongs to the *infected* component or that the antibody measurement was sampled from a truly infected individual (Nielsen et al. 2007). Thus, π can be interpreted as the prevalence in the population (Evans and Erlandson 2004). Note that in contrast with the direct approach discussed in Sect. 11.3 we do not focus on the mean antibody level $\mu(a)$ but we focus on the mixture probability π and leave $\mu(a)$ unspecified. At this stage we use predefined age groups and assume that the mixture probability π is constant across these age groups and that it follows a uniform distribution $\pi \sim U(0,1)$. Similar to Evans and Erlandson (2004) we assume that larger values of antibody levels indicate a positive status and therefore include order restriction $\mu_1 \leq \mu_2$ in the model. This can be done by assuming a constrained noninformative prior for μ_1:

$$\mu_1 \sim U(0,\mu_2),$$
$$\mu_2 = \mu_1 + \delta, \qquad (11.17)$$
$$\delta \sim U(0,C).$$

Here C is a relatively high constant. The parameter δ represents the shift of the mean antibody level between the two components of the mixture.

To complete the specification of the hierarchical model, the following (noninformative) hyperprior distributions are assumed:

$$\sigma_j^{-2} \sim \text{gamma}(0.0001,0.0001), \quad j = 1,2, \qquad (11.18)$$

where $\text{gamma}(\alpha,\beta)$ denotes a gamma distribution with mean equal to α/β and variance α/β^2. Hence, by choosing $\alpha = \beta = 0.0001$, the prior distribution for both precision parameters is a gamma distribution with mean 1 and variance 10,000 which reflects our uncertainty about the true values of the parameters (see,e.g., Gilks et al. 1996).

11.5.2 Age-Dependent Mixture Probability

As argued before, the mixture probability can be interpreted as the prevalence in the population. For many infectious diseases both the prevalence and the FOI are known to be age-dependent. In what follows we relax the assumption that π is constant across the age groups. In particular we assume that

$$\text{logit}(\pi(a)) = \gamma_0 + \gamma_1 \log(a) \; ; \; \gamma_1 > 0, \qquad (11.19)$$

which implies that

$$\pi(a) = \frac{\delta_0 a^{\gamma_1}}{1 + \delta_0 a^{\gamma_1}}, \qquad (11.20)$$

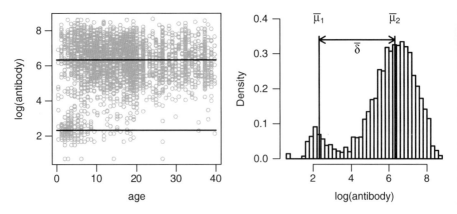

Fig. 11.6 The Belgian VZV dataset. *Left panel*: a scatterplot of the log(antibody level) and posterior means for the two components. *Right panel*: a histogram of the log(antibody level), $\bar{\delta}$ is the posterior mean difference

with $\delta_0 = \exp(\gamma_0)$. Note that the parametric structure of $\pi(a)$ implies a log-logistic distribution for the time spent in the susceptible class (Shkedy et al. 2003). The FOI, which is the rate at which individuals move from the susceptible component to the infected component of the mixture model, is given by

$$\lambda(a) = \frac{\gamma_1 \delta_0 a^{\gamma_1 - 1}}{1 + \delta_0 a^{\gamma_1}}. \tag{11.21}$$

We assume independent noninformative priors for γ_0 and γ_1:

$$\begin{aligned} \gamma_0 &\sim N(0, \tau_0^2), \\ \gamma_1 &\sim N(0, \tau_1^2)I(0,). \end{aligned} \tag{11.22}$$

Note that the prior distribution for γ_1 is truncated at zero to ensure that $\gamma_1 \geq 0$. The hyperparameters τ_0^2 and τ_1^2 were assumed to follow inverse gamma distributions, $\tau_0^{-2} \sim \text{gamma}(0.01, 0.01)$, $\tau_1^{-2} \sim \text{gamma}(0.01, 0.01)$.

11.5.3   Application to the Data

An MCMC simulation was conducted using WINBUGS 1.4. We run the model for 10,000 iterations from which the first 1,000 are used as burn-in period. Data and posterior means of the mean antibody levels are shown in Fig. 11.6 and Table 11.1. The posterior mean for the infected component is equal to 6.32 and higher than

Table 11.1 Posterior mean and 95% credible intervals for μ_i, σ_i^2, $i = 1, 2$ and δ

Parameter	Posterior means (Credible interval)
μ_1	2.326 (2.248,2.423)
μ_2	6.322 (6.278,6.362)
σ_1^2	0.326 (0.257,0.410)
σ_2^2	1.067 (1.001,1.130)
δ	4.002 (3.912,4.081)

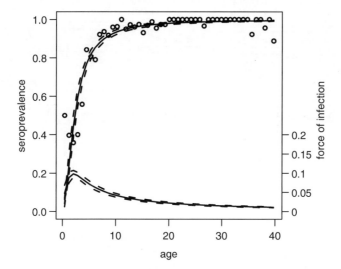

Fig. 11.7 The posterior mean (*solid line*) for the mixture probability at each age group with 95% credible intervals (*dashed lines*) together with the age-dependent FOI. The *dots* represent the estimated fraction seropositives in the sample

the posterior mean of the susceptible component 2.32. Posterior means for the variance of each component are equal to 1.067 and 0.326 for the infected and susceptible components, respectively. The posterior mean for the shift parameter δ equals 4.002 (95% credible interval: 3.912–4.081). Figure 11.7 shows the posterior mean for the mixture probability at each age group with 95% credible intervals together with the age-dependent FOI. The dots in Fig. 11.7 represent the estimated fraction seropositives in the sample which we will discuss in the following section.

11.5.4 Determining the Current Infection Status

As we mentioned in the previous section, the current infection status of each subject in the sample is unknown. The advantage of the hierarchical mixture model is that the current status of the individuals in the sample is not needed in order to

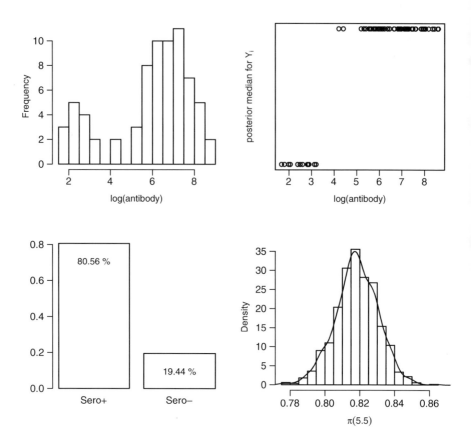

Fig. 11.8 *Upper left panel*: distribution of log(antibody level) at age 5.5 years. *Upper right panel*: log(antibody level) versus the posterior median of Y_i. *Lower left panel*: proportion of individuals being classified as seropositive (80.55%) and seronegative (19.45%) at age group 5.5. *Lower right panel*: density estimate for the posterior distribution of $\pi(5.5)$

estimate the prevalence and the FOI. However, in many cases, diagnosis at the individual level, i.e., the determination whether the ith individual is infected or not, is of primary interest. Classically, this can be done using the cutoff point method (Sect. 11.1). In this section we show that diagnosis at individual level can be based on the hierarchical mixture model without the necessity to use predefined or model-based cutoff points. In order to determine whether each individual in the sample has been infected or is susceptible we need to classify the individual into the two components of the mixture. For classification, we use the posterior median of the latent variable Y_i. If $Y_i = 1$, subject i has been infected before, if $Y_i = 0$, subject i is still susceptible.

The upper left panel in Fig. 11.8 shows the histogram for the log(antibody levels) in the age group with mid age 5.5 years. Posterior medians of Y_i in this age group are shown in the upper right panel of Fig. 11.8. Subjects for which $\bar{Y}_i = 0$ are classified as susceptible while subjects with $\bar{Y}_i = 1$ are classified as seropositive. Furthermore, once the classification is done, one can calculate the proportion seropositive at each age group by $\sum_{i=1}^{n(a)} \bar{Y}_i(a)/n(a)$.

For the age group with mid age 5.5 years the estimated proportion of seropositives in the sample equals 0.806. Note that this is not our estimate of the prevalence at this age group in the population but our estimate of the proportion of seropositive individuals in this age group under the assumption that the prevalence in the population is equal to $\pi(a)$. The estimated density for the posterior distribution of the prevalence in this age group $\pi(5.5)$ in the population is shown in Fig. 11.8. The posterior mean for the prevalence in this age group is equal to 0.819. Figure 11.7 shows the posterior mean for the prevalence (solid line) and the estimate for the proportion of seropositives in the sample (dots). We notice that the posterior mean of the prevalence should be monotonically increasing while the estimated proportion of seropositives can be non-monotone.

11.5.5 Implementation in Winbugs

The hierarchical mixture model discussed above was fitted in Winbugs 1.4. In the first part of the program we specify the normal likelihood in (11.15). The variable *Nsub* defined in the program is the total sample size.

```
for( i in 1 : Nsub )
{
Zi[i]~dnorm(mu[i],tau[i])
T[i]~dcat(P[agegr[i],])
Yi[i]=T[i]-1
mu[i]=mu1.y*Yi[i]+mu2.y*(1-Yi[i])
tau[i]=tau1.mu*Yi[i]+tau2.mu*(1-Yi[i])
```

Note that we specify the mean and the variance for the mixture model $Y_i\mu_1 + (1 - Y_i)\mu_2$ and $Y_i\sigma_1^2 + (1 - Y_i)\sigma_2^2$ by *mu[i]=mu1.y*Yi[i]+mu2.y*(1-Yi[i])* and *tau[i]= tau1.mu*Yi[i]+tau2.mu*(1-Yi[i])*, respectively. The variable *Yi* corresponds to the latent current status of the disease given in (11.16). There are several options to specify the binomial distribution for this latent variable. In this example we use a discrete categorical distribution using the Winbugs function *dcat(p[])*. We define a categorical variable *T[i]* that takes the values of 1 and 2 with probability $\pi(a_i)$ and $1 - \pi(a_i)$, respectively ($\pi(a_i)$ is the mixture probability of the age group to which the *i*th individual belongs). The current status of the disease is *Yi[i]=T[i]-1*. Next we specify prior distributions (11.17) and (11.18) for the mean and precision parameters of the two components.

```
mu2.y ~ dunif(0,mu1.y)
mu1.y = mu2.y+delta
delta ~ dunif(0,7)
tau1.mu   ~ dgamma(0.01,  0.01)
tau2.mu   ~ dgamma(0.01,  0.01)
sig1=1/tau1.mu
sig2=1/tau2.mu
```

The variables *sig1* and *sig2* correspond to σ_1^2 and σ_2^2, respectively. In the next stage of the program we define the age-dependent mixture probability given in (11.19) and (11.20) by

```
for(i in 1:Nage)
{
theta[i]=gamma0+gamma1*log(age1[i])
p.i[i]=1-exp(theta[i])/(1+exp(theta[i]))
foi[i]=exp(gamma0)*gamma1*pow(age1[i],gamma1-1)
            /(1+exp(gamma0)*pow(age1[i],gamma1))
}
gamma0 ~ dnorm(0,tau.gamma0)
tau.gamma0   ~ dgamma(0.01,  0.01)
gamma1 ~ dnorm(0,tau.gamma1)I(0,)
tau.gamma1   ~ dgamma(0.01,  0.01)
```

Lastly, we need to make the connection in the program between the mixture probability and the distribution of the latent variable *Yi*. We define a $K \times 2$ matrix P (K is the number of age groups) for which $[P]_{i1} = \pi(a_i)$ and $[P]_{i2} = 1 - \pi(a_i)$. Thus, the first column in P is the mixture probability for each age group and the second columns in the probability to be susceptible for each age group.

```
for(i in 1:Nage){
P[i,1]=p.i[i]
P[i,2]=1-p.i[i]
```

The variable *agegr[i]* is a categorical variable which represents the age group to which each subject belongs. Therefore, the mixture probability for the *i*th subject is given by *P[agegr[i],1]*. As mentioned above, we define a discrete categorical distribution for the latent categorical variable *T[i]*:

```
T[i]~dcat(P[agegr[i],])
Yi[i]=T[i]-1
```

This implies that

$$T[i] = \begin{cases} 1 & P[agegr[i],1], \\ 2 & P[agegr[i],2], \end{cases} \quad \text{and} \quad Yi[i] = \begin{cases} 0 & P[agegr[i],1], \\ 1 & P[agegr[i],2], \end{cases}$$

$$\text{or} \quad Y_i = \begin{cases} 1 & \pi(a_i), \\ 0 & 1 - \pi(a_i). \end{cases}$$

Hence, it $P[agegr[i],2]$ represents the probability to belong to the infected component or the prevalence.

11.6 Concluding Remarks

The question what the prevalence of a certain infectious disease is in the population is not straightforward to answer due to the uncertainty in the determination of a subject's current infection status when predefined manufacturer thresholds are used. In this chapter, we presented alternative methods to estimate the prevalence, the FOI and the current status of the diseases. Since both methods are based on mixture models, the current infection status is a latent variable and as a result both methods avoid the choice and use of any thresholds. The main strength of the direct method is based on combining a simple mean regression fit with a simple mixture fit. The main strength of the hierarchical Bayesian mixture model is due to the fact that the quantity of primary interest, the prevalence, is a central part of the model. The FOI can easily be derived in the same way as in the previous chapters. For the direct method we used monotone penalized splines to estimate $\mu(a)$. Of course the direct method could also be combined with a parametric model for the age-dependent mean antibody levels. For the hierarchical mixture model, we used a log-logistic model for the mixture probability. Depending on the setting, other parametric models can be used for the mean structure in (11.19) as well.

Chapter 12
Modeling Multivariate Serological Data

12.1 Introduction

For feasibility and economical reasons, serum samples are often tested for more than one antigen. Studying diseases with similar transmission routes can govern new insights for disease dynamics. In this chapter, we focus on two different methods to study the association between several infections using multisera data. We restrict attention to two infections but note that these methods can be extended towards three or more infections.

The first approach uses marginal and conditional models to study the association between past infection for both pathogens. The use of a bivariate model for this kind of data improves not only the efficiency, but it also allows us to study the association between infections. Next to the derivation of the age-dependent marginal FOI, we introduce new epidemiological parameters: the age-dependent joint and conditional FOI. These parameters allow one to study the association among the occurrence and acquisition of both infections. Moreover, these models allow for testing whether there exists an association and whether the infection-specific age-dependent FOI curves are proportional, indicating whether separable mixing in the population holds. The methodology as applied for multisera data was published by Hens et al. (2008b). These authors showed that the difference between marginal and conditional models diminishes when using semiparametric methods. In this chapter, we will focus on the bivariate Dale model (BDM) and smoothing splines as flexible modeling tools (see Sect. 8.2.1).

The second approach ascribes dependency to individual heterogeneity. The idea originates from Coutinho et al. (1999) and was first applied in the infectious disease setting by Farrington et al. (2001) and pursued by Farrington and Whitaker (2005); Kanaan and Farrington (2005), and Sutton et al. (2006), who proposed the use of this bivariate model to estimate the heterogeneity in acquisition for mumps and rubella, and hepatitis B and C, respectively. We do not focus on the relationship between heterogeneity in acquisition but the underlying mixing matrices here and refer to Chaps. 14 and 15.

N. Hens et al., *Modeling Infectious Disease Parameters Based on Serological and Social Contact Data*, Statistics for Biology and Health 63, DOI 10.1007/978-1-4614-4072-7_12, © Springer Science+Business Media New York 2012

In Sect. 12.2, we introduce the BDM as a marginal model and briefly indicate which conditional models can be used. We show its application to multisera data on rubella and mumps in the UK and data on the varicella zoster virus (VZV) and parvovirus B19 in Belgium (see Chap. 4). In Sect. 12.3, we introduce and apply a gamma frailty model to estimate the heterogeneity in acquisition for the two infections in each example.

12.2 Marginal and Conditional Models

Given bivariate binary dependent data on two infectious diseases (y_1, y_2) from a sample of individuals together with their age a, denote the joint probability $\pi_{j_1, j_2} = P(y_1 = j_1, y_2 = j_2)$, where the index $j_k, k = 1, 2$ corresponds to diseases 1 and 2, respectively, and $j_k = 1$ (0) indicating past or current infection (susceptibility) for disease $k = 1, 2$. Modeling such multivariate categorical data can be done using conditional or marginal models (Liang et al. 1992).

A first marginal model that can be considered is the bivariate Dale model (BDM, Dale 1986; Palmgren 1989). The BDM relates the probability of past or current infection for both diseases to the age at infection. The BDM consists of the following three models which are modeled simultaneously:

$$\begin{cases} \text{logit}(\pi_{1+}|a) = h_1(a), \\ \text{logit}(\pi_{+1}|a) = h_2(a), \\ \log(\text{OR}|a) = h_3(a). \end{cases} \tag{12.1}$$

Here OR denotes the age-dependent odds ratio $(\pi_{11}\pi_{00})/(\pi_{10}\pi_{01})$; π_{1+}, π_{+1} the marginal probabilities, and h_i, $i = 1, 2, 3$ smooth differentiable functions. Using (12.1), it is straightforward to write down the multinomial (log)likelihood in terms of h_i, $i = 1, 2, 3$ governing a maximum likelihood estimation procedure. Indeed, expressing the multinomial probabilities in terms of (12.1) is straightforward noting that, when OR $\neq 1$, $\pi_{11} = 1 + (\pi_{1+} + \pi_{+1})(\text{OR} - 1) - \{[1 + (\pi_{1+} + \pi_{+1})(\text{OR} - 1)]^2 + 4\text{OR}(1 - \text{OR})\pi_{1+}\pi_{+1}\}^{1/2}/(2(\text{OR} - 1))$, and when OR $= 1$, $\pi_{11} = \pi_{1+}\pi_{+1}$. Modeling the odds ratio allows us to describe the association between both diseases. An OR $= 1$ indicates both infectious disease processes to behave independently whereas OR $\neq 1$ indicates association between both diseases.

Hens et al. (2008b) suggested to use the multivariate extension of the smoothing spline approach, known as vector generalized additive models (Yee and Wild 1996). This extension is provided by considering $\ell(h_1, h_2, h_3; y) - \frac{1}{2}\sum_{i=1}^{3} \lambda_i \int \{h_i''(a)\}^2 da$, where $\ell(h_1, h_2, h_3; y)$ denotes the loglikelihood of the multivariate model, λ_i, $i = 1, 2, 3$ denote component-specific smoothing parameters, and $\int \{h_i''(a)\}^2 da$, $i = 1, 2, 3$ denote component-specific penalties. Determining the optimal values for λ_i, $i = 1, 2, 3$ is done by generalized cross-validation or alternatively a model selection criterion as BIC.

The implementation of the BDM with smoothing splines for the $h_i, i = 1, 2, 3$, in R is given through the "VGAM"-library (Yee and Wild 1996; Yee 2008). In the following code for *fit.dale1*, *cbind(NN, NP, PN, PP)* are the quadruples of numbers of negative–negative, negative–positive, positive–negative and positive–positive test results per (ordered) unique age value given by the vector a; *s(a,spar=sparopt)* refers to the smoothing spline with optimal smoothing parameter *sparopt* which can be chosen using, e.g., the BIC criterion (see Chap. 8). Note that specifying *spar=sparopt* chooses the same smoothing parameter for the three smooth components $h_i, i = 1, 2, 3$ in (12.1). Alternatively, *spar=c(sparopt1,sparopt2,sparopt3)* could be specified to select different smoothing parameters for the different components $h_i, i = 1, 2, 3$. The family *binom2.or(zero=NULL)* specifies the use of the Dale model (12.1). *fit.dale2* adapts the fit of *fit.dale1*, specifying a constant odds ratio by indicating that the smoothing spline is only used for the two first components *"s(a, spar = sparopt)"=diag(3)[,1:2]* whereas an intercept is specified for all components *"(Intercept)"=diag(3)*. If in addition to a constant odds ratio, *"(Intercept)"=diag(3)[1:2,]* is specified, the model assumes OR $= 1$ and thus independence. Whether or not the smooth components h_i are age-dependent can be tested using an F-test modification of the likelihood ratio test (Yee and Wild 1996), easily obtained in the code by requesting *summary(fit.dale1)*.

```
# R-code for the Bivariate Dale Model with Smoothing Splines
library(VGAM)
fit.dale1=vgam(cbind(NN,NP,PN,PP)~s(a,spar=sparopt),
        binom2.or(zero=NULL))
fit.dale2=vgam(cbind(NN,NP,PN,PP)~s(a,spar=sparopt),
        binom2.or(zero=NULL),constraints=list(
        "(Intercept)"=diag(3),
        "s(a, spar = sparopt)"=diag(3)[,1:2]))
```

As an alternative to the BDM, one can opt to use a bivariate probit model in which the odds ratio is replaced by the correlation coefficient and the logit links and the log link in (12.1) are replaced by probit-links and a rhobit-link, respectively. Both the BDM and the bivariate probit model are marginal models since their parameters characterize the marginal probabilities and the association is of secondary importance. Note that the marginal probabilities are reproducible using univariate analyses at the cost of efficiency. In contrast, conditional models focus on the association by looking at one variable conditional on the other. Examples include the baseline category logits model where one of the joint probabilities is used as a baseline and the other probabilities are modeled in relation to the baseline probability using a log link function and smooth differentiable functions $\tilde{h}_i$, $i = 1, 2, 3$. We note that, using smoothing splines as flexible functions $h_i, \tilde{h}_i, i = 1, 2, 3$ of age, the difference between marginal and conditional models diminishes. We refer to Hens et al. (2008b) for more on this matter.

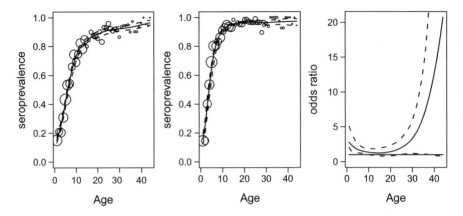

Fig. 12.1 The marginal prevalence curves for rubella (*first panel—solid line*) and mumps (*second panel—solid line*) together with the odds ratio (*third panel—solid line*) according to the spline-based BDM together with 95% bootstrap-based pointwise confidence intervals (*dashed lines*). The *horizontal line* in the *third panel* corresponds to an OR = 1

12.2.1 The Bivariate Dale Model Applied to Airborne Infections

We use data on rubella and mumps in the UK, previously analyzed by Farrington et al. (2001) and data on the VZV and parvovirus B19 (B19) in Belgium, previously analyzed by Hens et al. (2008b). We fit the BDM to both datasets and restrict attention to age > 6 months to omit seropositive individuals due to the presence of maternal antibodies. We monotonize the estimated age-dependent seroprevalence by applying the pool adjacent violator algorithm (PAVA, Chap. 9) to $\hat{\pi}_{11}, \hat{\pi}_{1+}$ and $\hat{\pi}_{+1}$ from which all other joint probabilities can be derived. Note that we use the nonparametric bootstrap approach to obtain 95% pointwise confidence intervals since this method allows the application of the PAVA.

In Figs. 12.1 and 12.2, the age-dependent prevalences for rubella and mumps and VZV and B19 together with the respective odds ratios according to the monotonized spline-based BDM are shown.

The summary of the BDM model as applied to the rubella and mumps data from the UK is given in the following output window. According to the BIC criterion, *sparopt* = 0.009 was the most optimal common smoothing parameter. Testing for a constant odds ratio using the F-test modification of the likelihood ratio test indicated a significant trend with age (p = 0.0011). The bootstrap-based confidence intervals in Fig. 12.1 confirmed the latter finding. Note that the odds ratio starts of above 1, indicating dependence in the occurrence of rubella and mumps infections for children younger than 12 years whereas from then on the 95% bootstrap-based confidence interval for the OR contains 1. This result can be interpreted as an indication of similarity in transmission for both infections and the very likely occurrence of acquiring either infection before the age of 12 years (0.79 and 0.94

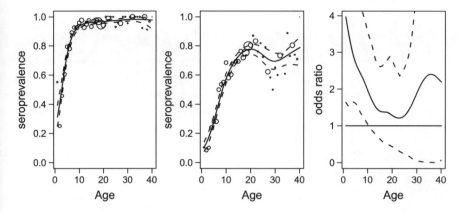

Fig. 12.2 The marginal prevalence-curves for VZV (*first panel—solid line*) and B19 (*second panel—solid line*) together with the odds ratio (*third panel—solid line*) according to the spline-based BDM together with 95% bootstrap-based pointwise confidence intervals (*dashed lines*)

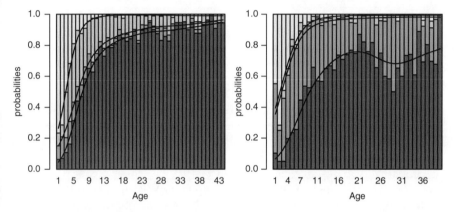

Fig. 12.3 The joint probabilities according to the spline-based BDM for both datasets. Observed proportions are shown from *dark gray* to *light gray* for p_{11}, p_{10}, p_{01}, and p_{00}, respectively. In the *left panel*: rubella and mumps, in the *right panel*: VZV and B19

for rubella and mumps, respectively, see Fig. 12.1). Note that the rise in odds ratio for adults is the result of the high prevalence for both rubella and mumps (0.92 and 0.96, respectively). Note that a deviance of 127.14 on 116.76 degrees of freedom indicates a good fit to the data as shown in the barplot (left panel) in Fig. 12.3.

```
Call:
vgam(formula = cbind(NN, NP, PN, PP) ~ s(a, spar = sparopt),
     family = binom2.or(zero = NULL))
```

(continued)

```
(continued)
Number of linear predictors:    3
Names of linear predictors: logit(mu1), logit(mu2), log(oratio)
Dispersion Parameter for binom2.or family:    1
Residual Deviance:   127.1351 on 116.764 degrees of freedom
Loglikelihood: -3195.352 on 116.764 degrees of freedom
Number of Iterations:  8


DF for Terms and Approximate Chi-squares for Nonparametric
Effects
                          Df Npar Df Npar Chisq     P(Chi)
(Intercept):1             1
(Intercept):2             1
(Intercept):3             1
s(a, spar = sparopt):1    1       4.1      184.36 0.00000000
s(a, spar = sparopt):2    1       3.3      333.77 0.00000000
s(a, spar = sparopt):3    1       1.8       13.00 0.00112071
```

The summary of the BDM for VZV and B19 is given next. Note that
sparopt=0.022 according to the BIC criterion. The deviance of 3,029.08 on 5,217.15
degrees of freedom indicates a good fit to the data. Testing for a constant odds ratio
using the BDM-models and the F-test modification of the likelihood ratio test
resulted in a constant odds ratio (p = 0.18). Bootstrap-based confidence intervals
confirmed the latter result (Fig. 12.2). Refitting the model while constraining the
odds ratio to be constant resulted in an estimated odds ratio of 2.09 with 95%
confidence interval (1.44,3.02), indicating significant dependency of VZV- and
B19-occurrence. Note that an odds ratio of 2.09 indicates that the odds of past
or current VZV(B19)-infection among the B19(VZV)-non-susceptible group is
2.09 times larger than the odds of past or current VZV(B19)-infection among the
B19(VZV)-susceptible group. Non-susceptibility is referring to past or current
infection.

```
Call:
vgam(formula = cbind(NN, NP, PN, PP) ~ s(a, spar = sparopt),
    family = binom2.or(zero = NULL), data = data)

Number of linear predictors:    3
Names of linear predictors: logit(mu1), logit(mu2),
    log(oratio)
Dispersion Parameter for binom2.or family:    1
Residual Deviance:   3029.082 on 5217.146 degrees of freedom
Loglikelihood: -1906.319 on 5217.146 degrees of freedom
Number of Iterations:  8

DF for Terms and Approximate Chi-squares for Nonparametric
Effects
```
(continued)

Fig. 12.4 Schematic representation of the flow of individuals among different stages. X_{ij} denotes the number of persons in class $\{i, j\}$, $i, j = 0, 1$ denoting whether infected (1) or not (0) for infection 1 (y_1) and infection 2 (y_2), respectively

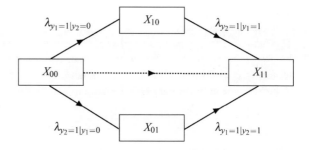

(continued)

	Df Npar	Df Npar	Chisq	P(Chi)
(Intercept):1	1			
(Intercept):2	1			
(Intercept):3	1			
s(a, spar = sparopt):1	1	1.9	87.748	0.00000
s(a, spar = sparopt):2	1	3.1	174.567	0.00000
s(a, spar = sparopt):3	1	0.9	1.626	0.17915

12.2.2   The Marginal, Conditional and Joint Force of Infection

Using the marginal prevalences derived from the spline-based BDM, the marginal FOI is easily derived by

$$\lambda_{1+}(a) = h_1'(a)\pi_{1+}(a) \quad \text{and} \quad \lambda_{+1}(a) = h_2'(a)\pi_{+1}(a). \tag{12.2}$$

However, using multisera data, one can analyze quantities like the prevalence and FOI for one infection conditional on being in a specific state for the second infection (Fig. 12.4). The potential interest in conditional prevalences and FOIs is not only related to quantifying the association between two or more infections (e.g., to evaluate the impact of combination vaccines) but could also be valuable to analyze chronic co-infections such as Human Papilomavirus (HPV), Human Immunodeficiency Virus (HIV) and hepatitis B (HBV) or C (HCV) virus where the acquisition of a second related infection could have a dramatic impact on the course of disease and infectiousness to others (Alberti and others (Jury Panel) 2005).

Suppose that conditional on a first infection, one is interested in the rate of acquiring a second infection. Thus one looks at the quantities

$$\lambda_{y_1=1|y_2=i} = \frac{\pi_{y_1=1|y_2=i}'}{1 - \pi_{y_1=1|y_2=i}}, \tag{12.3}$$

where $i = 1$ ($i = 0$) if the state for y_2 is (non-)infected (Fig. 12.4) and the derivative is taken with respect to age. Note that $\lambda_{y_1=1|y_2=1} = \lambda_{y_1=1|y_2=0} = \lambda_{y_1=1}$ if and only if y_1 and y_2 are independent and that in case of a positive dependence (OR >1), $\lambda_{y_2=1|y_1=1} > \lambda_{y_2=1|y_1=0}$. Similarly, one can be interested in looking at the rate of acquiring y_2 conditional on y_1 by interchanging the indices in (12.3).

Next to the conditional FOIs, looking at the quantity

$$\lambda_{y_1=1,y_2=1} = \pi'_{11}/(1 - \pi_{11}), \tag{12.4}$$

could be of interest. However, the interpretation of this joint FOI is tedious. The numerator indicates the proportion that is still susceptible for at least one of the two infections, while the denominator gives us the instantaneous rate at which persons, at least susceptible for one of both infections, go to the state of having (had) both infections. Since VZV and B19 have a short generation interval, simultaneous acquisition is unlikely to occur. Moreover, due to the discrete nature of the data; i.e. age at infection is measured in days; the contribution to this rate from individuals moving from a fully susceptible status to a fully infected status (see dashed arrow in Fig. 12.4) for both diseases should be interpreted as the rate of acquisition of both infections in one day.

In Fig. 12.5, the conditional and marginal prevalences and FOI curves for rubella and mumps and VZV and B19 are shown.

Looking at the multisera data on rubella and mumps, conditioning on occurrence (dashed line) results in moderately higher prevalence as compared to the marginal prevalence (solid line), whereas conditioning on non-occurrence (dotted line) results in a lower prevalence. In other words, a person who has been infected for either infection has a higher probability to have been infected for the other infection compared with persons who are still susceptible. This is translated on the scale of the FOI in that the age of maximal FOI is lower for seropositives as compared to seronegatives. A similar observation is made for VZV and B19. Since these infections are transmitted through similar routes, i.e., close contacts, it is more likely that a person who has already been infected with a first infection has had more close contacts than a person who has not been infected. Such a once infected person is also more likely to continue having more contacts through which a second, similarly transmitted infection, can be acquired, than a person who has not been infected yet. Note that these findings are again in accordance to the positive odds ratio in Sect. 12.2.1.

Figure 12.6 shows the joint probability and joint FOI for both datasets. Note that the joint FOI for rubella and mumps closely follows the conditional FOI for rubella given a past mumps infection, especially from 12 years onwards. Similarly the joint FOI for VZV and B19 closely follows the conditional FOI for parvovirus B19 given a past infection with VZV. This is not surprising given that the mumps infection and the VZV infection are the dominant infections and their acquisition is almost complete at 12 years of age. The contribution to the joint FOI thus merely comes

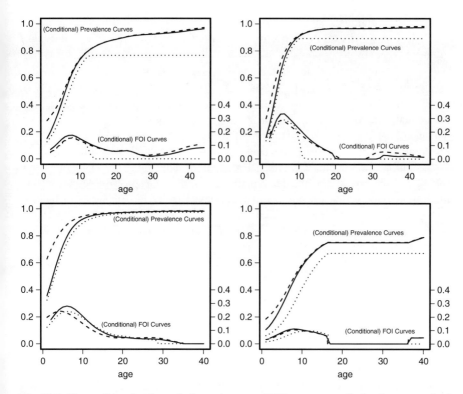

Fig. 12.5 The conditional and marginal prevalences and FOI-curves according to the monotonized spline-based BDM for rubella and mumps (*upper row*) and for the VZV and B19 (*lower row*). In the *upper left* and *right panel* conditioning is done on, respectively, mumps and rubella past occurrence (*dashed line*) and nonoccurrence (*dotted line*). In the *lower left* and *right panel* conditioning is done on, respectively, B19 and VZV past occurrence (*dashed line*) and non-occurrence (*dotted line*). The *solid lines* in all four panels correspond to the marginal prevalences and FOI curves

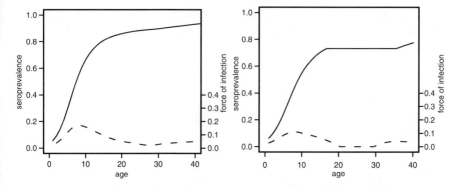

Fig. 12.6 The joint prevalence (*solid line*) and FOI (*dashed line*) for rubella and mumps (*left panel*) and VZV and B19 (*right panel*) according to the monotonized spline-based BDM

from those individuals infected by mumps and the VZV but still susceptible for rubella and parvovirus B19, respectively. Looking more carefully at the expressions of both FOIs in terms of prevalences, say y_1 is the dominant infection:

$$\pi'_{y_1=1,y_2=1}/(1 - \pi_{y_1=1,y_2=1}) \text{ and } \pi'_{y_2=1|y_1=1}/(1 - \pi_{y_2=1|y_1=1}), \tag{12.5}$$

near equality holds when $\pi_{y_1=1,y_2=1} \cong \pi_{y_2=1|y_1=1}$ or equivalently when $\pi_{y_1=1} \cong 1$ which is indeed the case for individuals from 12 years onwards. Moreover, this result indicates that acquiring both diseases on the same day is very unlikely.

In summary, using the BDM, it is shown that the acquisition of, on the one hand, rubella and mumps, and on the other hand, VZV and B19, is positively related, most likely, due to the similarity in transmission by close contacts. This was translated as well in the higher odds ratio for infants and preadolescents as compared to adults, albeit nonsignificantly for VZV and B19. Therefore, it is quite natural to ascribe dependency to heterogeneity in the acquisition of the infection.

12.3 Individual Heterogeneity

In its origin, studying individual differences was done in the context of susceptibility to death. In epidemic theory, Coutinho et al. (1999) were the first to systematically treat heterogeneity in the acquisition of infections. Individual heterogeneity has been shown to be a key factor in the estimation of the basic reproduction number R_0. We refer to Chaps. 14 and 15 for a more in depth discussion on the impact of heterogeneity on and the estimation of R_0.

Individuals are dissimilar in the way they acquire infections. Some individuals are more susceptible than others and will experience infection earlier. This can be expressed in terms of the age-dependent FOI by $\lambda(a,Z)$ where Z can be an individual-specific covariate or, alternatively, a random variable (Vaupel et al. 1979; Aalen 1988). Z is often referred to as the frailty and expresses to what extent an individual has a lower or higher risk of infection. $\lambda(a,Z)$ has a conditional interpretation, i.e., it denotes the FOI at age a conditional on the frailty Z. The corresponding conditional susceptible proportion is then given by

$$s(a|Z) = e^{-\int_0^a \lambda(t,Z)dt}, \tag{12.6}$$

which when combined with the proportional hazards assumption $\lambda(a,Z) = Z\lambda_0(a)$ becomes

$$s(a|Z) = e^{-Z\int_0^a \lambda_0(t)dt}, \tag{12.7}$$

where λ_0 is the baseline FOI. The unconditional susceptible proportion can be obtained by integrating out the random frailty Z using the Laplace transform L of Z:

$$s(a) = \mathrm{E}(s(a|Z)) = \mathrm{L}\left(\int_0^a \lambda_0(t)dt\right). \tag{12.8}$$

Since it is not possible to test the hypothesis that individual heterogeneity is present by using data from one serological survey without assuming specific functional forms for the baseline FOI, one mostly uses multisera data to estimate the heterogeneity. Assume that we have multisera data on two infections such as the rubella and mumps data from the UK and the VZV and B19 data from Belgium. Moreover, assume that we have frailty distributions $Z_i, i = , 1, 2$ for each infection, we can then express the conditional and unconditional susceptible proportion (12.6) by adding the necessary indices. We can than assume that (Z_1, Z_2) follows a bivariate frailty distribution, such as, e.g., a bivariate gamma distribution, where in addition to the baseline hazards and the heterogeneity parameters for both infections, a correlation parameter describes the dependency between the two frailty distributions and thus the dependency in acquisition of both infections. Assuming conditional independence, we can formulate the conditional bivariate proportion susceptible. Depending on the specific choice for the bivariate frailty distribution, either an explicit expression can be given for the unconditional bivariate proportion susceptible or numerical integration is required. In general, numerical integration with respect to the frailty, or random-effects, distribution is not straightforward but has become more accessible through the development of appropriate statistical software and reformulating non-normal random effects, as done by Nelson et al. (2006) and Liu and Yu (2007). However, here, we will focus on the gamma frailty distribution as the most often used frailty distribution because of its explicit solution for the unconditional bivariate proportion susceptible (see e.g. Hougaard 2000; Duchateau and Janssen 2008), which owes to conjugacy properties.

Again as in the univariate case (12.8), explicit expressions for the baseline FOIs are needed to be able to estimate the correlation between and heterogeneity for both infections (Hens et al. 2009a). This is the basic reason to assume a perfect correlation, which is tenable for similarly transmitted infections, since in that case nonparametric estimates can be used to model the baseline FOI.

Thus, starting from (12.7), assuming a common gamma frailty distribution, and using the Laplace transformation, the unconditional bivariate proportion susceptible is given by

$$\pi_{00}(a) = [s_1^{-1/\theta}(a) + s_2^{-1/\theta}(a) - 1]^{-\theta}, \qquad (12.9)$$

where θ denotes the shape parameter of the gamma frailty distribution $Z \sim \Gamma(\theta, 1/\theta)$. Since $E(Z) = 1$ and $Var(Z) = 1/\theta$, θ is the parameter describing the heterogeneity in acquisition of infection. The larger (smaller) θ, the smaller (larger) heterogeneity and thus people being more alike (different) in the way they acquire the infection. The joint probability of no previous infection (12.9) can be reparameterized in terms of the marginal FOIs, $\Lambda_i(a) = \int_0^a \lambda_i(s)ds, i = 1, 2$, and the corresponding loglikelihood $\sum_a \sum_{i,j=0}^1 n_{ija} \log\{\pi_{ij}(a)\}$, with n_{ija} the observed number of individuals in corresponding state $\pi_{ij}, i, j = 0, 1$ at age a and

$$\begin{cases} \pi_{00}(a) = \left(e^{\frac{\Lambda_1(a)}{\theta}} + e^{\frac{\Lambda_2(a)}{\theta}} - 1\right)^{-\theta}, \\ \pi_{10}(a) = e^{-\Lambda_2(a)} - \pi_{00}(a), \\ \pi_{01}(a) = e^{-\Lambda_1(a)} - \pi_{00}(a), \\ \pi_{11}(a) = 1 - \pi_{10}(a) - \pi_{01}(a) - \pi_{00}(a), \end{cases} \qquad (12.10)$$

can then be maximized to estimate the different parameters (Farrington et al. 2001; Sutton et al. 2006). The likelihood ratio test can be used to assess whether indeed heterogeneity is present. Note that

$$\lim_{\theta \to \infty} \pi_{00}(t) = \lim_{\theta \to \infty} \left(e^{\frac{\Lambda_1(t)}{\theta}} + e^{\frac{\Lambda_2(t)}{\theta}} - 1\right)^{-\theta} = e^{-\Lambda_1(t) - \Lambda_2(t)} = \pi_{0+}(t)\pi_{+0}(t),$$

(12.11)

indicating independence or since $\mathrm{Var}(Z) = 1/\theta \to 0$ homogeneity in acquisition of infection. Note that the discrepancies between the probabilities in (12.10) and the corresponding probabilities decrease as age increases, indicating that departures from independence are less evident in older individuals, a feature already observed in Sect. 12.2.1.

Although we can use nonparametric methods such as smoothing splines to model the marginal prevalences and thus the marginal FOIs, for convenience of programming, we use the gamma function (see e.g. Farrington et al. 2001) as a flexible parametric function for the FOI:

$$\lambda(a) = \alpha a^\beta \exp(-a/\gamma), \qquad (12.12)$$

where α, β, and γ are positive parameters. The following R-code shows how you can code the multinomial loglikelihood corresponding to (12.10) while using the gamma function with possibly different parameters for the FOI. To ensure positivity of the different parameters, we transform each parameter using the exponential function. The function *mle* is used to obtain the maximum likelihood estimates and standard errors for the different parameters. Since the symmetry, typically assumed when applying normal theory to the maximum likelihood estimate and standard errors to obtain confidence intervals, for the shape parameter of the gamma frailty, is untenable, we use the profile likelihood method (see Appendix B.3 for more details) to obtain 95% profile likelihood confidence intervals. This is easily achieved in R using the function *confint*.

```
# R-code for the gamma frailty model with gamma-shaped FOI
GF=function(alpha1eta=0.06,beta1eta=0.2,gamma1eta=0.005,
alpha2eta=0.06,beta2eta=0.2,gamma2eta=0.005,thetaeta=1){
```

(continued)

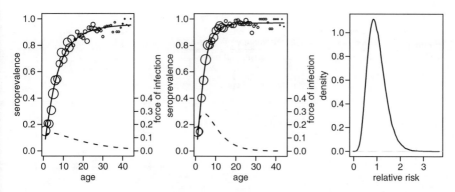

Fig. 12.7 The marginal prevalence and FOI-curves for rubella (*first panel—solid* and *dashed line*, respectively) and mumps (*second panel—solid* and *dashed line*, respectively) together with the density of the gamma frailty distribution with shape parameter $\hat{\theta}_{ML}$ (*third panel—solid line*) according to the model as proposed by Sutton et al. (2006) using a gamma function for the FOI (Farrington et al. 2001)

```
(continued)
alpha1=exp(alpha1eta);beta1=exp(beta1eta);gamma1=exp(gamma1eta)
alpha2=exp(alpha2eta);beta2=exp(beta2eta);gamma2=exp(gamma2eta)
theta=exp(thetaeta)

Lambda1=alpha1*gamma1^(beta1+1)
         *gamma(beta1+1)*pgamma(a/gamma1,beta1+1)
Lambda2=alpha2*gamma2^(beta2+1)
         *gamma(beta2+1)*pgamma(a/gamma2,beta2+1)

p00=(exp(Lambda1/theta)+exp(Lambda2/theta)-1)^(-theta)
p10=exp(-Lambda2)-p00
p01=exp(-Lambda1)-p00
p11=1-p00-p01-p10

return(-sum(PP*log(p11)+PN*log(p10)+NP*log(p01)+NN*log(p00)))
}

fit=mle(GF,start=list(rep(-1,7)))
summary(fit)
# The delta method to obtain ML-estimates and s.e.
cbind(exp(coef(fit)),sqrt(exp(coef(fit))^2*diag(vcov(fit))))
# 95% profile likelihood confidence intervals
confint(fit)
```

Figure 12.7 shows the marginal prevalences and FOIs for rubella (first panel) and mumps (second panel) in the UK. The 95% profile likelihood confidence interval for θ equals $(4.41, 12.91)$, whereas the corresponding interval for the variance parameter equals $(0.077, 0.227)$, indicating moderate, though significant,

Table 12.1 Overview of parameter estimates and 95% confidence intervals for the heterogeneity models applied to rubella and mumps and VZV and B19

		Likelihood		Profile likelihood	
Parameter	Estimate	lcl	ucl	lcl	ucl
Rubella and mumps					
α_1	0.12	0.11	0.14	0.11	0.14
β_1	0.27	0.08	0.46	0.09	0.47
γ_1	14.68	8.07	21.29	9.90	25.44
α_2	0.20	0.17	0.23	0.17	0.23
β_2	0.87	0.59	1.14	0.61	1.16
γ_2	4.82	3.52	6.13	3.72	6.41
θ	6.75	3.35	10.14	4.41	12.91
VZV and B19					
α_1	0.31	0.25	0.37	0.25	0.38
β_1	0.52	0.08	0.96	0.13	1.02
γ_1	5.67	2.64	8.70	3.46	10.39
α_2	0.04	0.02	0.07	0.03	0.07
β_2	1.45	0.80	2.10	0.87	2.12
γ_2	3.69	2.33	5.04	2.58	5.44
θ	7.74	1.41	14.07	4.11	31.86

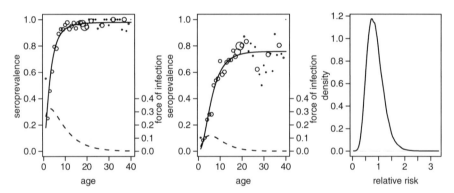

Fig. 12.8 The marginal prevalence and FOI curves for the varicella zoster virus (*first panel—solid* and *dashed line*, respectively) and parvovirus B19 (*second panel—solid* and *dashed line*, respectively) together with the density of the gamma frailty distribution with shape parameter $\hat{\theta}_{ML}$ (*third panel—solid line*) according to the model as proposed by Sutton et al. (2006) using a gamma function for the FOI (Farrington et al. 2001)

heterogeneity in the acquisition of rubella and mumps ($p = 5.5 \times 10^{-6}$ based on a 50:50-mixture of $\chi^2(0)$ and $\chi^2(1)$). Note that the BDM gave a similar result (see Sect. 12.2). The other parameter estimates together with their 95% confidence intervals are listed in Table 12.1. Note that there is only a moderate difference between the confidence intervals.

Figure 12.8 shows that the 95% profile likelihood confidence interval for θ equals $(4.11, 31.86)$, whereas the corresponding interval for the variance parameter equals

$(0.031, 0.243)$. Again, heterogeneity is shown to be significant ($p = 0.0039$), confirming the results in Sect. 12.2. The parameter estimates together with their 95% confidence intervals are listed in Table 12.1. Here the differences between the two likelihood methods to calculate the confidence intervals are somewhat more outspoken than for rubella and mumps.

Note that, as before, the conditional and joint FOI can easily be derived using the results outlined in this section.

12.4 Concluding Remarks

Whereas both the BDM and the heterogeneity model take into account the dependency between observations from the same individual, the philosophy behind these models differs. Using the odds ratio, the BDM studies the association in past acquisition of two infections, whereas the dependency in the heterogeneity model is ascribed to the heterogeneity in acquisition of infection which is assumed to be identical for both infections when using the shared frailty approach. We refer to Del Fava et al. (2012) for a more recent application of the BDM to model HCV and HIV. The motivation for the latter originates from the underlying transmission process. This transmission process will be the focus of Chaps. 14 and 15.

Chapter 13
Estimating Age-Time Dependent Prevalence and Force of Infection from Serial Prevalence Data

The use of serological surveys is nowadays a common way to study the epidemiology of many infections. In case a single cross-sectional survey is available, one needs to assume that the disease is in steady state. While reasonable for some infections, as illustrated in earlier chapters, this assumption might be untenable for other situations. In this chapter we address methods to estimate age- and time-specific prevalence and force of infection from a series of prevalence surveys. Models such as the proportional hazards model of Nagelkerke et al. (1999) are discussed and illustrated on hepatitis A and tuberculosis data.

13.1 Introduction

In previous chapters we mainly focused on a cross-sectional prevalence survey while assuming time homogeneity (stationarity) and lifelong immunity, leading to a simplified SIR model and equation

$$\frac{ds(a)}{da} = -\lambda(a)s(a),$$

or equivalently

$$s(a) = \exp\left\{ -\int_0^a \lambda(s)ds \right\}. \tag{13.1}$$

This stationarity assumption might be questionable or untenable. The force of infection may change with time, may increase or decrease, as a consequence of changes in the pathogen, in the treatment, outbreak occurrences, cohort effects, etc. Assuming stationarity in such cases would lead to a substantial to severe age-dependent bias in the estimation of the prevalence and the force of infection.

N. Hens et al., *Modeling Infectious Disease Parameters Based on Serological and Social Contact Data*, Statistics for Biology and Health 63, DOI 10.1007/978-1-4614-4072-7_13, © Springer Science+Business Media New York 2012

Following Becker (1989) and Keiding (1991), the generalization of equation (13.1) to an age- and time-specific prevalence and force of infection is given by (for an individual of age a at time t):

$$s(a,t) = \exp\left\{ - \int_0^a \lambda(s,t-a+s)ds \right\}. \tag{13.2}$$

Ades and Nokes (1993); Marschner (1996), and Nagelkerke et al. (1999) proposed several models to analyze serial prevalence data, varying from fully parametric to semi-parametric. Ades and Nokes (1993) proposed a piecewise linear model for the FOI as well as several parametric models, all assumed to be a product of a time function and an age function, including exponential polynomial models EP_I/EP_J of the form

$$\lambda(a,t) = \exp\left(\mu_0 + \sum_{i=1}^I \mu_i a^i + \sum_{j=1}^J \theta_j t^j \right), \; I,J = 1,2,\ldots.$$

Marschner (1996, 1997) subsequently proposed using a discrete time multiplicative model and a penalized spline approach to relax assumptions typically made by using parametric models. Nagelkerke et al. (1999) proposed a semiparametric model, based on a proportional hazards assumption.

Using serial seroprevalence data, several authors addressed the issue of differential selection, i.e., scenarios where disease-related mortality affects the interpretation of the observed serological profile (Ades and Medley 1994; Marschner 1997; Batter et al. 1994).

We will focus on non-differential selection, a plausible assumption for most childhood infections in developed countries and cast the aforementioned methods within the generalized additive model (GAM) framework as already done by Marschner (1997). We will illustrate these methods using hepatitis A data from Flanders (see Sect. 4.1.1) and the tuberculosis (TB) data (as listed in Appendix II of Nagelkerke et al. (1999) and Sect. 4.1.7).

For the TB data, on which we focus in the next sections, surveys of schoolchildren were carried out in the period 1966–1973 in the Netherlands. These children were tested by means of Tuberculin (PPD); indurations ≥ 10 mm were considered evidence of previous infection with *M. tuberculosis*. For more details on these data, we refer to Sutherland et al. (1984) and Nagelkerke et al. (1999).

Figure 13.1 shows the *design* of the serial survey. Note that the 1970-survey covered the full range of ages, from 6 to 18 years of age, whereas earlier surveys covered (part of) the older ages, and later surveys the opposite. Figure 13.2 shows the TB data as a bubble plot (data for females in the left panel, for males in the right panel), with age a on the horizontal axis, shifted year of birth $x = b - 48 = t - a - 48$ on the vertical axis (1948 was the lowest year of birth), and with bubble size proportional to the prevalence. The number of children in each (age × year of birth) combination varies from 794 to 76,069, the proportion positives from 0.0009

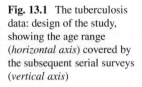

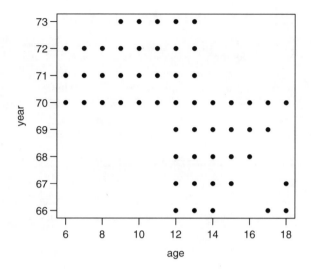

Fig. 13.1 The tuberculosis data: design of the study, showing the age range (*horizontal axis*) covered by the subsequent serial surveys (*vertical axis*)

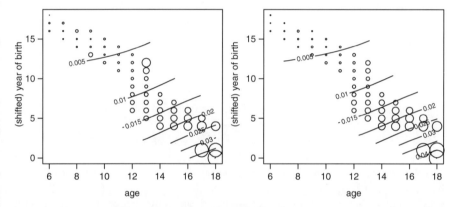

Fig. 13.2 The tuberculosis data: data on females in the *left panel*, on males in the *right panel*; age and (shifted) year of birth *bubble plot*, with size of bubbles proportional to samples taken. *Contours* represent the estimated prevalence according to model 6 (see Table 13.1)

to 0.0432. In the next sections we first introduce the proportional hazards model of Nagelkerke et al. (1999) as a semiparametric and next as a nonparametric model. We also consider a non-proportional hazards model and show that the proportional hazards assumption can be rejected for the TB data. The different models are fitted to the TB data using the *gam* function of the R package *mgcv*. The PAV algorithm was applied to assure monotonicity in the age dimension. In Sect. 13.5 the hepatitis A data are analyzed and the use of monotone penalized P-splines (see also Chap. 9) within the maximization–maximization (MM) algorithm of Nagelkerke et al. (1999) is illustrated using R code in Sect. 13.6.

13.2   Proportional Hazards Model

Nagelkerke et al. (1999) addressed the issue of estimating age- and time-specific FOI under the assumption that the FOI changes exponentially with time, but without any assumption about the age dependency. They showed that these assumptions lead to a proportional hazards semiparametric model, as introduced in the next section.

13.2.1   Semiparametric Model

Nagelkerke et al. (1999) assumed an exponential decline (or increase) in the force of infection, represented by the following identity (for two calendar times t_1 and t_2):

$$\lambda(a,t_2) = \exp(\beta(t_2 - t_1))\lambda(a,t_1). \tag{13.3}$$

Define $\lambda_b(a)$ as the age-specific force of infection experienced by a cohort born at calendar time b. As a cohort born at calendar time b has age a at calendar time $a + b$, we have that

$$\lambda_b(a) = \lambda(a, a + b).$$

The proportional hazards assumption (13.3) then translates into

$$\lambda_b(a) = \exp(\beta(b - b_0))\lambda_{b_0}(a), \tag{13.4}$$

where $\lambda_{b_0}(a) = \lambda(a, a + b_0)$ is the hazard at the baseline year of birth b_0.

Using an iterative MM algorithm, Nagelkerke et al. (1999) estimate $\lambda_b(a)$ in a semiparametric way, with a nonparametric isotonic stepwise estimate for the baseline hazard $\lambda_{b_0}(a)$ and a parametric proportionality factor $\exp(\beta(b - b_0))$. They also formulate the parametric part as function of other covariates next to year of birth such as gender. In the following section we reformulate this model as a GAM model.

13.2.2   Non-parametric Model

The semiparametric model (13.4) can be reformulated as a fully nonparametric proportional hazards model by writing

$$\lambda(a,t_2) = \exp(g(t_2 - t_1))\lambda(a,t_1), \tag{13.5}$$

where $g(t)$ is a smooth function with the constraint that $g(0) = 0$.

Substituting (13.5) in expression (13.2) leads to

$$s_b(a) = s(a, b+a) = \exp\{\exp(g(b-b_0))\log s_{b_0}(a)\},\tag{13.6}$$

where, with $\lambda_{b_0}(a) = \lambda(a, b_0+a)$,

$$s_{b_0}(a) = \exp\{-\int_0^a \lambda_{b_0}(u)du\}.$$

With $\pi_b(a) = 1 - s_b(a)$ the proportion subjects infected at age a or before, from the cohort with year of birth b, (13.6) can be written as a GAM for binary data with complementary log–log link function

$$\log(-\log(1-\pi_b(a))) = f_1(a) + f_2(b),\tag{13.7}$$

where

$$f_2(b) = g(b-b_0),$$

and

$$f_1(a) = \log(-\log(x_{b_0}(a))).$$

The corresponding force of infection for this cohort then equals

$$\lambda_b(a) = \frac{\pi_b'(a)}{1-\pi_b(a)} = \exp(f_2(b))\lambda_{b_0}(a),\tag{13.8}$$

with

$$\lambda_{b_0}(a) = \frac{\pi_{b_0}'(a)}{1-\pi_{b_0}(a)} = \frac{d}{da}\exp(f_1(a)).\tag{13.9}$$

Equation (13.7) shows that the proportional hazards model translates into an additive cloglog model for the seroprevalence status. This GAM approach can be generalized to include other subject-specific characteristics, net to year of birth, such as gender.

13.2.3 Example I: Tuberculosis

The first six rows of Table 13.1 show the effective degrees of freedom (edf), Akaike's information criterion (AIC), and Schwarz's Bayesian criterion (BIC) for fully parametric (models 1–3) and semiparametric models (model 4–6). Models 1–3 correspond to Ades and Nokes's exponential polynomial model of the type EP_1/EP_1; models 4–6 are analogous to those of Nagelkerke et al. (1999) using a spline smoother for the base hazard function $\lambda_{b_0}(a)$ (instead of the isotonic step function). The PPD binary response data were fit using the cloglog link and with thin plate regression splines as smoother (with appropriate smoothness for each applicable model term selected by GCV/UBRE, the default of the *gam* function), using R code such as

Table 13.1 The tuberculosis data. Results for different models: parametric models (model 1–3), semiparametric models (models 4–6), nonparametric models (models 7–9), non-proportional hazards models (models 10–12)

Model components	edf	AIC	rank	BIC	rank
Model 1: $a + b$	3	1,242.271	12	1,250.372	12
Model 2: $a + b + g$	4	1,149.267	9	1,160.069	8
Model 3: $a + b + g + (b \times g)$	5	1,120.103	8	1,133.605	3
Model 4: $s(a) + b$	10.65	1,202.249	11	1,231.013	11
Model 5: $s(a) + b + g$	11.65	1,114.943	7	1,146.388	6
Model 6: $s(a) + b + g + (b \times g)$	12.65	1,113.547	6	1,147.698	7
Model 7: $s(a) + s(b)$	18.48	1,177.402	10	1,227.323	10
Model 8: $s(a) + s(b) + g$	19.48	1,089.939	5	1,142.553	5
Model 9: $s(a) + s(b) + g + (s(b) \times g)$	22.20	1,075.008	3	1,134.950	4
Model 10: $s(a,b)$	28.20	1,089.034	4	1,165.188	9
Model 11: $s(a,b) + g$	29.20	1,001.643	2	1,080.475	2
Model 12: $s(a,b) + g + (s(a,b) \times g)$	33.54	987.776	1	1,078.342	1

The complexity of the model is reflected by its effective degrees of freedom (edf)
Note that the notation s in this table refers to the specification of a smooth term in the *mgcv*-library in R and that $s(a)$ and $s(b)$ imply two different smoothers

```
# R-code Ades and Nokes (1993) exponential polynomial model
# showing the edf, AIC and BIC value as depicted in the table
tbdata=read.table("tb.dat",header=T)
attach(tbdata)
a=AGE
x=BRTHYR-min(BRTHYR)
g=SEX
ts=a+BRTHYR
s=PPD
p=s/N
f=N-s
y=cbind(s,f)

# Fit of Model 2 as in table, x represents shifted year of
birth gamfit2=gam(y~a+x+g,family=binomial(link="cloglog"))
c(sum(gamfit2$edf),AIC(gamfit2),AIC(gamfit2, k = log(nrow(y))))

# R-code Nagelkerke et al. (1999) type of model based on
splines

# Fit of Model 6 as in table, x represents shifted year of
birth

gamfit6=gam(y~s(a)+x*g,family=binomial(link="cloglog"))
c(sum(gamfit6$edf),AIC(gamfit6),AIC(gamfit6, k = log(nrow(y))))
```

According to AIC, model 6 is the best choice within the family of models 1–6; BIC however indicates model 3 to be the best choice. Figure 13.2 shows contour curves for model 6 (for females in the left panel and for males in the right panel). These plots were produced by the R-code

```
# contour plots from model 6 for females (g=0) and males (g=1)
win.graph()
gamfit6=gam(y~s(a)+x*g,family=binomial(link="cloglog"))
vis.gam(gamfit6,view=c("a","x"),cond=list(g=0),type="response",
plot.type="contour",color="bw",too.far=0.10,main="prevalence")
points(a[g==0],x[g==0],cex=100*p[g==0])
vis.gam(gamfit6,view=c("a","x"),cond=list(g=1),type="response",
plot.type="contour",color="bw",too.far=0.10)
points(a[g==1],x[g==1],cex=100*p[g==1])
```

Rows 7–9 in Table 13.1 show edf, AIC, and BIC values for fully nonparametric GAM models based on thin plate regression splines for age a and year of birth b, and again with cloglog link function. According to AIC, model 9 is now the overall best choice; BIC however still indicates the simpler model 3 to be the best one.

In the next section we extend our family of candidate models with three further models, which are no longer proportional hazards models.

13.3   Non-proportional Hazards Model

A model containing the interaction of age a with year of birth b (or gender) leads to a non-proportional hazards model. Taking the GLM model with a two-dimensional smoother

$$\log(-\log(1 - \pi_b(a))) = f(a,b),$$

some straightforward calculus shows that

$$\frac{\lambda_b(a)}{\lambda_{b_0}(a)} = \{\exp(f(a,b) - f(a,0))\} \left\{ \frac{(\partial f(a,b)/\partial a)}{(\partial f(a,0)/\partial a)} \right\}. \tag{13.10}$$

The right-hand side of (13.10) is no longer independent of age a. Note that it reduces to (13.8) in case $f(a,b) \equiv f_1(a) + f_2(b)$.

Comparing a model with a (parametric or nonparametric) (age × year of birth) interaction term with the corresponding model with main effects only allows one to test the proportional hazards assumption. This is illustrated on the TB data in the next section.

13.4   The Tuberculosis Data Revisited

Rows 10–12 in Table 13.1 show edf, AIC, and BIC values for GAM cloglog-models with a two-dimensional smoother $s(a,b)$ and extended with two models including

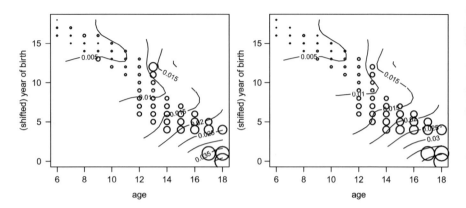

Fig. 13.3 The tuberculosis data: data on females in the *left panel*, on males in the *right panel*; age and (shifted) year of birth *bubble plot*, with size of bubbles proportional to samples taken. *Contours* represent the estimated prevalence according to model 12 (see Table 13.1)

a gender effect *g*. According to both criteria, model 12 is now the best model. Consequently the proportional hazards assumption can be rejected, as confirmed by an analysis-of-deviance using the chi-squared test (as considered most appropriate for binomial and Poisson models).

```
#contrasting best additive model with best non-additive model
#-------------------------------------------------------------#
bgamfit=gam(y~s(a,x)+g+s(a,x,by=g),family=binomial
                                    (link="cloglog"))
b1gamfit=gam(y~s(a)+x*g,family=binomial(link="cloglog"))
anova(b1gamfit,bgamfit,test="Chisq")

# OUTPUT
Analysis of Deviance Table

Model 1: y ~ s(a) + x * g
Model 2: y ~ s(a, x) + g + s(a, x, by = g)
  Resid. Df Resid. Dev      Df Deviance P(>|Chi|)
1    97.353    312.09
2    76.463    144.54  20.890   167.55 6.801e-25
```

Figure 13.3 shows the contour curves from model 12, separately for females and males. Comparing these curves with those of Fig. 13.2 indicates that model 12 mainly deviates from model 6 within the age range 6–14.

Figure 13.4 shows prevalence data and fitted prevalence curves, for each year in the study period 1966–1973, and for both gender groups separately (solid line for males, dashed line for females). The horizontal gray lines in corresponding line types indicate the estimates at the age of 12 (common to all study years). The curves

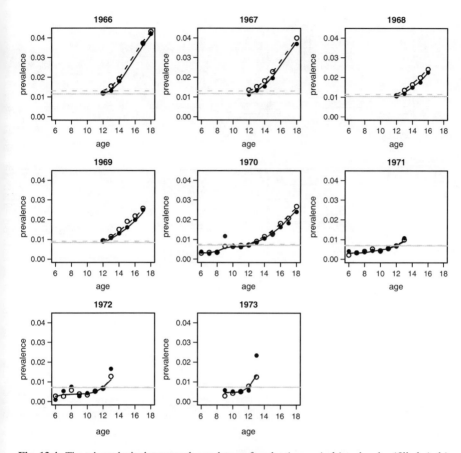

Fig. 13.4 The tuberculosis data: prevalence data on females (*open circle*) and males (*filled circle*) as a function of age, for the different survey years 1966–1973, together with the fitted prevalence curves from model 12 (see Table 13.1). *Dashed lines*: females, *solid lines*: males

seem to fit the prevalence data quite well. There are a few interesting observations from these plots, as also summarized indicatively by the horizontal dashed lines: (1) the prevalence decreases over the years from above 0.01 to below 0.01, (2) the difference in gender (higher for females) seems to disappear over the consecutive years.

Figures 13.5 and 13.6 show for each cohort ($1948 \leq b \leq 1966$) prevalence data, the fitted prevalence curves and the fitted force of infection curves, (lower curve in each panel). The PAV algorithm was applied to monotonize the prevalence curves, as a function of age a. Again the fitted prevalence curves seem to fit the data well. In general, the FOI curves indicate a maximum at the age of about 13 and 14, a bit varying over the different cohorts. Of course for the oldest cohorts, as well as for the youngest ones, there is a limited amount of direct information in the data.

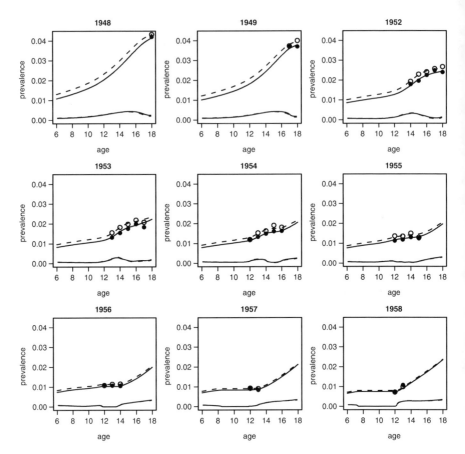

Fig. 13.5 The tuberculosis data: prevalence data on females (*open circle*) and males (*filled circle*) as a function of age, for the different cohorts (year of birth from 1948 to 1958, except for 1950 and 1951 as no data are available for these cohorts), together with the fitted prevalence curves and fitted force of infection curves from model 12 (see Table 13.1). *Dashed lines*: females, *solid lines*: males

13.5 Example II: Hepatitis A

The hepatitis A dataset is an interesting borderline situation, as it contains only two survey years 1993 and 2002 (see Sect. 4.1.1 for more details). The data for both years are shown in Fig. 13.7 together with fitted prevalence curves. Table 13.2 gives an overview of complexity and goodness of fit of five models: one parametric model (model 1), two semiparametric models (models 2 and 3), and two nonparametric models (models 4 and 5). Model 5 is a non-proportional hazards model. According to this table, and by both criteria AIC and BIC, model 4 is selected as the best model. Figure 13.7 shows the fitted prevalence curves of this best model as solid

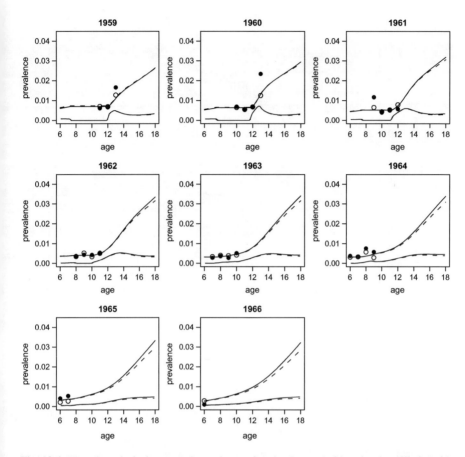

Fig. 13.6 The tuberculosis data: prevalence data on females (*open circle*) and males (*filled circle*) as a function of age, for the different cohorts (year of birth from 1959 to 1966), together with the fitted prevalence curves and fitted force of infection curves from model 12 (see Table 13.1). *Dashed lines*: females; *solid lines*: males

lines, overlaid with the fits of model 2 (a too simple model, as dashed lines), and with the fits of model 5 (a needless complicated model, as dotted lines).

```
# Testing for the proportional hazards assumption
#-------------------------------------------------#
anova(gamfit4,gamfit5,test="Chisq")

# OUTPUT
Analysis of Deviance Table
```

(continued)

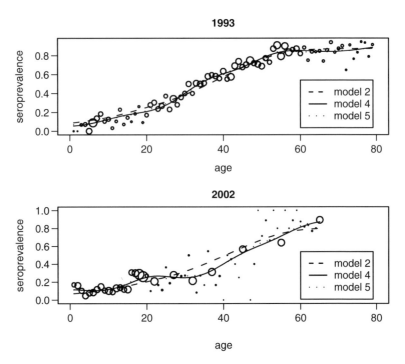

Fig. 13.7 The Belgian hepatitis A data. Bubble plot with fitted prevalence curves as a function of age, for each survey year, according to best model 4 (*solid line*), the too simple model 2 (*dashed line*), and the too complicated model 5 (*dotted line*)

Table 13.2 Models for the hepatitis A data from Flanders

Model components	edf	AIC	rank	BIC	rank
Model 1: $a + b$	3	6,062.03	5	6,082.07	5
Model 2: $s(a) + b$	10.03	5,976.90	4	6,043.94	3
Model 3: $a + s(b)$	10.55	5,958.68	3	6,029.17	2
Model 4: $s(a) + s(b)$	13.85	5,934.30	1	6,026.83	1
Model 5: $s(a,b)$	19.04	5,936.16	2	6,063.34	4

Results for different models: parametric model 1, semi-parametric models 2 and 3, nonparametric models 4 and 5

```
(continued)
Model 1: y ~ s(a) + s(x)
Model 2: y ~ s(a, x)
  Resid. Df Resid. Dev        Df Deviance P(>|Chi|)
1 5873.1493      5906.6
2 5867.9628      5898.1   5.1865      8.5       0.1
```

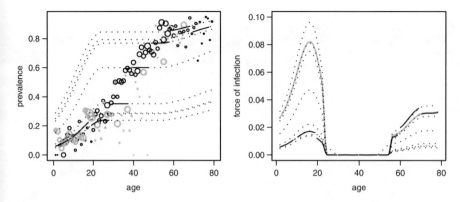

Fig. 13.8 The hepatitis A data. *Bubble plots* of the data (*black* for 1993, *gray* for 2002), with fitted cohort-specific prevalence curves as a function of age (*left panel*) and cohort-specific FOI curves as a function of age, both according to the best model 4. The *solid black* part of each curve refers to that region of the age range in which data are available; the *dotted* part of any curve is extrapolated from the model. The *gray* FOI curve in the *right panel* shows the baseline FOI $\lambda_{b_0}(a)$ from (13.9) for an assumed $b_0 = 1914$

Contrary to the TB data, the proportional hazards assumption seems to hold, as model 4 is selected above model 5. Also an analysis-of-deviance (*p*-value=0.1, see R output) confirms that there is no convincing evidence in the data to reject the proportional hazards assumption. One has to be cautious however with this hypothesis test and with the model selection procedure, as these are based on only data from two survey times, the minimum number to detect any time heterogeneity. Especially when extrapolating and considering concepts as proportionality of the hazards is a form of extrapolation, one has to be very careful. This latter concern is also visualized in both panels of Fig. 13.8. It shows fitted cohort-specific prevalence curves as a function of age (left panel) and cohort-specific FOI curves as a function of age (right panel), both according to the best model 4. The solid black part of each prevalence curve refers to that region of the age range in which data are available; the dotted part of any curve is extrapolated from the model. As shown by (13.7) for the nonparametric proportional hazards model, the cohort-specific age-dependent prevalence curves are parallel on the complementary log–log scale. Although the *p*-value of 0.1 indicates that the available data show no convincing evidence against the proportional hazards assumption, it should be repeatedly stressed that the model is only supported by the data on a small diagonal band in the age × cohort plane (see Fig. 13.9). The solid part of the curves does confirm that these parts of the model are supported by the corresponding part of the data. This discussion opens an interesting avenue for further research, namely how to design serial prevalence studies (number of survey times, sample size for each survey).

A similar story holds for the FOI curves in the right panel. The gray FOI curve in the right panel shows the baseline FOI $\lambda_{b_0}(a)$ from (13.9) for an assumed $b_0 = 1914$. The black (dotted) curves result from the gray curve by the proportionality factor $\exp(g(b - b_0))$ in (13.8).

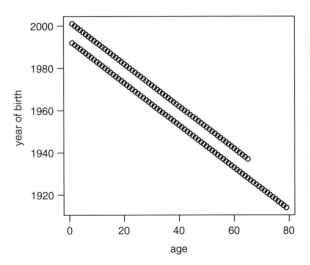

Fig. 13.9 The hepatitis A data. Part of the age × year of birth plane for which data are available

As a final exercise, we briefly discuss the issue of monotonicity in the next section. Up till now the PAV algorithm was used to assure that cohort-specific prevalence curves are monotone. An alternative and more direct way is to use the penalized spline methodology (see Chap. 9).

13.6   Monotonicity

In previous sections the PAV algorithms was applied to guarantee that cohort-specific prevalence estimates are nondecreasing in age. A more direct way is to fit the splines with an additional penalization against non-monotonicity. Although this is a more direct approach, it turns out to be more computationally involving as the fitting of both dimensions (age & birth of year) cannot be performed simultaneously in a straightforward way. As discussed in Nagelkerke et al. (1999), a simple but computationally expensive way is to alternate in (13.7) between (i) the estimation of $f_1(a)$ for given b and (ii) the estimation of $f_2(b)$ for given a, and (re)iterate until convergence has occurred (Nagelkerke et al. (1999) call this the MM algorithm in analogy with the EM algorithm). In our approach here, and in both steps, a penalized spline is used with penalizing for smoothness in the age direction (step (i)) or the birth of year direction (step (ii)). A second additional penalization is applied in step (i) in order to guarantee the cohort-specific prevalence curve to be a nondecreasing function of age.

The application of the R function *additive.mpspline.fitter* in both steps of the MM-algorithm to the hepatitis A data resulted in Fig. 13.10. The upper panels show that the fitted prevalence curves for both survey years are fitting well to the data. These curves are also close to the ones in Fig. 13.7. The dashed lines show pointwise

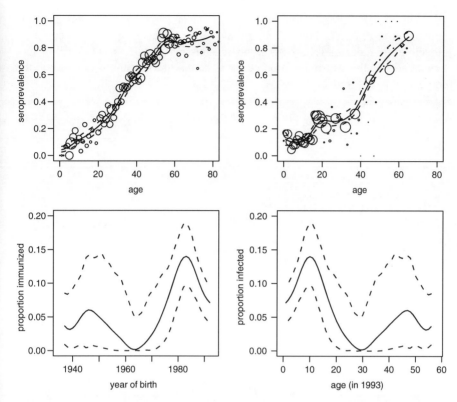

Fig. 13.10 The hepatitis A data. Fitted prevalence curves for survey year 1993 (*left upper panel*) and year 2002 (*right upper panel*). The proportion immunized between 1993 and 2002 is shown by year of birth (*left lower panel*) or by age in 1993 (*right lower panel*). *Dashed curves* represent pointwise 95% bootstrap confidence intervals

95% bootstrap confidence intervals. The lower panels show the proportion infected between 1993 and 2002 by year of birth (left) or by age in 1993 (right), again with bootstrap confidence intervals as dashed lines. Although this difference is more closely resembling the incidence rather than the FOI, the right lower panel qualitatively resembles the baseline FOI in the right panel of Fig. 13.8.

13.7 Concluding Remarks

In the last two chapters we discussed the modeling setting in which more than one serological sample is available. In Chap. 12 we modeled multivariate serological data and we focused on modeling the association between the two infections and individual heterogeneity in the population. In this chapter we discussed the setting in which several serological samples, for the same infection, sampled from the same population at different time points, are available. In this chapter we focused on modeling age-time trends (effects) of the transmission parameters. The topic of age-time effects on the transmission process will be discussed again in Chap. 16 in the context of the SIR model.

Part V
Estimating Mixing Patterns and the Basic Reproduction Number

The force of infection reflects the degree of contact with potential for transmission between susceptible and infected individuals. The mathematical relation between the force of infection and effective contact patterns is known as the mass action principle which yields the necessary information to estimate transmission rates from serological data. The traditional approach by Anderson and May (1991) is introduced and discussed in Chap. 14 whereas a recent approach based on social contact data is discussed in Chap. 15. We show how to estimate the basic reproduction number based on these mixing patterns.

Chapter 14
Who Acquires Infection from Whom?
The Traditional Approach

As mentioned in Sect. 3.5.2, the transmission process of an infection is governed by the mixing patterns in the population. In dynamic models of infectious disease transmission, typically various mixing patterns are imposed by the configuration of the so-called Who-Acquires-Infection-From-Whom matrix (WAIFW). In this chapter, we briefly summarize how transmission parameters can be estimated from serological data. We elaborate on the traditional approach as described by Anderson and May (1991) using the techniques of Farrington and Whitaker (2005).

14.1 Who Acquires Infection from Whom?

If mean duration of infectiousness D is short compared to the timescale on which transmission and mortality rate vary, the force of infection (FOI) $\lambda(a)$ can be approximated by (Anderson and May 1991):

$$\lambda(a) = D \int_0^\infty \beta(a,a')\lambda(a')S(a')da', \tag{14.1}$$

where $\beta(a,a')$ denotes the transmission rate, i.e., the per capita rate at which an individual of age a' makes an effective contact with a person of age a per year, and $S(a')$ denotes the number of susceptible persons of age a'. Formula (14.1) reflects the so-called "mass action principle", which implicitly assumes that infectious and susceptible individuals mix completely with each other and move randomly within the population. Note that (14.1) assumes that we are in endemic equilibrium.

When interest lies in the estimation of the age-dependent transmission rates, one can use the methodology described by Anderson and May (1991). They start from a discretization of (14.1) into J age categories yielding a system of J equations with $J \times J$ unknowns since $\beta(a,a')$ turns into an unknown $J \times J$ matrix. These authors propose to, based on imposing different mixing patterns on this so-called WAIFW

N. Hens et al., *Modeling Infectious Disease Parameters Based on Serological and Social Contact Data*, Statistics for Biology and Health 63, DOI 10.1007/978-1-4614-4072-7_14, © Springer Science+Business Media New York 2012

matrix hereby constraining the number of distinct elements for identifiability reasons, estimate the parameters from serological data.

Many authors, among whom among whom Greenhalgh and Dietz (1994), Farrington et al. (2001), and Van Effelterre et al. (2009) have elaborated on this approach of Anderson and May (1991). However, estimates of important epidemiological parameters such as the basic reproduction number R_0 turn out to be sensitive to the choice of the imposed mixing pattern (Greenhalgh and Dietz 1994).

An alternative method was proposed by Farrington and Whitaker (2005), where contact rates are modeled as a continuous contact surface and estimated from serological data. Clearly, both methods involve a somewhat ad hoc choice, namely the structure for the WAIFW-matrix and the parametric model for the contact surface.

14.2   Estimation from Serological Data

Setting the scene is done using a compartmental MSIR-model to describe the transmission dynamics (see Chap. 3). By doing so, we explicitly take into account the fact that, in a first phase, newborns are protected by maternal antibodies and do not take part in the transmission process. Assuming a closed population of size N and that we are in demographic and endemic equilibrium, the analytical solution for the proportion susceptibles of the corresponding set of differential equations is given by

$$s(a) = \left[\int_0^a \gamma(u) \exp \left(\int_0^u \lambda(v) - \gamma(v) dv \right) du \right] \exp \left(- \int_0^a \lambda(u) du \right). \quad (14.2)$$

Without loss of generality, we assume a prompt loss of maternal immunity at age A:

$$m(a) = \exp \left(- \int_0^a \gamma(u) du \right) = \begin{cases} 1, \text{ if } a \leq A \\ 0, \text{ if } a > A, \end{cases} \quad (14.3)$$

meaning that all newborns are protected by maternal antibodies until a certain age A after which they instantaneously move to the susceptible class. We will refer to this assumption as the Type I maternal antibody assumption. Under this assumption, the proportion of susceptibles becomes

$$s(a) = \exp \left(- \int_A^a \lambda(u) du \right), \quad \text{if } a > A, \quad (14.4)$$

where $\lambda(a)$ denotes the age-specific FOI, and $s(a) = 0$ if $a \leq A$.

Considering a large population of fixed size N with age-specific mortality rate $\mu(a)$ and with age density

$$L^{-1} \exp\left\{ -\int_0^a \mu(u)du \right\},\tag{14.5}$$

where L is the life expectancy, $S(a')$ in (14.1) can be rewritten as $S(a') = N/L \cdot s(a') \cdot m(a')$, where $s(a')$ and $m(a') = \exp\{ -\int_0^{a'} \mu(t)dt \}$ denote the proportion susceptible and the survival function at age a', respectively.

We illustrate how the survival function and mortality rate can be estimated from data on mortality from Belgium anno 2006. The following R-code displays how the survival function is obtained from data on the number of deaths ND per integer age value AGE and the population size PS. The model fitted here is a Poisson model with log link and offset term. To ensure flexibility we used a thin plate regression spline available through the gam-function in the R-package $mgcv$ (see Sect. 8.2.1).

```
library(mgcv)
demfit=gam(ND~s(AGE),offset=log(PS),family="poisson",
                                    link="log")
muy=predict(demfit,type="response")
My=exp(-cumsum(muy))
L=sum(My)
```

Figure 14.1 shows the survival function by age (solid line) and the mortality rate (dashed line) together with the observed death rate for Belgium. The mean life expectancy was estimated at 78.8 years.

Given the assumption of instantaneous loss of maternal immunity at age A, we proceed by following Diekmann et al. (1990); Farrington et al. (2001) and rewrite (14.1) as

$$\lambda(a) = \frac{ND}{L} \int_A^\infty \beta(a,a')\lambda(a')s(a')m(a')da',\tag{14.6}$$

for $a \geq A$. Assuming a short infectious period, the basic reproduction number R_0, i.e., the dominant eigenvalue of the next generation operator, can be related to $\beta(a,a')$ (Farrington et al. 2001): $R_0\ell(a') = ND/L\int_A^{+\infty} \ell(a)m(a)\beta(a,a')da$, where $\ell(a)$ denotes the leading left eigenfunction of $ND/Lm(a)\beta(a,a')$. Multiplying both sides with $\lambda(a')s(a')m(a')$, integrating over a', swapping the integration order, and using (14.6) result in the following expression for R_0:

$$R_0 = \frac{\int_A^\infty \ell(a)\lambda(a)m(a)da}{\int_A^\infty \ell(a)\lambda(a)s(a)m(a)da}.\tag{14.7}$$

Equation (14.7) shows that, given $\lambda(a)$, R_0 can only be estimated when $\ell(a)$ is identifiable. However, $\ell(a)$ depends on $\beta(a,a')$ which is unknown unless further

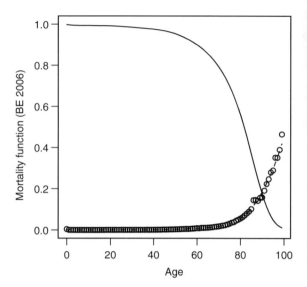

Fig. 14.1 The estimated survival function (*solid line*) and mortality rate (*dashed line*) with observed death rate (*dots*) for Belgium anno 2006

assumptions are made. The most restrictive assumption is that of homogeneous mixing where $\beta(a,a') = \beta \; \forall a,a'$. In that case, (14.7) simplifies to L/A^* where L is the life expectancy since loss of maternal immunity and A^* is the average time to removal by infection or death since loss of maternal immunity. When assuming separable mixing, $\exists\, u,v : \beta(a,a') = u(a)v(a')$, the left eigenfunction $l(a')$ is approximately proportional to $v(a')$ and $\lambda(a)$ is proportional to $u(a)$. This assumption is not sufficient for R_0 to be identifiable and the assumption of proportional mixing is often imposed: $\exists\, u : \beta(a,a') = u(a)u(a')$. Given the latter assumption (14.7) simplifies to (Dietz and Schenzle 1985; Hethcote and Van Ark 1987):

$$R_0 \approx \frac{\int_A^\infty \lambda(a)^2 m(a)da}{\int_A^\infty \lambda(a)^2 s(a)m(a)da}.$$ (14.8)

In case $\beta(a,a') \propto u(a)$ this equation simplifies by replacing $\lambda(a)^2$ by $\lambda(a)$.

Parvovirus B19 in Belgium

We illustrate the aforementioned methods by calculating R_0 for parvovirus B19 from Belgium (see Sect. 4.1.5). When homogeneous mixing is assumed $R_0 = 4.31$ with 95% bootstrap-based confidence interval $(4.09, 4.52)$; further assuming proportional mixing and susceptibility-dependent mixing using a gamma-shaped FOI (see Sect. 12.3) the resulting estimates decrease to $1.72(1.66, 1.78)$ and $1.93(1.87, 2.01)$, respectively. Note that the aforementioned estimates depend on the assumed parametric shape of the FOI. Indeed when using the monotonic P-spline estimates from Chap. 9, the resulting estimates of R_0 are $1.77(1.69, 2.01)$ and

2.06(1.88, 2.33) for proportionate and susceptible-specific mixing, respectively. The assumption of separable and thus also proportionate mixing seems hardly tenable for parvovirus B19 which is believed to be transmitted through similar routes as the varicella zoster virus (Hens et al. 2008b). As a result, more general mixing patterns should be envisaged.

14.2.1 The Discretized Mass Action Principle

As stated before, for general mixing patterns, estimating transmission rates using seroprevalence data cannot be done analytically since the integral equation (14.1) has no closed form solution. However, it is possible to solve this numerically by turning to a discrete age framework, assuming a constant FOI in each age class. Denote the first age interval $(a_{[1]}, a_{[2]})$ and the jth age interval $[a_{[j]}, a_{[j+1]})$, $j = 2, \ldots, J$, where $a_{[1]} = A$ and $a_{[J+1]} = L$. Making use of (14.4), the prevalence of immune individuals of age a in the jth age interval is now well approximated by (Anderson and May 1991):

$$\pi(a) = 1 - \exp\left(-\sum_{k=1}^{j-1} \lambda_k(a_{[k+1]} - a_{[k]}) - \lambda_j(a - a_{[j]})\right). \tag{14.9}$$

Note that the prevalence of immune individuals is allowed to vary continuously with age and that we do not summarize the binary seroprevalence outcomes into a proportion per age class. Further, the FOI for age class i equals ($i = 1, \ldots, J$):

$$\lambda_i = \frac{ND}{L} \sum_{j=1}^{J} \beta_{ij} \frac{\lambda_j}{\lambda_j + \mu_j} \left[\exp\left(-\sum_{k=1}^{j-1}(\lambda_k + \mu_k)(a_{[k+1]} - a_{[k]})\right) \right.$$
$$\left. - \exp\left(-\sum_{k=1}^{j}(\lambda_k + \mu_k)(a_{[k+1]} - a_{[k]})\right)\right], \tag{14.10}$$

where D denotes the mean duration of infectiousness and β_{ij} the per capita rate at which an individual of age class j makes an effective contact with a person of age class i, per year. The transmission rates β_{ij} make up a $J \times J$ matrix, the so-called WAIFW matrix.

Given the WAIFW matrix, following Diekmann et al. (1990), the basic reproduction number R_0 can be calculated as the dominant eigenvalue of the $J \times J$ next generation matrix with elements ($i, j = 1, \ldots, J$):

$$D\left(\int_{a_{[i]}}^{a_{[i+1]}} N(a)da\right)\beta_{ij}. \tag{14.11}$$

In case of Type I maternal antibodies, R_0 represents the number of secondary cases that are produced by a typical infected person during his or her entire period of infectiousness, when introduced into an entirely susceptible population with the exception of newborns who are passively immune through maternal antibodies.

14.2.2 Imposing Mixing Patterns: The Traditional Approach of Anderson and May (1991)

The traditional approach of Anderson and May (1991) imposes different mixing patterns on the WAIFW matrix in order to make the system (14.10) of J equations with $J \times J$ unknown parameters identifiable. Typically, J is chosen as small as 3–6 where the choice of the different age classes corresponds to mixing groups in the population as often largely inspired by the schooling system. Specific structures, often used in literature, are homogeneous mixing, proportional mixing, separable mixing (see Sect. 14.2), and the assumption of symmetry $(\beta(a,a') = \beta(a',a))$. Note that the latter two mixing assumptions require additional restrictions to be made. As illustrated by Greenhalgh and Dietz (1994), the structure imposed on the WAIFW matrix has a high impact on the estimate of R_0.

In this section, we considered the following WAIFW structures for six age classes. These structures are based on prior knowledge of social mixing behavior and were used before to estimate R_0 for VZV (Anderson and May 1991; Van Effelterre et al. 2009; Ogunjimi et al. 2009; Goeyvaerts et al. 2010):

$$
W_1 = \begin{pmatrix}
\beta_1 & \beta_6 & \beta_6 & \beta_6 & \beta_6 & \beta_6 \\
\beta_6 & \beta_2 & \beta_6 & \beta_6 & \beta_6 & \beta_6 \\
\beta_6 & \beta_6 & \beta_3 & \beta_6 & \beta_6 & \beta_6 \\
\beta_6 & \beta_6 & \beta_6 & \beta_4 & \beta_6 & \beta_6 \\
\beta_6 & \beta_6 & \beta_6 & \beta_6 & \beta_5 & \beta_6 \\
\beta_6 & \beta_6 & \beta_6 & \beta_6 & \beta_6 & \beta_6
\end{pmatrix}, \quad
W_2 = \begin{pmatrix}
\beta_1 & \beta_1 & \beta_3 & \beta_4 & \beta_5 & \beta_6 \\
\beta_1 & \beta_2 & \beta_3 & \beta_4 & \beta_5 & \beta_6 \\
\beta_3 & \beta_3 & \beta_3 & \beta_4 & \beta_5 & \beta_6 \\
\beta_4 & \beta_4 & \beta_4 & \beta_4 & \beta_5 & \beta_6 \\
\beta_5 & \beta_5 & \beta_5 & \beta_5 & \beta_5 & \beta_6 \\
\beta_6 & \beta_6 & \beta_6 & \beta_6 & \beta_6 & \beta_6
\end{pmatrix}
$$

$$
W_3 = \begin{pmatrix}
\beta_1 & \beta_1 & \beta_1 & \beta_4 & \beta_5 & \beta_6 \\
\beta_1 & \beta_2 & \beta_3 & \beta_4 & \beta_5 & \beta_6 \\
\beta_1 & \beta_3 & \beta_3 & \beta_4 & \beta_5 & \beta_6 \\
\beta_4 & \beta_4 & \beta_4 & \beta_4 & \beta_5 & \beta_6 \\
\beta_5 & \beta_5 & \beta_5 & \beta_5 & \beta_5 & \beta_6 \\
\beta_6 & \beta_6 & \beta_6 & \beta_6 & \beta_6 & \beta_6
\end{pmatrix}, \quad
W_4 = \begin{pmatrix}
\beta_1 & \beta_1 & \beta_1 & \beta_1 & \beta_1 & \beta_1 \\
\beta_2 & \beta_2 & \beta_2 & \beta_2 & \beta_2 & \beta_2 \\
\beta_3 & \beta_3 & \beta_3 & \beta_3 & \beta_3 & \beta_3 \\
\beta_4 & \beta_4 & \beta_4 & \beta_4 & \beta_4 & \beta_4 \\
\beta_5 & \beta_5 & \beta_5 & \beta_5 & \beta_5 & \beta_5 \\
\beta_6 & \beta_6 & \beta_6 & \beta_6 & \beta_6 & \beta_6
\end{pmatrix} \quad (14.12)
$$

$$
W_5 = \begin{pmatrix}
\beta_1 & \beta_6 & \beta_6 & \beta_6 & \beta_6 & \beta_6 \\
\beta_6 & \beta_2 & \beta_6 & \beta_6 & \beta_6 & \beta_6 \\
\beta_6 & \beta_6 & \beta_3 & \beta_6 & \beta_6 & \beta_6 \\
\beta_6 & \beta_6 & \beta_6 & \beta_4 & \beta_6 & \beta_6 \\
\beta_6 & \beta_6 & \beta_6 & \beta_6 & \beta_5 & \beta_6 \\
\beta_6 & \beta_6 & \beta_6 & \beta_6 & \beta_6 & \beta_5
\end{pmatrix}, \quad
W_6 = \begin{pmatrix}
\beta_1 & 0 & 0 & 0 & 0 & 0 \\
0 & \beta_2 & 0 & 0 & 0 & 0 \\
0 & 0 & \beta_3 & 0 & 0 & 0 \\
0 & 0 & 0 & \beta_4 & 0 & 0 \\
0 & 0 & 0 & 0 & \beta_5 & 0 \\
0 & 0 & 0 & 0 & 0 & \beta_6
\end{pmatrix}.
$$

In order to estimate the transmission parameters $\beta = (\beta_1, \ldots, \beta_6)^T$ from sero-prevalence data, we follow Anderson and Aitkin (1985) and Anderson and May (1991). Since (14.10) constitutes a system of six equations and six unknowns, there exists a unique matrix $\mathbf{D}(\lambda)$ such that (14.10) can be rewritten as $\lambda = \mathbf{D}(\lambda)\beta$. Conditional on $\mathbf{D}(\lambda)$ being invertible, the parameter vector β can be estimated by fitting a piecewise constant FOI to the seroprevalence data and using $\hat{\beta} = \mathbf{D}(\hat{\lambda})^{-1}\hat{\lambda}$. Whenever $\mathbf{D}(\hat{\lambda})^{-1}\hat{\lambda} \geq 0$, one says that W has a regular configuration for the data. The deviance is identical for all such configurations. For non-regular configurations estimation is constrained by the condition $\mathbf{D}(\hat{\lambda})^{-1}\hat{\lambda} \geq 0$.

As an example, we now derive $\mathbf{D}(\lambda)$ for W_3. Denote

$$
\Psi_j = \frac{ND}{L}\frac{\lambda_j}{\lambda_j + \mu_j}\left[\exp\left(-\sum_{k=1}^{j-1}(\lambda_k + \mu_k)(a_{[k+1]} - a_{[k]})\right)\right.
$$

$$
\left. - \exp\left(-\sum_{k=1}^{j}(\lambda_k + \mu_k)(a_{[k+1]} - a_{[k]})\right)\right], \qquad (14.13)
$$

for $j = 1, \ldots, J$, then $\lambda = \mathbf{D}(\lambda)\beta$ can be rewritten as $\lambda = \mathbf{W}\Psi^T$. More specifically, given W_3, $\mathbf{D}(\lambda)$ looks like

$$
\begin{pmatrix}
\sum_{j=1}^{3}\Psi_j & 0 & 0 & \Psi_4 & \Psi_5 & \Psi_6 \\
\Psi_1 & \Psi_2 & \Psi_3 & \Psi_4 & \Psi_5 & \Psi_6 \\
\Psi_1 & 0 & \Psi_2 + \Psi_3 & \Psi_4 & \Psi_5 & \Psi_6 \\
0 & 0 & 0 & \sum_{j=1}^{4}\Psi_j & \Psi_5 & \Psi_6 \\
0 & 0 & 0 & 0 & \sum_{j=1}^{5}\Psi_j & \Psi_6 \\
0 & 0 & 0 & 0 & 0 & \sum_{j=1}^{6}\Psi_j
\end{pmatrix}. \qquad (14.14)
$$

Similarly, $\mathbf{D}(\lambda)$ can be derived for the other WAIFW structures.

Until now, the FOI was assumed constant in each of the J age categories. However, a more general approach could be envisaged. Van Effelterre et al. (2009) suggested to use fractional polynomials to model the age-dependent seroprevalence (see 6.2) while assuming Type I mortality. Given the linear predictor $\eta = \eta_m(a, \beta, p)$ defined in (6.3) and assuming Type I mortality, Ψ_j, $j = 1, \ldots, J$, can be written as

$$
\Psi_j = \frac{(1 + e^{\eta(a_0)})(e^{\eta(a_j)} - e^{\eta(a_{j-1})})}{(1 + e^{\eta(a_{j-1})})(1 + e^{\eta(a_j)})}. \qquad (14.15)
$$

Note that obtaining and explicit expression is not always possible (for instance because of the untenable assumption of Type I mortality) and numerical approximation has to be used.

Numerical Approximation

Since the discretized mass action principle as given by (14.10) can be written down for any number of age classes J, one could opt to use one-year age- intervals yielding a numerical method to solve the mass action principle for all continuous functions λ, μ, and β as long as the functional form for β ensures identifiability.

Parvovirus B19 in Belgium

We illustrate the WAIFW approach on the parvovirus B19 data from Belgium (see Sect. 4.1.5). We use the estimated mortality function for Belgium anno 2006 and corresponding sample size $10,511,382$, the mean duration of infectiousness $D = 6/365$ for B19 and assume Type I maternal antibodies with age $A = 0.5$. Six age classes following the schooling system in Belgium were chosen (Van Effelterre et al. 2009): $(0.5, 2), [2, 6), [6, 12), [12, 19), [19, 31), [31, +\infty)$.

The R-code hereunder fits a piecewise constant FOI while ensuring a positive FOI. The function *pcwrate.fitter* uses as input a vector of binary values (*y.var*) denoting past infection by 1 and 0 otherwise and the corresponding vector of age values (*x.var*). Alternatively, the number of individuals *n.var*, their age *x.var*, and the number of individuals with past infection *y.var* can be used as input values too. The following ML-estimate for λ was obtained:

$$\hat{\lambda}^{ML} = (0.0576 \quad 0.0878 \quad 0.1138 \quad 0.0359 \quad 0.0000 \quad 0.0137)^{T}.$$

Figure 14.2 shows the fitted prevalence and FOI curves together with the observed seroprevalence.

These ML-estimates give rise to the estimated WAIFW matrices as long as they are regular. The assessment of regularity as well as invertibility of $\mathbf{D}(\hat{\lambda})$ based on the ML-estimate for the FOI is done using the R-code *waifw.6parms*. If regular, *waifw.6parms* determines the estimated WAIFW matrices and corresponding R_0 estimate. Note that *muhat* is the piecewise constant mortality rate, *Lmax* is the maximum age, N is the population size, and D is the mean infectious period.

```
# R-code
# Function code to fit WAIFW structures (see book's website)
foi.fit=pcwrate.fitter(y.var=y,x.var=a,breaks=breakpoints)
foihat=foi.fit$ratevec
waifw=waifw.6parms(foihat=foihat,muhat=muhat,breaks=breakpoints,
            N=N,D=D,Lmax=Lmax)
```

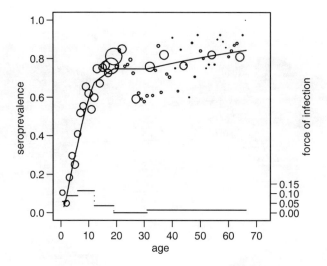

Fig. 14.2 The piecewise constant FOI and corresponding prevalence for Parvovirus B19 in Belgium. The *dots* are the observed seroprevalence per integer age value with size proportional to the number of samples taken

From the six WAIFW matrices in Sect. 14.2.2, W_4 and W_5 were found to be regular whereas W_2 and W_3 were irregular and therefore fitted under constrained optimization ensuring $\mathbf{D}(\hat{\lambda})^{-1}\hat{\lambda} \geq 0$. For W_1 and W_6, $\mathbf{D}(\hat{\lambda})$ was not invertible and therefore left from further consideration.

The following R-code fits the irregular WAIFW structures under constrained optimization. The function *waifw.6parms.irr* requires the choice of WAIFW matrix as input value (*waifw.choice*) and uses as starting values the parameters from *waifw.6parms* (with negative values put to zero).

```
# R-code
# Function code to fit surface model (see book's website)
waifw.6parms.irr=waifw.fitter(a=a,y=y,waifw.choice,
    breaks=breakpoints,N=N,D=D,Lmax=Lmax,plots="TRUE")
```

Table 14.1 and Fig. 14.3 summarize the WAIFW results. The AIC value for the regular matrices equalled 3,452.11. Note that the fit of the two regular WAIFW-matrices is equal in terms of AIC and thus provide no basis to guide the choice of mixing pattern whereas the estimated basic reproduction numbers differ considerably. The large variation of R_0 and the different mixing patterns question the appropriateness of the assumed mixing patterns.

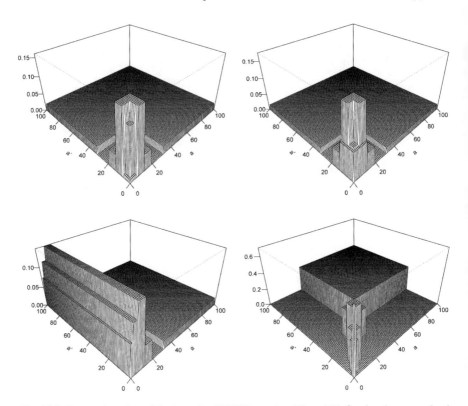

Fig. 14.3 Perspective plots of the irregular WAIFW matrices W_2 and W_3 fitted under constrained optimization (*upper row*, *left* and *right panel*, respectively) and of the regular WAIFW matrices W_4 and W_5 (*lower row*, *left* and *right panel*, respectively) for Parvovirus B19 in Belgium

Table 14.1 Overview of WAIFW matrices, AIC values and estimated basic reproduction numbers for the Belgian Parvovirus B19

WAIFW	Invertible	Regular	$\hat{R}_0$	AIC
1	Not invertible	–	–	–
2	Invertible	Irregular	2.00	3,454.44
3	Invertible	Irregular	1.89	3,463.53
4	Invertible	Regular	2.33	3,452.11
5	Invertible	Regular	14.80	3,452.11
6	Not invertible	–	–	–

14.2.3 Exploiting an Underlying Continuous Mixing Surface

Whereas, in the previous section $\beta(a,a')$ was discretized taking $J = 6$ age classes and thus constituting a matrix, it is quite natural to assume a low-dimensional bivariate parametric model. Farrington and Whitaker (2005) proposed to use a bivariate function that incorporates qualitative epidemiologic knowledge about the contacts in the population. Their idea originated from Massad et al. (1994) and Eichner et al. (1996) who used a contact surface to describe the transmission of rubella and measles, respectively. These authors however did not focus on the estimation of the surface as such, whereas Farrington and Whitaker (2005) put this in the heart of the estimation problem. Denoting $u = (a + a')/\sqrt{2}$ and $v = (a - a')/\sqrt{2}$, the model for $\beta(a, a')$ can be written as

$$\beta(a, a') = \kappa(\gamma(u) \times b(v|u) + \delta), \qquad (14.16)$$

where

$$\gamma(u; \mu, v) = c^{-1} u^{v-1} \exp\left(-\frac{vu}{\sqrt{2}\mu}\right),$$

$$b(v|u; \alpha, \beta) = \frac{(u+v)^{\alpha-1}(u-v)^{\beta-1}}{u^{\alpha+\beta-2}},$$

with $c = \{\sqrt{2}\mu(1 - 1/v)\}^{v-1} e^{1-v}$ to ensure $\gamma(u; \mu, v) = 1$ at the mode when it exists. They suggest to constrain the model for symmetry $\alpha = \beta$ and to reparameterize the model using $\gamma = (\alpha + \beta + 1)^{-1}$ and $\sigma = v^{-2}$, leaving the five parameters κ, μ, σ, γ, and δ to estimate.

Note that the reparameterization of (a, a') into (u, v) facilitates a geometric interpretation. Whereas u looks in the direction of the main diagonal, v looks into the direction of the antidiagonal (the diagonal perpendicular to the main diagonal). $\gamma(u; \mu, \sigma)$ is a function which specifies a distribution over the diagonal with mean μ and shape parameter σ whereas $b(v|u; \gamma)$ is a symmetric function and γ determines the width of the assortative component; δ serves as a background transmission parameter. Figure 14.4 shows two example surfaces indicating the unimodal but relatively flexible shape of (14.16). The surfaces take on an assortative structure thought to be predictive for the observed serological profiles of most common childhood infections.

The implementation of this continuous parametric surface can be done using the discretization as in (14.10) for one-year age intervals. Although we developed R-code for this, we note that the numerical optimization procedure was found sensitive towards starting values and therefore different starting values have been used. We illustrate the code with the serological data on parvovirus B19 in Belgium.

Parvovirus B19 in Belgium

We use the following R-code to fit the low-dimensional bivariate parametric model as proposed by Farrington and Whitaker (2005) to the Belgian parvovirus B19 data. The function *surface.fitter* fits the surface to the serological data. The option *plots="TRUE"* shows the fitted prevalence and FOI during iterations and the resulting mixing surface as a perspective and contourplot.

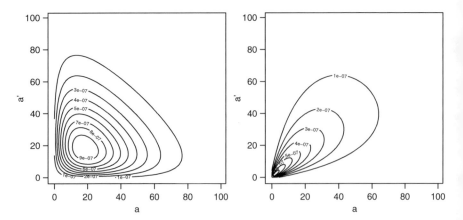

Fig. 14.4 Contourplot of two surface examples. For the first surface (*left panel*) the parameters were chosen as ($\kappa = 1e - 6, \mu = 25, \sigma = 1, \gamma = 0.1, \delta = 0$), whereas for the second surface (*right panel*) parameters were chosen as ($\kappa = 1e - 6, \mu = 25, \sigma = 0.5, \gamma = 0.2, \delta = 0$)

```
# R-code
# Function code to fit surface model (see book's website)
surface.fitter(a=a,y=y,muy=muy,Lmax=Lmax,N=N,D=D,plots="TRUE")
```

Figure 14.5 shows the resulting surface and fit towards the seroprevalence data. The corresponding AIC of 3461.00 is slightly higher as the AIC values for the different WAIFW matrices (Sect. 14.2.2) and R_0 was estimated at 1.76. The ML-estimates for the surface parameters was $\hat{\kappa} = 9.6e - 5, \hat{\mu} = 7.65, \hat{\sigma} = 0.50, \hat{\gamma} = 0.12$, and $\hat{\delta} = 0.04$. The observed mixing surface shows a peak at 5 years of age indicating that most transmission occurs in primary school as is also reflected in the FOI which is maximal at 5 years of age.

14.3   Topics in Estimating WAIFW Matrices

We briefly mention some topics related to the estimation of WAIFW matrices as presented in the literature.

14.3.1   Model Selection

Whereas we have used the AIC-criterion to decide on the most appropriate WAIFW-matrix amongst the set of candidate matrices for the observed serological profile

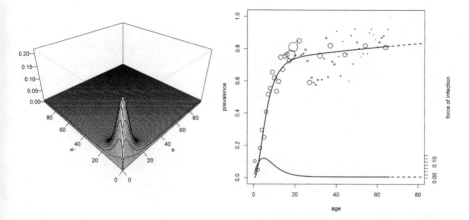

Fig. 14.5 Perspective plot of the fitted transmission surface (*left panel*) and resulting prevalence fit and force of infection (*right panel*) for Parvovirus B19 in Belgium

of Parvovirus B19 (Table 14.1), Farrington et al. (2001) proposed to augment the estimation using serological data from another infection with similar transmission route thereby allowing to impose more complex structures for the WAIFW matrices under the assumption of direct proportionality of the WAIFW structures for both infections. However, since this approach relies on making the assumption of direct proportionality, the authors suggested to use a different approach to assess goodness of fit amongst a candidate set of WAIFW matrices by assuming WAIFW parameters for the different infections to be "close" to each other and using Bayes factors to favour one matrix over the other. Since their method is an alternative to using the AIC-criterion to select the most appropriate WAIFW matrix amongst a set of candidate WAIFW matrices, we will refrain from its discussion and implementation and refer the reader to Farrington et al. (2001) for more details. We would like to note that the reader should take care when using the Bayes factor approach because of the assumed relationship between the two infections.

14.3.2   Lifelong Immunity

The aforementioned methods focus on infections that govern lifelong immunity. In case no immunity is conferred by infection, the susceptible–infective–susceptible (SIS) representation is often used and provided the infectious period is short on the timescale on which the FOI and mortality vary, serological data can be used to estimate the FOI as $\pi(a) \approx D\lambda(a)$, with D the mean infectious period. Farrington et al. (2001) showed that minimal knowledge (symmetry) of $\beta(a,a')$ is required to estimate R_0 without estimating $\beta(a,a')$ itself. Estimating $\beta(a,a')$ itself is however possible using the mass action principle as stated in (14.1) and the relation between the FOI and serological data.

Using serological data for an SIR infection, R_0 can be approximated without estimating $\beta(a,a')$ provided serological data on a SIS infection with similar infection route is available. In a similar way age-specific incidence data on a newly emerging pathogen can provide the essential information to estimate R_0 for any SIR infection with similar transmission route without the need to estimate $\beta(a,a')$. Indeed, starting from (14.7), assuming $A = 0$ and replacing $l(a)$ by $\lambda_{SIS}(a)$ (or alternatively the age-specific relative incidence), one obtains

$$R_0 \approx \frac{\int_0^\infty \lambda_{SIS}(a)\lambda_{SIR}\exp\{-\int_0^a \mu(u)du\}da}{\int_0^\infty \lambda_{SIS}(a)\lambda_{SIR}\exp\{-\int_0^a \lambda_{SIR}(u)+\mu(u)du\}da}.$$

14.4   Concluding Remarks

In this chapter, we have shown how transmission parameters can be estimated from serological data by imposing specific structures on the so-called WAIFW matrix . We used serological data on parvovirus B19 from Belgium and employed the AIC-criterion to quantify the appropriateness of the different WAIFW structures among the set of candidate structures. The result is somewhat discomforting since no clear distinction among the different WAIFW-matrices can be made. This is however inherent to the use of serological data since these data only provide information on immunity resulting in the necessity to impose identifiable WAIFW structures.

Chapter 15
Informing WAIFW with Data on Social Contacts

In the previous chapter we have shown how the basic reproduction number can be estimated using serological data and an *assumed* social contact pattern in the population (either discrete or continuous). Such an approach does not take into account the underlying contact mixing pattern in the population but assumes that the configuration of contact patterns is known and estimated the transmission parameters under a specific configuration. In this chapter, we present an alternative approach in which transmission parameters can be estimated from serological data augmented with social contact data when dealing with airborne infections.

15.1 Estimation from Serological Data and Data on Social Contacts

In general, the choice of the structures as well as the choice of the age classes and the bivariate mixing surface are somewhat ad hoc. Since evidence for mixing patterns is thought to be found in social contact data, i.e., governing contacts with high transmission potential, an alternative approach to estimate transmission parameters could be based on data of social contacts (Wallinga et al. 2006). In this section, we use social contact data from Belgium (Mossong et al. 2008b; Hens et al. 2009b) and contrast those to the serological data on parvovirus B19 from Belgium. We first address the social contact hypothesis (Wallinga et al. 2006) and then present some refinements to this hypothesis.

15.1.1 The Social Contact Hypothesis

In Wallinga et al. (2006), it was argued that $\beta(a,a')$ is proportional to $c(a,a')$, the per capita rate at which an individual of age a' makes contact with a person of age

N. Hens et al., *Modeling Infectious Disease Parameters Based on Serological and Social Contact Data*, Statistics for Biology and Health 63, DOI 10.1007/978-1-4614-4072-7_15, © Springer Science+Business Media New York 2012

a, per year:

$$\beta(a,a') = q \cdot c(a,a'), \tag{15.1}$$

with q a constant proportionality factor.

Wallinga et al. (2006) used data on whether or not people had a conversation as a proxy of those contacts with high transmission potential. By assuming q constant, it is assumed that those conversational contact data are proportional to these high transmission contacts. It is therefore referred to as the "social contact hypothesis."

We illustrate the social contact hypothesis using serological data on parvovirus B19 and social contact data from Belgium (Mossong et al. 2008b; Hens et al. 2009b) (Sect. 4.3). We estimate age-specific contact rates using a smoothing approach, which allows estimating the entire "contact surface" exploiting the continuous nature of contact behavior at the population level (Hens et al. 2009b; Goeyvaerts et al. 2010). We briefly explain the principle behind this estimation technique.

Estimating Contact Rates

Consider the random variable Y_{ij}, i.e., the number of contacts in age class j during one day as reported by a respondent in age class i $(i,j = 1,\ldots,J)$, which has observed values $y_{ij,t}$, $t = 1,\ldots,T_i$, where T_i denotes the number of participants in the contact survey belonging to age class i. Now define $m_{ij} = E(Y_{ij})$, i.e., the mean number of contacts in age class j during one day as reported by a respondent in age class i. The elements m_{ij} make up a $J \times J$ matrix, which is called the "social contact matrix." Now, the contact rates c_{ij} are related to the social contact matrix as follows:

$$c_{ij} = 365 \cdot \frac{m_{ji}}{w_i},$$

where w_i denotes the population size in age class i, obtained from demographical data. When estimating the social contact matrix, the reciprocal nature of contacts needs to be taken into account (Wallinga et al. 2006):

$$m_{ij}w_i = m_{ji}w_j, \tag{15.2}$$

which means that the total number of contacts from age class i to age class j must equal the total number of contacts from age class j to age class i.

Wallinga et al. (2006) used a weighted negative binomial model with reciprocal constraint to estimate a discrete bivariate contact function whereas Mossong et al. (2008b); Goeyvaerts et al. (2010); Hens et al. (2009b), and Ogunjimi et al. (2009) used a two-dimensional continuous function over age of respondent and contact, giving rise to a "contact surface." The basis is a tensor-product spline derived from two smooth functions of the respondent's and contact's age, ensuring flexibility. We briefly mention the results presented by Goeyvaerts et al. (2010) where both estimation methods were compared for the Belgian contact survey (Hens et al. 2009b) conducted as part of the POLYMOD project (Mossong et al. 2008b).

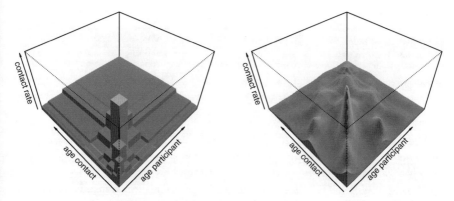

Fig. 15.1 Perspective plots of the estimated contact rates c_{ij} obtained with maximum likelihood estimation following Wallinga et al. (2006) (*left panel*) and Goeyvaerts et al. (2010) (*right panel*). The X- and Y-axes represent age of the respondent and age of the contact, respectively. Source: Goeyvaerts et al. (2010)

On the left side of Fig. 15.1, the estimated contact structure following the methodology used by Wallinga et al. (2006) is shown. Clearly, the high rates are observed on the diagonal indicating that people mostly mix with people of the same age class. On the right side of Fig. 15.1, the estimated contact surface obtained with the bivariate smoothing approach is shown. The smoothing approach seems better able to capture important features of human contacting behavior. Three components are apparent in the smoothed contact surface. First of all, the assortative structure on the diagonal is again clear. Second, an off-diagonal parent–child component is observed, reflecting a very natural form of contact between parents and children, which might be important in modeling infections such as Parvovirus B19, likely transmitted from child to mother (Mossong et al. 2008a). Finally, there seems to be evidence for a grandparent–grandchild component. Except for the assortativeness, these features are not reflected by the imposed WAIFW structures nor by the parametric surface.

Contrasting Contact Rates to Seroprevalence Data on Parvovirus B19

Given the estimated contact rates, under the social contact hypothesis (15.1), we are able to estimate the transmission function $\beta(a, a')$ for parvovirus B19 using serological data. Keeping the estimated contact rates fixed, we estimate the proportionality factor q from serological data using (14.9) and (14.10). As before we use 1-year age intervals as a numerical approximation to solving the integral equation explicitly. Consequently, one can estimate the transmission rates β_{ij} and the basic reproduction number R_0.

Table 15.1 Overview of
various types of contacts
contrasted to the Belgian
parvovirus B19 serology
using the social contact
hypothesis

Table 15.1 Overview of various types of contacts contrasted to the Belgian parvovirus B19 serology using the social contact hypothesis

Contact type	$\hat{q}$	$\hat{R}_0$	AIC
All contacts	0.0320	3.99	3,812.52
Close contacts	0.0474	3.20	3,637.01
Close contacts > 15 min	0.0536	2.84	3,581.78
Close contacts > 1 h	0.0708	2.47	3,531.63
Close contacts > 4 h	0.1030	2.19	3,489.22

The participants were also asked to register the location, duration, frequency, and whether the contact involved skin-to-skin touching, enabling the stratification of contacts into various types of contacts. By contrasting these various types of contacts to serology, it is believed that insight is gained into the transmission process of nonsexual close contact infections transmitted from person to person. We now show how combining duration and whether or not a contact involved skin-to-skin touching predicts the observed serological profile for parvovirus B19 in Belgium.

The following R-code fits the contact data to the serological data. The function *contact.fitter* requires the specification of a matrix *rij* which is the smoothed contact matrix obtainable form the book's web site. Since contacts were only registered up to 85 years of age, we choose *Lmax* = 85. The resulting *fit* contains *deviance, aic, bic*, and R_0 enabling us to compare the fitted profiles for various types of contacts.

```
# R-code (see book's website)
# Function to fit the contact data using the social
# contact hypothesis
fit=contact.fitter(a=a,y=y,rij,muy=muy,N=N,D=D,
                   Lmax=85,plots="TRUE")
```

Table 15.1 shows different types of contacts thought to be predictive for those contacts constituting transmission. From the AIC values of the different types of contacts, it is seen that close contacts lasting 4 h or more are best capable of describing the observed serological profile.

Figure 15.2 shows the fitted transmission surface and resulting FOI and prevalence. When comparing the fitted prevalence to the observed prevalence, there is a clear indication that the social contact hypothesis is not tenable for the types of contacts under consideration. This is also reflected in the AIC values of the different fits being considerably higher than the AIC values obtained by imposing mixing structures using WAIFW-matrices (3,452.11) or the mixing surface (3,461.00). We therefore illustrate some recent refinements towards the social contact hypothesis (Ogunjimi et al. 2009; Goeyvaerts et al. 2010).

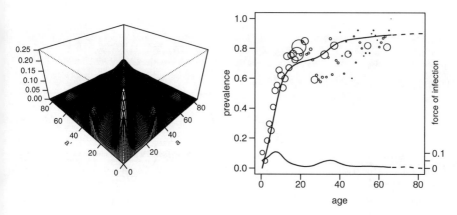

Fig. 15.2 Perspective plot of the transmission surface for close contacts lasting at least 4 h (*left panel*) together with the fitted FOI and prevalence (*right panel*)

15.1.2   Refinements to the Social Contact Data Approach

Although the social contact hypothesis is intuitively appealing, several questions remain. Is the assumed type of contact a good proxy of the contact with high transmission potential or do different types of contacts contribute differently to the transmission process? Is the proportionality factor not only reflecting infectivity and susceptibility but potentially also underreporting of contacts truly age-independent? Some of the refinements focusing on these specific questions are briefly touched upon in this section.

15.1.2.1   The Identification of Contacts with High Transmission Potential

A first refinement to the social contact hypothesis addresses the potential of different types of social contacts to contribute to transmission, possibly at their own level (Ogunjimi et al. 2009). Therefore, we adapt the social contact hypothesis by considering

$$\beta(a,a') = \sum_l q_l \cdot c_l(a,a'),$$ (15.3)

where the index l refers to the different stratification levels of the contacts.

Consider location as the stratification variable with levels "home,", "school", "work" and "other." We use the function *contact.fitter.location* which uses the corresponding contact rates r_{ijk}, $k = 1,\ldots 4$ as input variables.

```
# R-code (see book's website)
# Function to fit the contact data using stratification
                                                    (continued)
```

(continued)
```
fit=contact.fitter.location(a=a,y=y,rij1,rij2,rij3,rij4,
                            muy=muy,N=N,D=D,Lmax=85,L=L,plots="TRUE")
```

The ML-estimate of $q = (q_1 \dots q_4)^T$ was $\hat{q}_{ML} = (0.055\ 0.048\ 0.000\ 0.000)^T$ with standard errors $(0.012\ 0.009\ 0.011\ 0.047)^T$ indicating that both home and school contacts are most predictive for the observed serological profile of parvovirus B19. Note that we did not consider the stratification levels "leisure" and "transport" because of their collinearity with "home" contacts.

The AIC value was 3,549.32 providing no improvement over the social contact hypothesis and being considerably higher than the AIC values as obtained from the methods imposing specific mixing structures.

15.1.2.2   Age-Dependent Proportionality of the Transmission Rates

Whereas in the previous section, refinement was based on stratification, we now focus on close contacts lasting at least 15 min and argue that the proportionality factor q might depend on several characteristics related to susceptibility and infectiousness, which could be ethnic-, climate-, disease-, or age-specific. Examples of age-specific characteristics related to susceptibility and infectiousness include the mean infectious period, mucus secretion, and hygiene. In the situation of seasonal and pandemic influenza this has been established before (see, e.g., Cauchemez et al. (2004) and Longini et al. (2005)).

Furthermore, the conversational and physical contacts reported in the diaries are just proxies of those events by which an airborne infection can be transmitted. For example, sitting close to someone in a bus without actually touching each other may also lead to transmission of infection. If these discrepancies are age-dependent, then q can be considered as an age-specific adjustment factor which relates the true contact rates underlying infectious disease transmission to the social contact proxies.

In view of this, we will explore whether q varies with age, an assumption we will refer to as "age-dependent proportionality"

$$\beta(a,a') = q(a,a') \cdot c(a,a'). \tag{15.4}$$

Again we use a numerical approximation by one-year age intervals to estimate $q(a,a')$.

Following Goeyvaerts et al. (2010), loglinear regression models are considered for $q(a,a')$, from the expectation of an exponential decline of q over a due to hygienic habits as well as an exponential decline of q over a' due to decreasing mucus secretion. The following loglinear model was fitted to the data

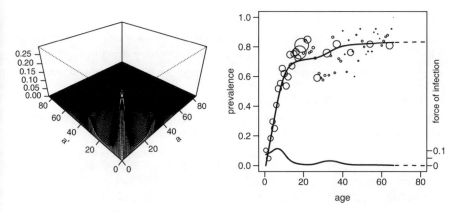

Fig. 15.3 Perspective plot of the transmission surface for close contacts lasting at least 4 h with age-dependent proportionality factor (*left panel*) together with the fitted FOI and prevalence (*right panel*)

$$\log\{q(a,a')\} = \gamma_0 + \gamma_1(a+a').$$

Note that we assumed a symmetric model for $q(a,a')$ motivated by the observation that in practice the function relating the q-parameter to infectiousness cannot be uniquely identified when estimated from serological data Goeyvaerts et al. (2010). Whereas $c(a,a')$ is symmetric due to reciprocity of contacts, in general $q(a,a')$ isn't.

```
# R-code (see book's website)
# Function to fit the contact data using stratification
contact.fitter.loglinear(a=a,y=y,rij=rij,int=F,muy=muy,
        N=N,D=D,Lmax=85,plots="TRUE",startpar=c(-2.3,0,0))
```

The resulting transmission surface and fitted prevalence and FOI are shown in Fig. 15.3. R_0 was estimated at 1.90 and the AIC value of 3,457.96 shows an improvement over the social contact hypothesis and is comparable to the imposed mixing structure approaches.

15.2 The Bootstrap and Multi-model Inference

In previous sections, we focused on the estimation of transmission parameters and consequently R_0. Equally important is the assessment of variability, not only with respect to the estimated parameters but also with respect to model selection. In this section we briefly indicate how proper inferences for the various methods in this chapter can be achieved.

15.2.1   The Nonparametric Bootstrap

When considering the methods that impose a specific mixing structure on $\beta(a, a')$, a nonparametric bootstrap approach on the serological samples can be used to obtain 95% confidence intervals. The use of the nonparametric bootstrap in this setting is beneficial since it allows the use of constraints in the optimization routines. Moreover, a nonparametric bootstrap does not rely on any symmetry property as normal theory does (see Sect. B.4).

Whereas the only source of variability is the serological sample for the methods based on imposed mixing patterns, the use of social contact data introduces a second source of variability since it is estimated from data itself. Goeyvaerts et al. (2010) assessed the sampling variability for the social contact data and the serological data using an extended nonparametric bootstrap approach. Furthermore, these authors build in a randomization process to account for the uncertainty when reporting the age of the contacted person (Mossong et al. 2008a). Concerning the age of contacts, an upper and lower age limit is given by the respondents. Instead of using the mean value of these age limits, a random draw is now taken from the uniform distribution on the corresponding age interval. In summary, these authors propose to use the following bootstrap cycle:

1. Randomize ages in the social contact data and the serological dataset.
2. Take a sample with replacement from the respondents in the social contact data.
3. Recalculate diary weights based on age and household size of the selected respondents.
4. Estimate the social contact matrix.
5. Rake a sample with replacement from the serological data.
6. Estimate the transmission parameters and R_0.

This bootstrap approach allows to calculate bootstrap confidence intervals for the transmission parameters and for the basic reproduction number, while taking into account all sources of variability.

15.2.2   Multi-model Inference

In this chapter, various methods to estimate transmission parameters and the basic reproduction number have been proposed. Selecting the most appropriate model among the candidate set of models under consideration can be done using the AIC-criterion. Once the best model has been selected, it can be used to estimate the parameter of interest and the above bootstrap approach governs the necessary inferences. However, the selection of the best model form the set of candidate models ignores the model selection uncertainty. A model producing a different fit with similar AIC could be lost from consideration and thus too strong conclusions can be drawn from what seems to be the best model based on AIC. Moreover,

Table 15.2 Overview of the different fitted models to the parvovirus B19 data from Belgium with estimated R_0, AIC value, and Akaike weight

Structure	$\hat{R}_0$	AIC	w_k
WAIFW-W_2	2.00	3,454.44	0.131
WAIFW-W_3	1.89	3,463.53	0.001
WAIFW-W_4	2.33	3,452.11	0.420
WAIFW-W_5	14.80	3,452.11	0.420
Mixing surface	1.76	3,461.00	0.005
All contacts	3.99	3,812.52	0.000
Close contacts	3.20	3,637.01	0.000
Close contacts $> 15\,\text{min}$	2.84	3,581.78	0.000
Close contacts $> 1\,\text{h}$	2.47	3,531.63	0.000
Close contacts $> 4\,\text{h}$	2.19	3,489.22	0.000
Stratification of contacts by location	2.68	3,549.32	0.000
Age-dependent proportionality factor	1.87	3,457.96	0.023

realizing that the best models for parvovirus B19 were the WAIFW matrices W_4 and W_5 resulting in the same AIC value, there is no guide to select the best model among two or more equally well fitting models. Therefore, multi-model inference is a valuable tool to consider (Burnham and Anderson 2002).

For each model, the AIC value, AIC difference $\Delta_k = \text{AIC}_k - \text{AIC}_{\min}$, and the Akaike weight

$$w_k = \frac{\exp(-\frac{1}{2}\Delta_k)}{\sum_\ell \exp(-\frac{1}{2}\Delta_\ell)},$$

can be calculated following Burnham and Anderson (2002). Here $\text{AIC}_{\min}$ corresponds to the model with the smallest AIC value. A given Akaike weight w_k is considered as the weight of evidence in favor of a model k being the actual Kullback–Leibler best model for the situation at hand, given the data and the set of candidate models considered (Burnham and Anderson 2002). Table 15.2 summarizes the different models fitted to the Belgian parvovirus B19 data in this chapter. The WAIFW structures W_2, W_4, and W_5 have the largest Akaike weights whereas assuming close contacts lasting at least $4\,\text{h}$ as proxies for contacts with high transmission potential in combination with an age-dependent proportionality factor does give some evidence of a good fit and avoids the choice of the somewhat ad hoc WAIFW structures.

Based on these results, one could argue that the use of social contact data to estimate transmission parameters based on serological data for parvovirus B19 in Belgium is of limited interest. However, one has to realize that the candidate set of models under consideration is rather limited and further research is needed to identify those contacts with high transmission potential. Indeed, it could be a combination of specific features of the social contact data and the age-dependent proportionality factor that explains the observed serological profile. In their paper, Goeyvaerts et al. (2010) studied the estimation of transmission parameters

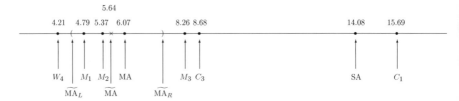

Fig. 15.4 Graphical representation of the estimates of R_0 for the models fitted to serological data on varicella-zoster virus in Belgium as reported by Goeyvaerts et al. (2010). Source: Goeyvaerts et al. (2010)

based on the same social contact data and serological data on the varicella zoster virus in Belgium. They found that a combination of close contacts that last 15 min or more in combination with an asymmetric age-dependent proportionality factor explained the observed serological profile much better than the WAIFW matrices.

Figure 15.4 shows the estimates of R_0 for the various models considered by Goeyvaerts et al. (2010): a contact-saturated model (SA) as proposed by Wallinga et al. (2006) assuming constant proportionality, a contact-bivariate smoothing model with constant proportionality with C_1 and C_3 considering all and close contacts longer than 15 min, respectively; three discrete age-dependent proportionality models M_1, M_2 and M_3 and model averaged estimates for R_0 (MA and $\widetilde{MA}$) together with 95% bootstrap-based percentile confidence interval limits for the model averaged estimate $(\widetilde{MA}_L, \widetilde{MA}_R)$. We refer to Goeyvaerts et al. (2010) for more details underlying these estimates.

Figure 15.4 illustrates the influence of the selected model on the estimation of R_0. Multi-model inference provides a way to incorporate model selection uncertainty in the estimation of parameters such as the basic reproduction number R_0.

15.3   Concluding Remarks

In this chapter, we have shown how based on serological data—possibly augmented with social contact data—transmission parameters can be estimated under the endemic equilibrium assumption. We distinguished between two estimation methods. The first method assumes somewhat ad hoc mixing structures for the transmission function whereas the second method uses social contact data to inform the structure of the transmission function. Whereas the use of social contact data looks promising further research should aim at identifying those contacts with high transmission potential. Since the proportionality factor reflects factors such as infectivity, susceptibility but potentially also underreporting in the social contact study and violations to the assumption of endemic equilibrium further research should be aimed at disentangling these different effects.

It is clear that the assumed model influences the estimation of the basic reproduction number and it is therefore essential to take model selection uncertainty into account.

Kretzschmar et al. (2010) and Goeyvaerts et al. (2011) have used a similar approach, assuming time equilibrium while considering several other underlying compartmental models such as SIS, SIRS, and SIRWb, where the latter model refers to a model which includes waning and boosting. Whereas Kretzschmar et al. (2010) focused on pertussis, Goeyvaerts et al. (2011) focused on parvovirus B19, including the same data as used in the illustration throughout this and previous chapter, but exploiting different compartmental models to explain the decrease in the age-specific seroprevalence between 20 and 30 years of age (see Chap. 9 and Hens et al. 2010b).

Note that we did not address the estimation of transmission parameters in combination with heterogeneity as done by Farrington et al. (2001) and Farrington and Whitaker (2005) using multisera data and predefined ad hoc mixing structures. Further research is needed to investigate how these approaches can be augmented with social contact data.

Part VI
Integration of Statistical Models into the Mathematical Model Framework

The main purpose of this part is to integrate the flexible models and methods described in the pervious parts of the book into the mathematical model framework. This part briefly illustrates the impact of modern flexible models to estimate the age-dependent force of infection (typically from serological data), the contact surface (from contact surveys), etc. on the mathematical model. In this way the book closes as it started, with mathematical models.

Chapter 16
Integrating Estimated Parameters in a Basic SIR Model

16.1 Introduction

The dynamics, prevention, and control of infectious diseases can be simulated by means of mathematical models. Many options have been described to formulate such models (for an overview see e.g. Capasso 2008). In general, a set of partial differential equations (PDEs) can be used to describe the mathematics of the model. Consider for instance the basic SIR model (Sect. 3.1.1):

$$\begin{cases} \frac{\partial S(a,t)}{\partial a} + \frac{\partial S(a,t)}{\partial t} = -(\lambda(a,t) + \mu(a))S(a,t), \\ \frac{\partial I(a,t)}{\partial a} + \frac{\partial I(a,t)}{\partial t} = \lambda(a,t)S(a,t) - (\nu + \mu(a))I(a,t), \\ \frac{\partial R(a,t)}{\partial a} + \frac{\partial R(a,t)}{\partial t} = \nu I(a,t) - \mu(a)R(a,t), \end{cases} \quad (16.1)$$

with $S(0,t) = B(t)$ the number of newborns at time t. Note that in (16.1) μ is assumed age-dependent whereas the recovery rate ν is assumed constant. We further assume no disease-related mortality. For the force of infection we distinguish between three different models: (1) the static model; (2) a dynamic model using WAIFW structures; and (3) a dynamic model using the social contact hypothesis.

1. *The Static Model:* In the static model, one assumes $\lambda(a,t) \equiv \lambda(a)$ where $\lambda(a)$ is estimated from serological data under the assumption of endemic equilibrium (see Chaps. 5–11).
2. *The Dynamic WAIFW Model:* In the dynamic WAIFW model, the force of infection is given by the mass action principle: $\lambda(a,t) = \int_0^{+\infty} \beta(a,a',t)I(a',t)da'$, where $\beta(a,a',t) \equiv \beta(a,a')$ is a WAIFW matrix estimated from serological data under endemic equilibrium (see Chap. 14).
3. *The Dynamic Social Contact Model:* In the dynamic social contact model, again the mass action principle is used: $\lambda(a,t) = \int_0^{+\infty} \beta(a,a',t)I(a',t)da'$, where $\beta(a,a',t) = \beta(a,a') = q(a,a')c(a,a')$ with $c(a,a')$ estimated from social contact data and $q(a,a') = q$ following the social contact hypothesis (see Chap. 15).

N. Hens et al., *Modeling Infectious Disease Parameters Based on Serological and Social Contact Data*, Statistics for Biology and Health 63, DOI 10.1007/978-1-4614-4072-7_16, © Springer Science+Business Media New York 2012

Solving a set of PDEs is not straightforward and depends on specific assumptions made for the different model parameters. In practice most PDE models are approximated using different methods in order to reduce the PDE model to a more solvable and workable model. In Sect. 3.5.2 the set of PDEs was replaced with a set of ordinary differential equations (ODEs) by considering K compartmental models representing K age groups and using continuous transitions from one age group to the next. Using this continuous age-structured model (CAS-model) has the disadvantage of allowing people to grow old instantaneously since rates represent exponential distributions and thus some individuals (in the tail of the distribution) will experience a high rate and quickly move to the next age group whereas other individuals (at the lower end of the exponential distribution) will only move to the next age group after a considerable amount of time.

Because of these disadvantages associated with continuous aging, we illustrate the integration of the estimated FOI, WAIFW structures, and contact mixing matrices into an age-time SIR model using a realistic age-structured model (RAS-model). A RAS-model allows individuals to change status from S to I and from I to R during 1 year (assuming age groups of 1 year) after which they instantaneously move to the next age group. It is often said that a RAS-model better reflects infectious disease dynamics because children switch grades in school generally at the same moment during the year and only once per year (Schenzle 1984). For a more in depth discussion about the advantages and disadvantages of the different methods to discretize age-structured models we refer to Capasso (2008); Keeling and Rohani (2008), and Vynnycky and White (2010).

The RAS-Model

The RAS-model consists of the following two-step iteration: Assuming 1-year age groups, let $\{S_i(t), I_i(t), R_i(t)\}$ denote the number of susceptible, infected, and recovered individuals of age $i = 0, \ldots, K-1$ at time t (in years).

Step 1: Given initial values $\{S_i(t), I_i(t), R_i(t)\} = \{S_i(t_0), I_i(t_0), R_i(t_0)\}, i = 0, \ldots, K-1$ we solve the following set of ODEs:

$$\begin{cases} \frac{dS_i(t)}{dt} = -(\lambda_i(t) + \mu_i)S_i(t), \\ \frac{dI_i(t)}{dt} = \lambda_i(t)S_i(t) - (\nu + \mu_i)I_i(t), \\ \frac{dR_i(t)}{dt} = \nu I_i(t) - \mu_i R_i(t), \end{cases} \quad (16.2)$$

to obtain $\{S_i(t+1), I_i(t+1), R_i(t+1)\}, i = 0, \ldots, K-1$ after 1 year.

Step 2: Individuals are then shifted by 1 year: $\{S_i(t+1), I_i(t+1), R_i(t+1)\} \to \{S_{i+1}(t+1), I_{i+1}(t+1), R_{i+1}(t+1)\}, i = 0, \ldots, K-2$ and all newborns B are assumed susceptible to infection: $\{S_0(t+1), I_0(t+1), R_0(t+1)\} = \{B, 0, 0\}$.

This process is iterated throughout the time period of interest.

Whereas time homogenous but age-dependent mortality rates μ_i and a constant number of newborns B were used in the description above, other demographic models can be used as well. Note that with the latter assumption $N_i(t)$ declines with time after which the last cohort $N_{K-1}(t)$ promptly dies at the end of the year and B newborns are added to the population. One commonly used age distribution is the rectangular distribution (Type I mortality) where $\mu_i = 0$ for $i = 0, \ldots, K-1$ and $B = N_{K-1}(t)$.

For the specific application here, we refer to Ogunjimi et al. (2009) and Brisson et al. (2010) who used RAS-models to model the transmission dynamics of varicella-zoster virus, focusing on the clinical disease chickenpox alone, and in combination with herpes zoster, respectively.

16.2 Application

We illustrate these approaches for varicella ignoring the herpes zoster component. We therefore assume $v = 1/(7/365)$ corresponding to an infectious period of 7 days. We use $\mu_i(t) \equiv \mu_i$ which we estimate from mortality data from Belgium anno 2005.

We first run the RAS-model until we reach endemic equilibrium after which we include a simple vaccination strategy in our model (see Chap. 3) by putting $S(0) = (1-p)B$ and $R(0) = pB$ for specific values of p. This corresponds to immunizing newborns at birth with coverage probability p.

Running the mathematical model can be done using the following R-code.

```
# Start loop RAS-ODE version of the PDEs
for (initrun in Tinit[1]:Tinit[2])
{
  # Some starting parameters
  print(paste("Year=",as.character(initrun),sep=""))
  states = ifelse(states < tol, 0, states)
  # moving everyone, one state forward
if (initrun!=Tinit[1]){
for (j in 99:1)
     {
        states[j+  1]= states[j    ]
          states[j+101]= states[j+100]
        states[j+201]= states[j+200]
        }
states[1]    = (1-p)*cohort.size # completely susceptible for p=0
states[101] = 0
states[201] = p*cohort.size
}
  # Time steps determined by resolution
```

(continued)

```
(continued)
times  = seq(0, 1, length=resolution)
params = matrix(c(mu = mu, betas = betas, nu=nu))
  # Output of the system of ODEs
out = as.data.frame(lsoda(states, times, ODE, params))
states=as.matrix(out[resolution,])[-1]
}
# End loop
```

For the three different approaches, the ODE function is given by

```
# static RAS model
#------------------
ODE = function(t, states, params)
  {
  S = states[  1:100]
  I = states[101:200]
  R = states[201:300]
  mu     = params[1:100]
  betas = matrix(params[101:10100],100,100)
  nu = params[10101]
  dS = - (foi+mu)*S        # Susceptibles
  dI = +foi*S -(nu+mu)*I        # Infection
  dR = +nu*I-mu*R        # Immune
  list(c(dS,dI,dR))
  }

# RAS model with WAIFW matrices
#------------------------------
ODE = function(t, states, params)
  {
  S = states[  1:100]
  I = states[101:200]
  R = states[201:300]
  mu     = params[1:100]
  nu = params[10101]
  dS = -(apply(W2*I,2,"sum")+mu)*S        # Susceptibles
  dI = +apply(W2*I,2,"sum")*S-(nu+mu)*I   # Infection
  dR = +nu*I-mu*R        # Immune
  list(c(dS,dI,dR))
  }

# RAS model with contact matrices
#--------------------------------
ODE = function(t, states, params)
```

(continued)

(continued)
```
{
S = states[   1:100]
I = states[101:200]
R = states[201:300]
mu     = params[1:100]
betas = matrix(params[101:10100],100,100)
nu = params[10101]
dS = -(apply(betas*I,2,"sum")+mu)*S    # Susceptibles
dI = +apply(betas*I,2,"sum")*S-(nu+mu)*I # Infection
dR = +nu*I-mu*R                         # Immune
list(c(dS,dI,dR))
}
```

For the static model, we use the FOI estimate based on a penalized spline FOI model (Chap. 9). For the dynamic WAIFW model, we use WAIFW matrix W2 and for the dynamic social contact model we rely on the social contact hypothesis and use close contacts lasting at least 15 min (Chap. 15, Goeyvaerts et al. 2010).

16.2.1 Model Comparison

First, we compare the three different approaches. Figure 16.1 shows the incidence in three age groups (in years): "0–12," "13–18," and "19+" over a course of 20 years after reaching endemic equilibrium. Both dynamic models clearly show periodicity over the course of 3 years whereas the static model, i.e., the penalized spline model, doesn't show any periodicity, as expected. In epidemic years the dynamic social contact data model reaches an incidence of about 119,130 infections per year in a population of about ten million people.

Figure 16.2 shows the age-specific prevalence, force of infection, and incidence using the dynamic social contact model, the dynamic WAIFW model, and static model. We averaged curves over the 3 year period over which a periodic behavior was observed (see Fig. 16.1).

For both dynamic models, only small differences on the scale of the prevalence and incidence can be observed whereas on the scale of the force of infection, these differences are more pronounced with a clear second and third peak at ages 35 and 60 for the dynamic social contact model. These three peaks originate from the social contact hypothesis and the high contact intensity between children and adults— presumably their parents and grandparents. The jigsaw behavior for the dynamic social contact model is a result of the abrupt aging in the RAS-model. By using a smaller age-grid this effect diminishes. The static model clearly shows a different behavior on all three epidemiological parameters.

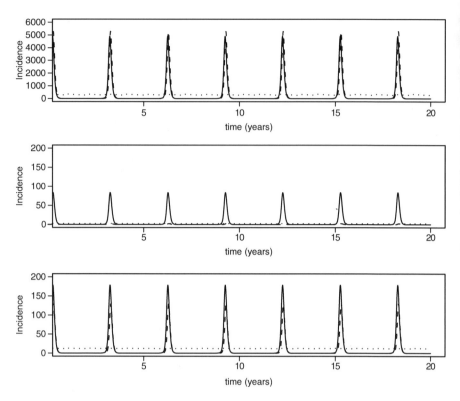

Fig. 16.1 Number of infected individuals over 20 years for age categories 0–12 years (*first panel*), 13–18 years (*second panel*), and 19 years and above (*third panel*) following the dynamic social contact data model (*solid line*), the dynamic WAIFW model (*dashed line*), and the static model (*dotted line*)

16.2.2   Uncertainty

While we have previously illustrated the impact of the chosen model on the resulting estimates, we now illustrate the impact of data uncertainty for the dynamic contact model. We follow the approach by Goeyvaerts et al. (2010) and resampled both contact data and serological data. Figure 16.3 shows the resulting uncertainty in the age-specific incidence.

Whereas the yearly incidence averaged over a period of 3 years yields 119,130 cases for a population of about ten million people, the 95%-bootstrap-based confidence interval ranges from 43,642 cases to 231,615 cases, showing a substantial amount of uncertainty.

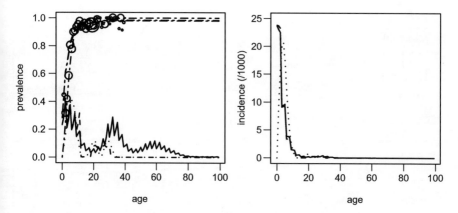

Fig. 16.2 Prevalence, force of infection (*left panel*), and yearly incidence averaged over a period of 3 years (*right panel*) by age following the dynamic social contact data model (*solid line*), the dynamic WAIFW model (*dashed line*), and the static model (*dotted line*). The observed age-specific prevalence for VZV is shown in the *left panel* with size proportional to the number of samples taken

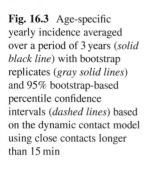

Fig. 16.3 Age-specific yearly incidence averaged over a period of 3 years (*solid black line*) with bootstrap replicates (*gray solid lines*) and 95% bootstrap-based percentile confidence intervals (*dashed lines*) based on the dynamic contact model using close contacts longer than 15 min

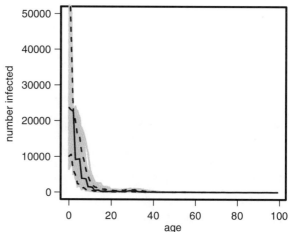

16.2.3 Vaccination

Finally, we illustrate the impact of vaccinating newborns. We first run all three models to reach endemic equilibrium. We then assume that newborns directly move to the immune state and are not subject to a susceptibility gap between birth and immunization. We illustrate the behavior of the incidence over 50 years after introducing an immunization programme with coverage 33%.

Figure 16.4 illustrates the herd-immunity effect associated with both dynamic models most strikingly for age categories "13–18" and "19+," in which the incidence

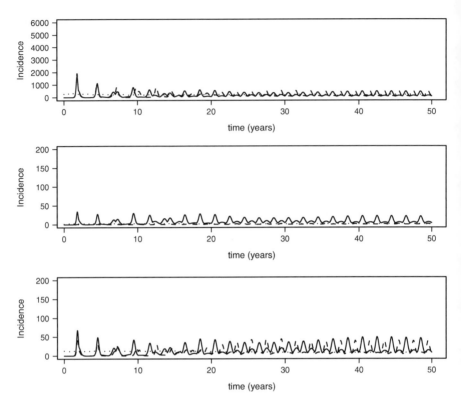

Fig. 16.4 Impact of introducing an immunization programme for newborns with 33% coverage: number of infected individuals for age categories 0–12 years (*first panel*), 13–18 years (*second panel*), and 19 years and above (*third panel*) following the dynamic social contact data model (*solid line*), the dynamic WAIFW model (*dashed line*), and the penalized spline model (*dotted line*). The dynamic behavior is illustrated for the first 50 years after introducing vaccination

declines quite rapidly after the immunization programme is implemented. For the static model, incidence decreases after following the immunized cohort.

Figure 16.5 illustrates the critical immunization coverage attained when vaccinating 75% of newborns for the three different models. For the dynamic WAIFW model with $R_0 = 3.5$, the infection is eliminated at 75% vaccine uptake because this allows to reach the critical effective immunization coverage. Since $R_0 = 8.2$ for the dynamic social contact data model, the infection cannot be eliminated. In addition to declining incidence in the various age groups, and the associated increase in the average age at infection, it is noteworthy that the interepidemic period also increases as a consequence of vaccination (see also Fig. 16.5). This phenomenon has previously been described (see Chapter 3 and e.g. Anderson and May 1991), and observed in postvaccination surveillance data.

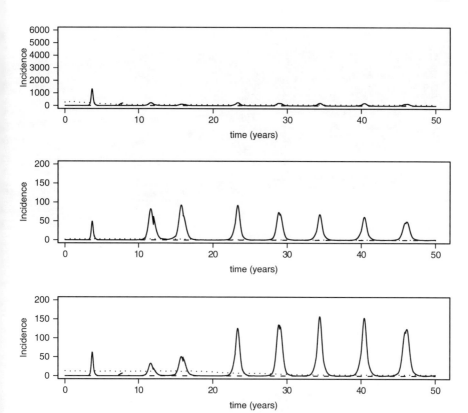

Fig. 16.5 Impact of introducing an immunization programme for newborns with 75% coverage: Number of infected individuals for age categories 0–12 years (*first panel*), 13–18 years (*second panel*), and 19 years and above (*third panel*) following the dynamic social contact data model (*solid line*), the dynamic WAIFW model (*dashed line*), and the penalized spline model (*dotted line*). The dynamic behavior is illustrated for the first 50 years after introducing vaccination

16.3   Discussion

In this chapter, we have shown how an age-time dependent model, often described by a system of partial differential equations, can be implemented in R using the realistic age-structured model (RAS-model). We illustrated the difference in applying either a static or a dynamic model. We considered two dynamic models, one based on the "traditional" WAIFW-approach and the other on the recent social contact data approach. The impact of using either one is clear from the resulting time-specific incidence in different age groups not only because of the higher R_0 for the social contact data approach but also because of the underlying social contact process. For a more elaborate discussion and illustration of how uncertainty with respect to parameter and model choice can be dealt with, we refer to Ogunjimi et al. (2009); Goeyvaerts et al. (2010), and Brisson et al. (2010). Note that, whereas the static model doesn't incorporate herd-immunity effects, both dynamic models do.

Appendix A
A Note on the R Environment

R is an open environment for data manipulation, graphical display, and interactive data analysis. It is available as Free Software under the terms of the Free Software Foundation's GNU General Public License in source code form. It compiles and runs on a wide variety of UNIX platforms and similar systems (including FreeBSD and Linux), Windows and MacOS.

R can be downloaded from http://www.r-project.org/. R can be extended (easily) via packages, available through the CRAN family of Internet sites covering a very wide range of modern statistics.

A.1 Data Structures in R

R operates on so-called objects. Examples are *vectors* or *matrices* (or *arrays*) of numeric values, logical values, or character strings. These are known as atomic structures since their components are all of the same type or mode.

R also operates on objects called *lists*. These are ordered sequences of objects which individually can be of any mode. Lists are known as recursive rather than atomic structures since their components can themselves be lists in their own right.

But the most relevant type of object for statistical data analysis is the *dataframe*. A dataframe is a special class of lists, but less technically, a dataframe is a type of table where the typical use employs the rows as observations and the columns as variables. Contrary to a matrix, the columns of a dataframe can be of different types.

In the following example two vectors are defined, one numeric with the age values of five subjects and one logical with their infection status; next both vectors are stored together in a dataframe.

N. Hens et al., *Modeling Infectious Disease Parameters Based on Serological and Social Contact Data*, Statistics for Biology and Health 63, DOI 10.1007/978-1-4614-4072-7, © Springer Science+Business Media New York 2012

```
> age=c(10, 25, 42, 16, 31)
> status=c(F, T, T, T, F)
> mydataset=data.frame(age,status)
> mydataset
  age status
1  10  FALSE
2  25   TRUE
3  42   TRUE
4  16   TRUE
5  31  FALSE
```

A.2   Reading and Writing Data

Large data objects will usually be read from external files rather than from
the keyboard. An entire dataset can be read directly into a dataframe with the
read.table() function, e.g.:

```
> mydataset=read.table("c:\\directorystructure\\data.dat")
```

Note the double backslashes to define the directory structure. You can read
"comma separated value" files using *read.csv()*, "delimiter separated value" files
with `read.delim()` and Microsoft Excel files with `read.xls()` (needs package *gdata*). Data can also be viewed, changed, or added via the spreadsheet
interface, using `edit(mydataset)`.

Data in R can also be exported, e.g., to a comma separated value file "tb.csv" in
the subdirectory "temp":

```
> write.table(mydataset,file="C:\\temp\\tb.csv",sep=",")
```

A.3   Graphical Procedures

There are very versatile graphical facilities in the R environment. Basic graphics
functions include:

- `plot(x), plot(x,y)`
- `points(x,y), lines(x,y)`
- `pairs(X), coplot(a b|c)`

- qqnorm(x), qqline(x), qqplot(x,y)
- hist(x), dotchart(x)
- image(x,y,z), contour(x,y,z), persp(x,y,z)

Text and legends can be added using text(x,y,labels, ...) and legend(x,y,legend,...).

A.4   Statistical Models in R

The basic structure of most function calls to fit models to data follows the example below (for logistic regression):

```
> myfit=glm(status~age,family=binomial,data=mydataset)
> summary(myfit)
Call:
glm(formula = status ~ age, family = binomial,
    data = mydataset)

Coefficients:
            Estimate Std. Error z value Pr(>|z|)
(Intercept) -1.07144    2.31866  -0.462    0.644
age          0.06161    0.09126   0.675    0.500
```

For more information about the specific output, one can look up the details of a function using help.

```
> help(glm)
```


A.5   Packages

The standard (or base) packages are considered part of the R source code. They contain the basic functions that allow R to work, as well as standard statistical and graphical functions and some datasets. They should be automatically available in any R installation. There are thousands of contributed packages for R. Some of these packages implement specialized statistical methods, others give access to data or hardware, and others are designed to complement textbooks. Most packages are available from CRAN (http://CRAN.R-project.org/ and its mirrors). Within the R environment, packages can be installed, updated, and loaded by clicking the "packages" button on the top bar.

A.6   References

There are many introductory and more advanced manuals and textbooks on R. Just have a look at the documentation available on http://www.r-project.org/.

Appendix B
Statistical Inference

The following sections summarize some basic concepts of statistical estimation and inference with illustrations on the VZV data (see Chap. 4). We focus on estimation, testing hypotheses, and the construction of confidence intervals for two types of data, normally distributed and binary data.

B.1 Maximum Likelihood Estimation and Likelihood Inference

We are interested in inference on the prevalence π and on the mean antibody activity level (on log scale) μ for VZV in Belgium. Denote $z_1, \ldots, z_n$ the sample of independent and identically distributed observations of the antibody activity level z on log scale and $d_1, \ldots, d_n$ the corresponding dichotomized infection indicators where $d_i = 1$ if $z_i > \tau_u$ for a particular upper threshold and 0 if $z_i < \tau_\ell$ (and missing for the equivocal area $[\tau_\ell, \tau_u]$).

Next we are also interested in the dependency of the antibody level z or infection status d on a covariate, for instance the age a; or in statistical terms we are interested in the conditional distribution of z or d given a. In what follows we use a generic notation $(x_1, y_1), \ldots, (x_n, y_n)$ where y refers to our response variable (such as z or d) and x to a covariate or explanatory variable (such as a). We are interested in modeling the distribution of y and in modeling the conditional distribution $y|x$. In such models θ refers to our parameter of interest (possibly vector valued). Nuisance parameters are denoted as η and their notation will be suppressed when not important or not applicable.

The likelihood function equals the joint density of $y_1, \ldots, y_n$, as a function of the unknown parameters θ and η:

$$L(\theta, \eta) = \prod_{i=1}^{n} f(y_i; \theta, \eta),$$

N. Hens et al., *Modeling Infectious Disease Parameters Based on Serological and Social Contact Data*, Statistics for Biology and Health 63, DOI 10.1007/978-1-4614-4072-7, © Springer Science+Business Media New York 2012

where $f(y_i; \theta, \eta)$ represents the density or mass function. The likelihood principle states that, for inference about θ and η, given $y_1, \ldots, y_n$, all information is contained in the likelihood function $L(\theta, \eta)$. Note that any dependency of the density function on covariates x has been suppressed for ease of presentation.

The maximum likelihood estimator (MLE) is defined as the value for θ, η that maximizes the likelihood $L(\theta, \eta)$ or equivalently the loglikelihood

$$\ell(\theta, \eta) = \sum_{i=1}^{n} \log(f(y_i; \theta, \eta)).$$

For instance, assuming the y_i are normally distributed with mean μ_i and variance σ_i^2, the loglikelihood equals

$$\ell(\mu; \sigma^2) = -\frac{n}{2} \log(2\pi) - \sum_{i=1}^{n} \log \sigma_i - \frac{1}{2} \sum_{i=1}^{n} \left(\frac{y_i - \mu_i}{\sigma_i} \right)^2.$$

In this case μ_i is typically the parameter of interest and σ_i a nuisance parameter. Assuming homoscedasticity $\sigma_i = \sigma$, maximization of $\ell(\mu; \sigma^2)$ with respect to μ_i is independent of the value of σ and reduces to minimization of the least-squares criterion $\sum_{i=1}^{n} (y_i - \mu_i)^2$. For $\mu_i = \mu$ the solution equals the sample mean $\bar{y} = (\sum_{i=1}^{n} y_i)/n$. When modeling the conditional distribution of y given a covariate x, the choice $\mu_i = E(y_i|x_i) = \beta_0 + \beta_1 x_i$ for the conditional mean, expressing the loglikelihood as a function of the regression coefficient β_0 and β_1, leads to classical linear regression.

For binary data y_i we get the following expression for the loglikelihood

$$\ell(\pi) = \sum_{i=1}^{n} y_i \log(\pi_i) + \sum_{i=1}^{n} (1 - y_i) \log(1 - \pi_i). \tag{B.1}$$

Note that there is no nuisance parameter in this case, as variance equals $\pi_i(1 - \pi_i)$. For $\pi_i = \pi$ the loglikelihood $\ell(\pi)$ is maximized at the overall proportion. When considering a model for the conditional distribution of y given a covariate x, the choice

$$\pi_i = \frac{e^{\beta_0 + \beta_1 x_i}}{1 + e^{\beta_0 + \beta_1 x_i}}, \tag{B.2}$$

for the conditional probability, or equivalently

$$\text{logit}(\pi_i) = \log \left(\frac{\pi_i}{1 - \pi_i} \right) = \beta_0 + \beta_1 x_i, \tag{B.3}$$

leads to logistic regression. In this case the loglikelihood (B.1) is again reexpressed as a function of the regression coefficients β_0 and β_1.

Figure B.1 visualizes the maximization of the loglikelihood curves for the Belgian VZV data, assuming the logarithm of the antibody levels z is normally

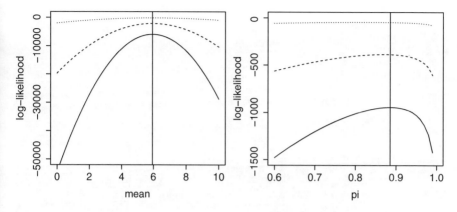

Fig. B.1 Belgian VZV data. Curves (*solid lines*) of the loglikelihood function for the mean antibody level μ (*left panel*) and prevalence π (*right panel*). *Vertical lines* visualize the respective MLEs. The *dashed* and *dotted lines* show similar loglikelihood functions for subsamples of size 1,000 and 100, respectively

distributed (left panel) and for the infection statuses d (right panel). The solid curves are based on samples of size 2,761 for z and size 2,656 for d (as 105 observations were classified as equivocal and omitted). The normal loglikelihood is maximized at the sample mean $\bar{z} = 5.933$; the Bernoulli loglikelihood is maximized at the sample proportion $\bar{d} = 0.886$. Both estimates are represented by vertical lines in the respective panels of Fig. B.1.

Figure B.1 also shows dashed and dotted curves in both panels. These correspond to loglikelihood functions based on a random subsample of size 1,000 (dashed curve) and size 100 (dotted curve). Although the vertical position of the curves cannot be directly interpreted or compared, as they are based on different samples, the curvature of the plots has an interesting interpretation. Indeed the curvature of the loglikelihood can be quantified through the second derivative of the loglikelihood. The observed Fisher information is defined as $-\partial^2 \ell(\theta)/\partial\theta^2$ and is inversely related to the standard error of the ML-estimate $\hat{\theta}$. Figure B.1 shows the decrease in curvature in the loglikelihood function, reflecting a decrease in information and corresponding increase in standard errors when sample sizes reduce to 1,000 and further to 100.

The following R-code fits the logistic regression model (B.3) for VZV infection status d and covariate *age*:

```
# Illustration of ML for logistic regression

# Using the glm function
fit=glm(d~age,family=binomial)
summary(fit)
```

(continued)

```
(continued)
logLik(fit)

# Using the optimization function nlm
# Defining -(loglikelihood)
minuslogll_lr=function(beta){
n=length(d)
p=exp(beta[1]+beta[2]*age)/(1+exp(beta[1]+beta[2]*age))
-(sum(d*log(p))+sum((1-d)*log(1-p)))
}
# Calling nlm (nonlinear minimization with Newton-type
   algorithm)
nlmfit=nlm(minuslogll_lr,c(mean(d),0),hessian=T)
beta_est=nlmfit$estimate
beta_se=sqrt(diag(solve(nlmfit$hessian)))
# showing estimates and corresponding se-estimates
round(cbind(beta_est,beta_se),5)
```

There are no longer explicit solutions for the estimates, and one has to rely on numerical methods such as the Newton–Raphson algorithm (or alternatively Fisher scoring or iterative reweighted least squares). For this purpose one can use the *nlm* function in R. As this function is a nonlinear minimizer rather than a maximizer we use $-\ell(\beta_0, \beta_1)$. The hessian matrix is also part of the output. The inverse of this matrix (using the R function *solve*) contains estimated variances on the diagonal.

```
# Using the glm function
> summary(fit)
Coefficients:
              Estimate Std. Error z value Pr(>|z|)
(Intercept) -0.07016    0.11629   -0.603    0.546
age          0.18889    0.01216   15.527   <2e-16 ***
Number of Fisher Scoring iterations: 6
> logLik(fit)
'log Lik.' -732.5021 (df=2)
# Using the optimization function nlm
> round(cbind(beta_est,beta_se),5)
     beta_est beta_se
[1,] -0.07015 0.11634
[2,]  0.18888 0.01218
```

The function *glm* uses Fisher scoring whereas *nlm* uses a Newton-type algorithm, resulting in estimates, which can be considered as identical for all practical purposes. Figure B.2 shows the contours of the loglikelihood function $\ell(\beta_0, \beta_1)$ with a horizontal and vertical line indicating the position of the solution $\hat{\beta}_0 = 0.0702$ and $\hat{\beta}_0 = 0.1889$.

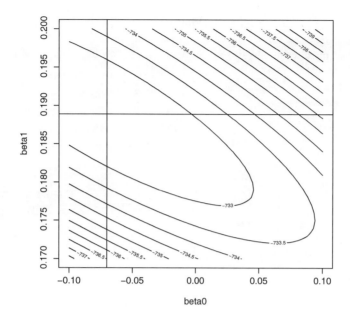

Fig. B.2 Belgian VZV data. Contour plot of the loglikelihood function $\ell(\beta_0, \beta_1)$ for the logistic regression model (B.3). The *horizontal* and *vertical line* visualize the MLEs $\hat{\beta}_0$ and $\hat{\beta}_1$

Testing hypotheses in the maximum likelihood paradigm is based on possibly three approaches: (1) a standardized difference between the values of the loglikelihood at its maximum for a full and a reduced model, defining the likelihood ratio test (LRT); (2) the standardized value of the evaluation of the derivative of the loglikelihood at the hypothesized value, leading to the score test; (3) the square of a t-type of test $(\hat{\theta}/\hat{se}(\hat{\theta}))^2$, leading to the Wald test. All three test statistics are asymptotically equivalent under the null hypothesis yielding a χ^2 distribution. Confidence regions and intervals can be defined by inverting these test procedures, or in the more classical way as $[\hat{\theta} - z_{\alpha/2}\hat{se}(\hat{\theta}), \hat{\theta} + z_{\alpha/2}\hat{se}(\hat{\theta})]$, where $z_{\alpha/2}$ is a critical point from the standard normal distribution. When focusing on one particular parameter of interest (considering the others as nuisance), profile methods can be used (see the next section). In this section we limit ourselves to an illustration of the LRT, the Wald test, and the Wald type confidence intervals.

As an example we consider the LRT for the null hypothesis $H_0 : \beta_1 = 0$ in the logistic regression model (B.3) with π_i the probability $P(d_i = 1)$ to be infected with VZV and with age a_i as a covariate. The LRT for this null hypothesis contrasts the value of the maximized loglikelihood of the full model with both parameters β_0, β_1 with that of the reduced model or *null* model with only an intercept β_0 and with $\beta_1 = 0$, more precisely

$$\text{LRT} = 2 \left\{ \max_{\beta_0, \beta_1} \ell(\beta_0, \beta_1) - \max_{\beta_0} \ell(\beta_0, 0) \right\}.$$

If the null hypothesis is true, the maximized loglikelihood of the reduced model is expected to be close to that of the full model and the value of the LRT is expected to be small, as described by the χ_1^2 distribution. The Wald statistic is defined as

$$\text{Wald} = \left\{ \frac{\hat{\beta}_1}{\hat{se}(\hat{\beta}_1)} \right\}^2,$$

also having a χ_1^2 null distribution. The R-code below illustrates the computation of both test statistics, their p-values, and a 95% Wald type confidence interval for β_1.

```
# Testing slope beta1=0
# LRT
lrt=2*(logLik(glm(d~age,family=binomial))
      -logLik(glm(d~1,family=binomial)))[[1]]
c(lrt,1-pchisq(lrt,1))
# Wald
wald=(beta_est[2]/beta_se[2])^2
c(wald,1-pchisq(wald,1))
# CI
c(beta_est[2]-1.96*beta_se[2],beta_est[2]+1.96*beta_se[2])
```

The R output below clearly shows, as expected, that the probability to be infected by VZV depends on age (at 5% level of significance).

```
# LRT
[1] 424.6611    0.0000
> # Wald
[1] 240.5193    0.0000
> # CI
[1] 0.1650135 0.2127564
```

Hypotheses testing can also be used to select a final model from a set of candidate models, at least if these candidate models are nested models. In general, however, we recommend to use genuine model selection criteria such as the well-known Akaike's Information Criterion (AIC, Akaike 1973). Such criteria also allow to compare non-nested models and models that differ in any ML model component.

The AIC-criterion originates from information theory and is defined as

$$\text{AIC} = -2\ell(\widehat{\theta}, \widehat{\eta}) + 2K, \tag{B.4}$$

with $\ell(\theta, \eta)$ the loglikelihood of the model and $(\widehat{\theta}, \widehat{\eta})$ the MLE of (θ, η). Here K stands for the total number of estimated parameters, nuisance parameters included. From a set of candidate models, the model with the lowest AIC is selected as the best model, as the best compromise between accuracy and complexity. The first loglikelihood based term measures how accurate the model fits to the data and will be smallest for the most complex model. The second term however penalizes for complexity and will be largest for the most complex model. The model that balances accuracy with complexity in an optimal way is chosen as best model. The AIC was designed to be an approximately unbiased estimator of the expected *Kullback-Leibler* (KL) information, which can be interpreted as the information loss as a consequence of using a candidate model to approximate the true unknown model. And that information loss should be minimized.

Let us reconsider the logistic regression model for VZV infection status d and covariate *age*, as a first candidate model. As a second candidate model we extend that model with an additional quadratic term age^2. These two models are nested, and the best model could be selected based on a test for the quadratic age-effect. As a third model we reconsider the model with only a linear age-effect, but with a probit link instead of logit link. This third model is non-nested with the two first models. The following R-code illustrates the fits of all three candidate models whereas the *(AIC)* function enables us to compute the corresponding AIC values for these models.

```
> # a first candidate model: linear in dose with logit link
> logitfit1=glm(d~age,family=binomial)
> print(c(AIC(logitfit1),-2*logLik(logitfit1)[1]+2*2))
[1] 1469.004 1469.004
>
> # a second candidate model: quadratic in dose with logit link
> logitfit2=glm(d~age+I(age^2),family=binomial)
> print(c(AIC(logitfit2),-2*logLik(logitfit2)[1]+2*3))
[1] 1420.795 1420.795
> summary(logitfit2)

Call:
glm(formula = d ~ age + I(age^2), family = binomial)

Deviance Residuals:
    Min       1Q    Median       3Q       Max
-3.0207   0.1491   0.2346   0.4380    3.3123

Coefficients:
              Estimate Std. Error z value Pr(>|z|)
(Intercept) -0.6050146  0.1510592  -4.005 6.20e-05 ***
age          0.3175378  0.0273750  11.600  < 2e-16 ***
I(age^2)    -0.0048546  0.0008926  -5.439 5.37e-08 ***
```
(continued)

```
(continued)
- - -
Signif. codes:  0 *** 0.001 ** 0.01 * 0.05 . 0.1   1

(Dispersion parameter for binomial family taken to be 1)

    Null deviance: 1889.9  on 2656  degrees of freedom
Residual deviance: 1414.8  on 2654  degrees of freedom
AIC: 1420.8

Number of Fisher Scoring iterations: 7

>
> # a third candidate model: linear in dose with probit link
> probitfit=glm(d~age,family=binomial(link="probit"))
> print(c(AIC(probitfit),-2*logLik(probitfit)[1]+2*2))
[1] 1508.195 1508.195
```

Comparing the first two logit models, both approaches indicate that the second model is a better model. Indeed, the AIC value 1,420.795 for the second model is smaller than the value 1,469.004 for the first model. The summary of the fit of the second model also indicates that the quadratic age-effect is highly significant, confirming again that the second model is better. The third probit model cannot be compared to these first two models by a test. But the AIC value of 1,508.195 clearly shows that this third model is no improvement. Conclusion is that the best model is the second model. A warning however is at its place here. Selecting the best model from a set of candidate models does not guarantee that this best model is a good model. Indeed, selecting the best model from a set of poor candidate models will still result in a poor final model. Having selected a best model from a set of candidate models can be followed next by a formal lack-of-fit test. If such a formal lack-of-fit test does not show any evidence from the data against the final model, one can decide to stop the search for a good model. For lack-of-fit tests in the ML setting, see, e.g., Aerts et al. (1999, 2000).

B.2   Generalized Linear Models

Linear regression models and logistic regression models are special cases of GLMs. Three components specify a GLM: the *random component*, the *linear predictor* or the *systematic component*, and the *link function* relating the random with the systematic component.

Let $y_1, \ldots, y_n$ denote a sample of a response variable y and $x_{1j}, \ldots, x_{nj}$ the corresponding values of p covariates $x_1, \ldots, x_j, \ldots, x_p$. The *random component* refers to the distribution of $y|x$ to be selected from the exponential family. This

Table B.1 Canonical link functions for the normal, Bernoulli, and Poisson members of the exponential family

Distribution	Mean μ_i	Natural parameter θ_i θ_i	Dispersion parameter ϕ	Link function $g(\mu_i)$	Regression model
Normal	μ_i	μ_i	σ^2	μ_i	$\mu_i = \sum_{j=0}^{p} \beta_j x_{ij}$
Bernoulli	π_i	$\log(\frac{\pi_i}{1-\pi_i})$	1	$\log(\frac{\mu_i}{1-\mu_i})$	$\log(\frac{\pi_i}{1-\pi_i}) = \sum_{j=0}^{p} \beta_j x_{ij}$
Poisson	μ_i	$\log(\mu_i)$	1	$\log(\mu_i)$	$\log(\mu_i) = \sum_{j=0}^{p} \beta_j x_{ij}$

family includes many of the most common distributions: continuous distributions (normal, exponential, gamma, …) as well as discrete distributions (Bernoulli, binomial, Poisson, …). An exponential family distribution for y_i has one natural parameter θ_i and might have an additional dispersion parameter ϕ. Its density can be written in the "exponential" form

$$f(y_i, \theta_i, \phi) = \exp\left\{ [y_i \theta_i - b(\theta_i)] / a(\phi) + c(y_i, \phi) \right\}.$$

The *systematic component* defines a linear combination of the p covariates

$$\eta_i = \sum_{j=0}^{p} \beta_j x_{ij},$$

with $x_{i0} = 1$ for all i, representing the intercept. Finally, the third component, the *link function*, connects the mean $\mu_i = E(y_i)$ to the covariate values x_{ij} by the formula

$$g(\mu_i) = \eta_i,$$

where the link function g is a monotonic and differentiable function. The link function that transforms the mean to the natural parameter is called the *canonical link*.

Table B.1 shows the canonical link functions for three popular models: the linear regression model, the logistic regression model, and the Poisson regression model (or the loglinear model). But other link functions can be chosen: a log link for the normal distribution, the probit link for logistic regression, etc.

GLMs provide a unifying theory of modeling and share many convenient properties of linear models, such as a concave optimization (loglikelihood) function implying that there is a unique MLE. A (small) price to pay however is that the likelihood equations for GLMs are usually nonlinear in the regression parameters $\beta_0, \ldots, \beta_p$, and hence no explicit analytical solutions are available. Iterative numerical methods are needed for solving the estimating equations and obtaining numerical values for the estimates (Newton–Raphson, Fisher scoring, iterative reweighted least squares). Further details can be found in several standard textbooks on ML estimation and inference for GLM, including McCullagh and Nelder (1989); Dobson (2002), and Agresti (2002).

One can fit GLMs easily in R using the *glm()* function. All three GLM-components have to be specified, if deviating from the default choices (normal distribution, identity link). The following simple simulation example illustrates the use of a Poisson regression model in R:

```
> # setting the 25 values of a single binary covariate x
> # (e.g. 0=low or 1=high socio-economic status)
> x=c(rep(0,20),rep(1,5))
> print(x)
 [1] 0 0 0 0 0 0 0 0 0 0 0 0 0 0 0 0 0 0 0 0 1 1 1 1 1
>
> # define the predictor 3-1*x
> # so the true values are beta0=3 and beta1=-1
> eta=3-1*x
> print(eta)
 [1] 3 3 3 3 3 3 3 3 3 3 3 3 3 3 3 3 3 3 3 3 2 2 2 2 2
>
> # use the inverse link function to define the mean
> mu = exp(eta)
> print(mu)
 [1] 20.085537 20.085537 20.085537 20.085537 20.085537 20.085537
 [7] 20.085537 20.085537 20.085537 20.085537 20.085537 20.085537
[13] 20.085537 20.085537 20.085537 20.085537 20.085537 20.085537
[19] 20.085537 20.085537  7.389056  7.389056  7.389056  7.389056
[25]  7.389056
>
> # generate Poisson response values (e.g. number of HIV cases
> # in a particular time period within a particular population)
> y=rpois(25,mu)
> print(y)
 [1] 25 20 15 12 22 20 15 30 22 21 23 17 17 13 22 22 15 19 19 27
[21]  4 10  8  8  3
>
> # using the glm function to fit the GLM to the data y and x
> myfit=glm(y~x,family=poisson(link="log"))
>
> # compare the estimates for intercept and slope
> # with the true value 3 and -1
> summary(myfit)

Call:
glm(formula = y ~ x, family = poisson(link = "log"))

Deviance Residuals:
    Min       1Q    Median        3Q       Max
-1.89246  -1.09261   0.04487   0.52721   2.12860

Coefficients:
              Estimate Std. Error z value Pr(>|z|)
```

(continued)

```
(continued)
(Intercept)   2.98568      0.05025   59.414  < 2e-16 ***
x            -1.09861      0.18119   -6.063 1.33e-09 ***
---
Signif. codes:  0 *** 0.001 ** 0.01 * 0.05 . 0.1   1

(Dispersion parameter for poisson family taken to be 1)

    Null deviance: 76.604  on 24  degrees of freedom
Residual deviance: 26.332  on 23  degrees of freedom
AIC: 144.74

Number of Fisher Scoring iterations: 4
```

The R output shows that the estimates 2.98568 and -1.09861 are quite close to the true values of the regression parameters $\beta_0 = 3$ and $\beta_1 = -1$. Further output includes deviance residuals (extending the classical residuals) and goodness-of-fit measures such as the residual deviance and AIC value. It also indicates that Fisher scoring was used and four iterations were needed to obtain convergence.

B.3   Profile Likelihood and Other Likelihoods

The likelihood paradigm has been extended in various ways leading to: composite likelihood, conditional likelihood, empirical likelihood, h-likelihood, marginal likelihood, nonparametric likelihood, partial likelihood, penalized likelihood, profile likelihood, pseudo likelihood, quasi likelihood, ..., Part of these extensions relax assumptions and cover extensions to multivariate response data but are no longer genuine likelihood methods, such as composite likelihood, pseudo likelihood, and quasi likelihood, etc. Others are likelihood methods that eliminate nuisance parameters: conditional likelihood, marginal likelihood, profile likelihood, and partial likelihood.

In what follows we briefly introduce the profile likelihood approach, and the construction of profile likelihood confidence intervals.

B.3.1   Profile Likelihood Estimation

Let $\ell(\theta, \eta)$ denote the loglikelihood for a parameter of interest θ and a nuisance parameter η. The profile likelihood for θ is

$$L_P(\theta) = L(\theta, \hat{\eta}(\theta)),$$

where $\hat{\eta}(\theta)$ is maximizing $L(\theta, \eta)$ for a fixed θ. So, $L_P(\theta) = \max_\eta L(\theta, \eta)$.

The profile likelihood estimator $\hat{\theta}_P$ for θ maximizes the profile likelihood or loglikelihood $\ell_p(\theta) = \log(L_P(\theta))$. Under certain conditions, the maximum profile likelihood estimator is equal to the ML estimator.

B.3.1.1   Profile Likelihood Estimator for μ for Normally Distributed Data

For fixed $\mu = \mu_{fixed}$, the MLE for σ^2 maximizing $\ell(\mu_{fixed}, \sigma^2)$ is

$$\hat{\sigma}^2(\mu_{fixed}) = \frac{1}{n} \sum_{i=1}^{n} (y_i - \mu_{fixed})^2.$$

Thus, the profile loglikelihood is given by

$$\ell_P(\mu) = \ell(\mu, \hat{\sigma}^2(\mu)) = -\frac{n}{2} \log(2\pi) - \frac{n}{2} \log\left(\frac{1}{n} \sum_{i=1}^{n} (y_i - \mu)^2\right) - \frac{n}{2}$$

which is maximized at $\hat{\mu}_P = \bar{y}$, which is also the MLE.

B.3.1.2   Profile Likelihood Estimator for the Slope β_1 for Logistic Regression

In this situation the intercept β_0 is considered as the nuisance parameter, and we use the profile loglikelihood function

$$\ell_P(\beta_1) = \max_{\beta_0} \ell(\beta_0, \beta_1).$$

This maximization requires us to fix β_1 and to maximize the loglikelihood over β_0. This can be done in R using the optimize function, as shown in the R-code below.

```
# Illustration profile likelihood for binary logistic regression
# using the optimize function

# defining the full loglikelihood
flogll=function(beta0,beta1){
n=length(d)
p=exp(beta0+beta1*age)/(1+exp(beta0+beta1*age))
sum(d*log(p))+sum((1-d)*log(1-p))
}
# defining the profile -(loglikelihood) for fixed beta1f
plogll=function(beta1f){
plogllh=function(beta0) -flogll(beta0,beta1f)
```

(continued)

```
(continued)
 optimize(plogllh,beta0,lower=-10,upper=10)$objective
}

# minimizing the profile -(loglikelihood) for beta1f
optimize(plogll,beta1f,lower=-0.2,upper=0.5)

# plotting the profile likelihood curve
betagrid=seq(0.13,0.25,by=0.001)
plogllgrid=rep(NA,length(betagrid))
for (i in (1:length(betagrid)))plogllgrid[i]=-plogll(betagrid[i])
plot(betagrid,plogllgrid,xlab="beta1",
                         ylab="profile loglikelihood",type="n")
lines(betagrid,plogllgrid)
fit=glm(d~age,family=binomial)
hatbeta1=fit$coef[2]
# plotting the estimate as a vertical dotted line
abline(v=hatbeta1,lty=3)
```

The R output shows the result of optimizing the profile loglikelihood for β_1 and Fig. B.1 shows the profile function $\ell_P(\beta_1)$ for $\beta_1 \in [-0.14, 0.24]$.

```
> optimize(p2logll,beta1f,lower=-0.2,upper=0.5)
$minimum
[1]  0.1888923
$objective
[1]  732.5021
```

B.3.2   Profile Likelihood Confidence Intervals

In general notation, the null hypothesis about the parameter of interest $H_0, \theta = \theta_0$ will not be rejected at the α level of significance if and only if

$$2\{\ell(\hat{\theta}, \hat{\eta}) - \ell(\theta_0, \hat{\eta}_0)\} = 2\{\ell(\hat{\theta}, \hat{\eta}) - \ell_p(\theta_0)\} < \chi^2_{1-\alpha}, \qquad (B.5)$$

where $\hat{\theta}$ and $\hat{\eta}$ are the MLEs for the full model, $\hat{\eta}_0$ for the reduced model with $\theta = \theta_0$, and $\chi^2_{1-\alpha}$ is that critical point of the χ^2_1-distribution with an area $1 - \alpha$ to the left or α to the right. Expression (B.5) can be expressed equivalently as

$$\ell_p(\theta_0) > \ell(\hat{\theta}, \hat{\eta}) - (\chi^2_{1-\alpha})/2. \qquad (B.6)$$

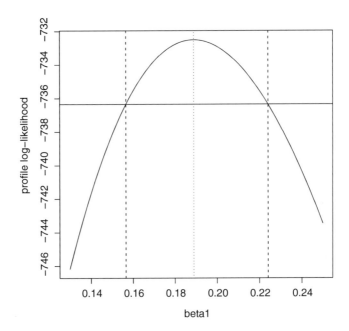

beta1

Fig. B.3 Belgian VZV data. Profile loglikelihood curve for the slope β_1 in the logistic regression model (B.3). The *dotted vertical line* represents the MLE. The *horizontal line* the threshold value defining the limits for the profile likelihood CI for β_1, given by the *dashed vertical lines*

A $(1 - \alpha)100\%$ confidence interval for θ can be defined by inverting the LRT: the CI equals the set of values θ_0 for θ that cannot be rejected as a null hypothesis $H_0 : \theta = \theta_0$. So the set of values θ_0 satisfying (B.6) defines the profile likelihood CI for θ.

The following R-code illustrates the computation of the profile likelihood confidence interval using the *uniroot* function, as well as its computation through the function *confint*. Figure B.3 shows the construction in a graphical way.

```
# computing the profile confidence interval for beta1f
cithreshold=logLik(fit)[1]-qchisq(0.95,1)
abline(h=cithreshold)

# profile confidence intervals using the confint function
confint.glm(fit,level=.95)
# for comparison, Wald type confidence intervals
confint.default(fit,level=.95)

profileci=function(beta1) -plogll(beta1)-cithreshold
pcil=uniroot(profileci,c(hatbeta1,hatbeta1+0.5))$root
pcir=uniroot(profileci,c(hatbeta1,hatbeta1-0.5))$root
```
                                                                    (continued)

```
(continued)
# plotting the confidence limits as dashed vertical lines
abline(v=pcil,lty=2)
abline(v=pcir,lty=2)
```

The corresponding R output

```
> confint(glm(d~age,family=binomial),level=.95)
Waiting for profiling to be done\ldots
                2.5 %      97.5 %
(Intercept) -0.2985224 0.1575799
age          0.1657261 0.2134456
```

B.4   The Bootstrap

Bootstrap methods are simulation based *resampling* techniques for assessing distributional properties of an estimator, such as bias, variability, quantiles, and percentiles. They are particularly useful when standard maximum likelihood inference is complex or unavailable, but they can also be applied to verify standard approximations (normal, χ^2, ...).

Consider the simple setting of a sample $y_1, \ldots, y_n$ from an unknown underlying distribution F. Interest is on estimation and inference about a parameter θ. A key principle, the bootstrap or *plug-in* principle, is to replace the unknown F with its known estimate $\hat{F}$, to imitate the original data generating mechanism ($y_1, \ldots, y_n$ from F) by generating, simulating bootstrap data, denoted as $y_1^*, \ldots, y_n^*$ from $\hat{F}$, and to recompute the estimate for this bootstrap sample, denoted by $\hat{\theta}^*$. As $\hat{F}$ is known, we can simulate such bootstrap data repeatedly (say $B = 999$ times), get B copies $\hat{\theta}_1^*, \ldots, \hat{\theta}_B^*$, and empirically observe distributional characteristics. It has been shown that in many cases, this bootstrap approximation is an appropriate approximation of the true distribution, and that it might even be superior to the typical normal or χ^2 approximation. It has also been illustrated however that there are settings in which the standard application of the bootstrap principle fails. In the next section, we briefly introduce and illustrate the nonparametric and parametric bootstrap in R using the *boot* function.

The bootstrap can be used to simulate the null distribution of certain test statistics, or to compute confidence intervals for a particular parameter. We will focus on the latter. For more reading on this topic, we refer to Davison and Hinkley (1997); Efron and Tibshirani (1993), and for a more mathematical survey to Shao and Tu (1995). Hall (1992) describes the underlying theory.

B.4.1   Bootstrap Confidence Intervals

The simplest type of bootstrap CI is the *normal bootstrap* CI, which in its most basic form replaces the normal critical points by quantiles of the simulated normal distribution. It might also include a bias correction and a studentization. The $(1 - \alpha)100\%$ *basic bootstrap* CI uses the confidence limits

$$\hat{\theta} - (\hat{\theta}^*_{((R+1)(1-\alpha/2)} - \hat{\theta}), \hat{\theta} - (\hat{\theta}^*_{((R+1)\alpha/2)} - \hat{\theta}),$$

where $\hat{\theta}^*_{(1)} < \ldots < \hat{\theta}^*_{(B)}$ are the sorted $\hat{\theta}^*$'s. The *percentile bootstrap* CI is given by

$$\hat{\theta}^*_{((R+1)\alpha/2)}, \hat{\theta}^*_{((R+1)(1-\alpha/2)}.$$

The percentile bootstrap CI shares, together with its improved version, the *bias-corrected adjusted bootstrap* CI, the attractive property of invariance to transformations of the parameters. For more discussion on the pros and cons of the different bootstrap CI, we refer to Davison and Hinkley (1997).

B.4.2   Nonparametric Bootstrap

In the nonparametric bootstrap, we generate bootstrap data $y_1^*, \ldots, y_n^*$ from the empirical distribution function (EDF) $\hat{F}_{EDF}$. This estimate $\hat{F}_{EDF}$, which puts mass $1/n$ on each of the observed y_i, is a nonparametric estimator for the unknown distribution function F. It is known to be a consistent estimator for F (under some mild regularity conditions). Generating data from the EDF is nothing else than sampling from the original data $y_1, \ldots, y_n$ with replacement, so it is *resampling* the original sample (a bit as recycling). In R it is easy to resample data using the *sample* function, but the *boot* function does it all for you, including the computation of bootstrap confidence intervals.

The following R-code provides confidence intervals for the mean antibody level, the prevalence for VZV, as well as for the slope parameter in the logistic regression model (B.3) with covariate age. The number of bootstrap replicates was taken as $B = 999$. For the estimation of quantiles of the distribution F, $B = 999$ bootstrap runs is considered to be a minimum number. For the estimation of moments such as the variance, 500 or even 250 runs could be sufficient.

```
# nonparametric bootstrap
library(boot)

# for the mean antibody level
meanstat=function(data,indices){
```

(continued)

```
(continued)
 data=data[indices]
 mean(data)
}
mub=boot(z,meanstat,R=999)
boot.ci(mub,type = c("norm","basic","perc"))

# for the prevalence
pib=boot(d,meanstat,R=999)
boot.ci(pib,type = c("norm","basic","perc"))

# for the effect of age
slope=function(data,indices){
 data=data[indices,]
 d=data[,2]
 age=data[,1]
 fit=glm(d~age,family=binomial)
 fit$coef[2]
}
data=data.frame(cbind(age,d))
slopeb=boot(data,slope,R=999)
boot.ci(slopeb,type = c("norm","basic","perc"))
```

The R output

```
> boot.ci(mub,type = c("norm","basic","perc"))
BOOTSTRAP CONFIDENCE INTERVAL CALCULATIONS
Based on 999 bootstrap replicates
CALL :
boot.ci(boot.out = mub, type = c("norm", "basic", "perc"))
Intervals :
Level      Normal                Basic             Percentile
95%   ( 5.872,  5.994 )    ( 5.869,  5.993 )   ( 5.874,  5.997 )
Calculations and Intervals on Original Scale

> boot.ci(pib,type = c("norm","basic","perc"))
BOOTSTRAP CONFIDENCE INTERVAL CALCULATIONS
Based on 999 bootstrap replicates
CALL :
boot.ci(boot.out = pib, type = c("norm", "basic", "perc"))
Intervals :
Level     Normal                Basic             Percentile
95%    (0.8735,  0.8977)   (0.8739,  0.8980)   (0.8731,  0.8972)
Calculations and Intervals on Original Scale
```

(continued)

```
(continued)
> boot.ci(slopeb,type = c("norm","basic","perc"))
BOOTSTRAP CONFIDENCE INTERVAL CALCULATIONS
Based on 999 bootstrap replicates
CALL :
boot.ci(boot.out = slopeb, type = c("norm", "basic", "perc"))
Intervals :
Level       Normal                 Basic                Percentile
95%    (0.1537,  0.2222)     (0.1503,  0.2202)     (0.1576,  0.2275)
Calculations and Intervals on Original Scale
```

B.4.3   Parametric Bootstrap

In contrast to the nonparametric bootstrap, one has to assume a particular parametric distribution (with estimated parameters) $\hat{F}$ to generate the bootstrap data. In the R-code below we illustrate two parametric bootstrap applications: $z_1^*, \ldots, z_n^*$ when generated (1) from the $N(\bar{z}, s_{\bar{z}}^2)$ distribution, and (2) from the Uniform$(0, \bar{z})$ distribution. The first choice is a reasonable one, the second one clearly not. The choice of an appropriate distribution is of course crucial, and misspecification of the generating distribution might lead to substantial bias. The text file C:/Bayeslogistic.txt contains the R code for the logistic regression model (in winbugs type of programming syntax).

```
# parametric bootstrap for the mean antibody level

# Function to generate normal data; mle will contain
# the mean and standard deviation of the original data
z.rg1=function(data,mle){
out=data
out=rnorm(length(out),mle[[1]],mle[[2]])
out
}
mub=boot(z,meanstat,sim="parametric",ran.gen=z.rg1,
         mle=list(mn=mean(z),sd=sqrt(var(z)))  ,R=999)
boot.ci(mub,type = c("norm","basic","perc"))

# Function to generate uniform data, obviously a bad choice!
z.rg2=function(data,mle){
out=data
out=runif(length(out),0,mle)
out
}
mub=boot(z,meanstat,sim="parametric",ran.gen=z.rg2,
                        mle=mean(z),R=999)
boot.ci(mub,type = c("norm","basic","perc"))
```

The R output for the normal distribution is in line with earlier results

```
> boot.ci(mub,type = c("norm","basic","perc"))
BOOTSTRAP CONFIDENCE INTERVAL CALCULATIONS
Based on 999 bootstrap replicates
CALL :
boot.ci(boot.out = mub, type = c("norm", "basic", "perc"))
Intervals :
Level       Normal                Basic                 Percentile
95%    ( 5.875,  5.992 )     ( 5.876,  5.990 )     ( 5.877,  5.991 )
Calculations and Intervals on Original Scale
```

which is clearly not the case when assuming a totally wrong uniform distribution.

```
> boot.ci(mub,type = c("norm","basic","perc"))
BOOTSTRAP CONFIDENCE INTERVAL CALCULATIONS
Based on 999 bootstrap replicates
CALL :
boot.ci(boot.out = mub, type = c("norm", "basic", "perc"))
Intervals :
Level       Normal                Basic                 Percentile
95%    ( 8.840,  8.965 )     ( 8.841,  8.968 )     ( 2.898,  3.025 )
Calculations and Intervals on Original Scale
```

B.4.3.1 Other Bootstraps

Next to the nonparametric and parametric bootstrap schemes, there are several other options, including semiparametric bootstrap, wild bootstrap, residual bootstrap, smoothed bootstrap, Bayesian bootstrap, iterated bootstrap, weighted bootstrap, etc. Further information, details, and examples can be found in Davison and Hinkley (1997).

B.5 Bayesian Methodology

Whereas frequentist methods assume that unknown parameters are fixed constants, Bayesian methods offer an alternative approach by treating parameters as random variables such that one can make probability statements about parameters. Probabilities are not interpreted as limiting relative frequencies but rather as *degrees of belief*. A Bayesian is a scientist who believes that a parameter θ cannot be determined exactly, but he can represent his prior information on the parameter by a *prior probability distribution*, can update this prior information by combining it with the data through the calculation of a *posterior distribution*. The key to combine prior distribution(s) with data is Bayes' theorem. An elaborate discussion about Bayesian analysis and hierarchical Bayesian modeling can be found in Gelman et al. (2010) and Gilks et al. (1996).

Consider again that you have data $y = (y_1, \ldots, y_n)$ and that you are interested in estimating a parameter θ. The essential components of a Bayesian analysis are:

The prior: specification of a prior distribution $f(\theta)$ for θ. This prior ranges from very informative to noninformative (also called "vague," "diffuse," or "flat"). A noninformative prior assigns equal likelihood on all possible values of the parameter, whereas an informative prior can have a substantial to major impact on the posterior distribution. Jeffreys' prior provides a way to define an optimal noninformative prior for a parametric model. If informative, prior distributions have to be selected with care, but proper use of prior information is the power of Bayesian methods. Some of the prior distributions are conjugate, such that the posterior distribution belongs to the same family as the prior distribution. These types of priors are computationally convenient to obtain the posterior, but are not central to posterior sampling.

The data: specification of a model $f(y|\theta)$ for the data y given θ: **the likelihood**.

The update to the posterior: combining prior with data by Bayes' theorem

$$f(\theta|y) = \frac{f(y|\theta)f(\theta)}{\int f(y|\theta)f(\theta)d\theta},$$

or, posterior is proportional to likelihood $\times$ prior:

$$f(\theta|y) \propto L(\theta)\pi(\theta).$$

All inferences follow from the posterior distribution $f(\theta|y)$ (posterior mean, posterior mode, and credible intervals), but most analyses require Markov Chain Monte Carlo (MCMC) for sampling from posterior distributions in order to compute posterior quantities of interest. To minimize the effect of initial values, the practice of burn-in discards the initial portion of the chain.

In Bayesian statistics, *credible intervals* play a similar role as confidence intervals in the frequentist paradigm. A $(1 - \alpha)100\%$ credible interval for θ is defined as a set I such that

$$P(\theta \in I|y) = \int_I f(\theta|y)d\theta = 1 - \alpha.$$

It can be constructed to have equal tails through the $(\alpha/2)100\%$ and $(1-\alpha/2)100\%$ quantiles of the posterior distribution $f(\theta|y)$. This approach has the nice property to be invariant under monotone transformations. Another choice is the highest posterior density interval which leads to the smallest intervals.

Bayesian Estimation of Binomial Parameter

Consider again the estimation of the probability π to be infected with VZV, but now in the Bayesian way. A natural (conjugate) prior for π is the beta distribution with parameters $\alpha, \beta > 0$:

$$f(\pi) \propto \pi^{\alpha-1}(1-\pi)^{\beta-1}.$$

A beta distribution with parameters α and β has mean $\alpha/(\alpha+\beta)$, variance $\alpha\beta/[(\alpha+\beta)^2(\alpha+\beta+1)]$ and reaches a single mode at $(\alpha-1)/(\alpha+\beta-2)$. The likelihood, given the data $(y_1,\ldots,y_n)$, is given by

$$L(y|\pi) \propto \pi^{\Sigma_i y_i}(1-\pi)^{n-\Sigma_i y_i},$$

which combined with the prior leads to the posterior

$$f(\pi|y) \propto \pi^{\alpha-1}(1-\pi)^{\beta-1}\pi^{\Sigma_i y_i}(1-\pi)^{n-\Sigma_i y_i},$$

or

$$f(\pi|y) \propto \pi^{\Sigma_i y_i+\alpha-1}(1-\pi)^{n-\Sigma_i y_i+\beta-1}.$$

This is again a beta distribution with parameters $\Sigma_i y_i + \alpha$ and $n - \Sigma_i y_i + \beta$. The following table gives an overview of the MLE, the standard error of the MLE, the posterior mode (also called the generalized MLE), the posterior mean, and the standard deviation of the posterior describing the accuracy. Table B.2 shows these estimates in general for a general beta prior and for the special case of the uniform prior ($\alpha = \beta = 1$). For the uniform prior, this table shows that the posterior mode coincides with the MLE and that the posterior mean and variance are different, but the differences are negligible for n large. When letting $\alpha \to \infty$, the beta prior gets very informative with a value approaching the value of 1. In this case the prior dominates the data, as posterior mode, posterior mean both tend to 1 (whatever the data are), and the posterior variance tends to zero. So the posterior fully follows the prior.

Table B.3 shows estimates for the VZV infection indicator for which $\Sigma_i d_i = 2{,}352$ and $n = 2{,}656$. All results are strikingly similar, even for a very informative prior with $\alpha = 100$ en $\beta = 1$ (mean prior is 0.99 with variance 0.000096). The reason that the prior does not dominate the data in the VZV example is the very large sample size. So the impact of the prior not only depends on the prior itself but also on the particular sample at hand and its size.

Table B.2 Estimation of a binomial parameter: comparison between the MLE and Bayesian estimates for the probability of success

Maximum likelihood estimate	$p = \frac{\sum_i y_i}{n}$	
Variance of MLE	$\frac{p(1-p)}{n}$	
Bayes estimates	$\alpha, \beta > 0$	$\alpha = \beta = 1$
Posterior mode	$\frac{\sum_i y_i + \alpha - 1}{n + \alpha + \beta - 2}$	$p = \frac{\sum_i y_i}{n}$
Posterior mean	$\frac{\sum_i y_i + \alpha}{n + \alpha + \beta}$	$\frac{p + 1/n}{1 + 2/n}$
Posterior variance	$\frac{(\sum_i y_i + \alpha)(n - \sum_i y_i + \beta)}{(n+\alpha+\beta)^2(n+\alpha+\beta+1)}$	$\frac{(p+1/n)(1-p+1/n)}{(n+2)^2(n+3)/n}$

The left lower part shows Bayesian estimates for an arbitrary beta prior; the right part for the uniform prior

Table B.3 Belgian VZV data. Estimation of the probability to be infected by VZV: comparison between the MLE and Bayesian estimates for the probability of success

Maximum likelihood estimate	0.8855	
Variance of MLE	0.000038	
Bayes estimates	$\alpha = 100, \beta = 1$	$\alpha = \beta = 1$
Posterior mode	0.8897	0.8855
Posterior mean	0.8894	0.8853
Posterior variance	0.000036	0.000038

The left lower part shows Bayesian estimates for the highly informative beta prior with $\alpha = 100, \beta = 1$; the right part for the flat uniform prior

We end this section with an illustration of the dependency of the probability to be infected with VZV on age by means of a logistic regression model (as before). The R-code below illustrates the use of the packages *rjags* and *R2jags*. These packages provide an interface to the JAGS MCMC library. JAGS is *Just Another Gibbs Sampler*. It is a program for analysis of Bayesian hierarchical models using MCMC simulation similar to BUGS. In the application the priors for the regression parameters β_0 and β_1 are taken as uninformative normal priors with mean 0 and very large variance 10^6.

```
library(rjags)
library(R2jags)

model.file="C:/Bayeslogistic.txt"

beta0i=mean(d)
beta1i=0
inits=function(){list(beta0=beta0i,beta1=beta1i)}
```
                                                                  (continued)

```
(continued)
N=length(d)
data=list("d","age","N")
parameters=c("beta0","beta1")
set.seed(1234)
jagsfit = jags(data=data, n.chains=2, inits=inits, parameters,
               n.burnin=5000, n.iter=10000, n.thin=5, n.sims = 2000,
               model.file=model.file)

traceplot(jagsfit)
jagsfit$BUGSoutput$summary
```

The file *C:/Bayeslogistic.txt* contains the logistic regression model. specification (in winbugs type of programming language).

```
model {
for( i in 1 : N) {
d[i] ~ dbern(p[i])
logit(p[i]) = beta0 + beta1 * age[i]
           }
beta0 ~ dnorm(0.0,1.0E-6)
beta1 ~ dnorm(0.0,1.0E-6)
}
```

The R output shows the following estimates for the slope β_1: posterior mean 0.1895 and posterior standard deviation 0.0121, which are very close to the corresponding MLEs; posterior mode 0.1893 and 95% credible interval [0.1661,0.2136], also very close to the profile likelihood CI.

```
> jagsfit$BUGSoutput$summary
               mean          sd         2.5%          25%          50%
beta0   -0.0723162  0.11494075   -0.3068040   -0.1471738   -0.07228818
beta1    0.1895055  0.01207152    0.1661102    0.1812876    0.18928988
               75%         97.5%        Rhat    n.eff
beta0  0.007902071   0.1454689    1.001606    1400
beta1  0.197191626   0.2135639    1.000550    2000
```

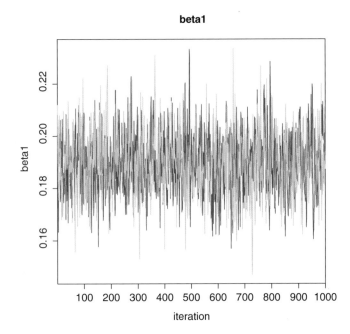

beta1

Fig. B.4 Belgian VZV data. Trace plots of two chains of the Bayesian application of the logistic regression model (B.3)

Figure B.4 shows traceplots for part of the two chains as a diagnostic way to check convergence of the MCMC algorithm. Similar analysis can be conducted using the R package R2WinBUGS Sturtz et al. (2005).

References

Aalen O (1988) Heterogeneity in survival analysis. Stat Med 7:1121–1137

Ades A, Medley G (1994) Estimates of disease incidence in women based on antenatal or neonatal seroprevalence data: HIV in New York City. Stat Med 13:1881–1894

Ades AE, Nokes DJ (1993) Modeling age- and time-specific incidence from seroprevalence:toxoplasmosis. Am J Epidemiol 137(9):1022–1034

Aerts M, Claeskens G, Hart J (1999) Testing the fit of a parametric function. J Am Stat Assoc 94:869–879

Aerts M, Claeskens G, Hart J (2000) Testing lack of fit in multiple regression. Biometrika 87(2):405–424

Agresti A (2002) Categorical data analysis, 2nd edn. Wiley, Hoboken,

Akaike H (1973) Information theory and an extension of the maximum likelihood principle. In: Petrov B, Csaki F (eds) 2nd international symposium on information theory, pp 267–281. Akademia Kiado, Budapest

Alberti A, and others (Jury Panel) (2005) Short statement of the first European consensus conference on the treatment of chronic hepatitis B and C in HIV-co-infected patients. J Hepatol 42:615–624

Anderson R (1988) The epidemiology of HIV infection: variable incubation plus infectious period and heterogeneity in sexual activity. J Roy Stat Soc B 151:66–93

Anderson D, Aitkin M (1985) Variance component models with binary response: interviewer variability. J Roy Stat Soc B 47:203–210

Andersson H, Britton T (2000) Stochastic epidemic models and their statistical analysis. In: Lecture notes in statistics, vol 151. Springer, Berlin

Anderson R, May R (1991) Infectious diseases of humans: dynamics and control. Oxford University Press, Oxford

Bailey N (1975) The mathematical theory of infectious diseases and its applications. Charles Griffin and Company, London

Baker R (2002) Natural history of hepatitis C. Technical report, NIH consensus report on hepatitis C, Bethesda, Maryland

Barlow RE, Bartholomew DJ, Bremner JM, Brunk HD (1972) Statistical inference under order restrictions. Wiley, New York

Batter V, Matela B, Nsuami M, MT, Kamenga M, Behets F, Ryder R, Heyward W, Karon J, St Louis M (1994) High HIV-1 incidence in young women masked by stable overall seroprevalence in young childbearing women in Kinshasa, Zaire: estimating incidence from seroprevalence data. AIDS 8:811–817

Becker NG (1989) Analysis of infectious disease data. Chapman and Hall, London

N. Hens et al., *Modeling Infectious Disease Parameters Based on Serological and Social Contact Data*, Statistics for Biology and Health 63, DOI 10.1007/978-1-4614-4072-7, © Springer Science+Business Media New York 2012

Bernoulli D (1766) Essai d'une nouvelle analyse de la mortalité causée par la petite vérole et des advantages de línoculation pour la prévenir. Mém Math Phys Acad Roy Sci pp 1–45

Beutels P, Shkedy Z, Mukomolov S, Aerts M, Shargorodskaya E, Plotnikova V, Molenberghs G, Van Damme P (2003) Hepatitis B in St Petersburg, Russia (1994–1999): incidence, prevalence and force of infection. J Viral Hepat 10:141–149

Beutels P, Shkedy Z, Aerts M, Van Damme P (2006) Social mixing patterns for transmission models of close contact infections: exploring self-evaluation and diary-based data collection through a web-based interface. Epidemiol Infect 134:1158–1166

Beutels M, Van Damme P, Aelvoet W, Desmyter J, Dondeyne F, Goilav C, Mak R, Muylle L, Pierard D, Stroobant A, Van Loock F, Waumans P, Vranckx R (1997) Prevalence of hepatitis A, B and C in the Flemish population. Eur J Epidemiol 13:275–280. doi: 10.1023/A: 1007393405966

Bollaerts K, Aerts M, Hens N, Shkedy Z, Faes C, Van Damme P, Beutels P (2012) Estimating the force of infection directly from antibody levels. Technical report, Center for Statistics, Hasselt University. In press by Statistical Modelling

Bollaerts K, Eilers P, Van Mechelen I (2006) Simple and multiple P-spline regression with shape constraints. Br J Math Stat Psychol 59:451–469

Bordes L, Chauveau D, Vandekerkhove P (2007) A stochastic EM algorithm for a semiparametric mixture model. Comput Stat Data Anal 51:5429–5443

Bowman A, Azzalini A (1997) Applied smoothing techniques for data analysis: the kernel approach with S-plus illustrations. Oxford University Press, Oxford

Breslow N, Clayton D (1993) Approximate inference in generalized linear mixed models. J Am Stat Assoc 88:9–25

Brisson M, Edmunds WJ, Gay NJ, Law B, De Serres G (2000) Modelling the impact of immunization on the epidemiology of varicella zoster virus. Epidemiol Infect 125, 651–669

Brisson M, Melkonyan G, Drolet M, Serres GD, Thibeault R, Wals PD (2010) Modeling the impact of one- and two-dose varicella vaccination on the epidemiology of varicella and zoster. Vaccine 28(19):3385–3397. doi: 10.1016/j.vaccine.2010.02.079

Broliden K, Tolfvenstam T, Norbeck O (2006) Clinical aspects of parvovirus B19 infection. J Intern Med 260:285–304

Burnham K, Anderson D (2002) Model selection and multi-model inference: a practical information-theoretic approach. Springer, New York

Capasso V (2008) Mathematical structures of epidemic systems. Springer, Berlin

Cauchemez S, Carrat F, Viboud C, Valleron AJ, Boëlle PY (2004) A Bayesian MCMC approach to study transmission of influenza: application to household longitudinal data. Stat Med 23: 3469–3487

Chambers J, Hastie T (1992) Statistical models in S. Wadsworth & Brooks, Belmont, CA

Congdon P (2003) Applied Bayesian modeling. Wiley, Chichester

Coutinho F, Massad E, Lopez L, Burattini M, Struchiner C, Azevedo-Neto R (1999) Modelling heterogeneities in individual frailties in epidemic models. Math Comput Model 30:97–115

Cruz-Medina I, Hettmansperger T, Thomas H (2004) Semiparametric mixture models and repeated measures: the multinomial cut point model. Appl Stat 53:463–474

Currie I, Durban M (2002) Flexible smoothing with P-splines: an unified approach. Stat Model 4:333–349

Dale JR (1986) Global cross-ratio models for bivariate, discrete, ordered responses. Biometrics 42:909–917

d'Alembert J (1761) Opuscules Mathématiques t. 2, David, Paris, Sur l'application du calcul des probabilités à l'inoculation de la petite vérole, p 26

Daley D, Gani J (1999) Epidemic modelling: an introduction. Cambridge University Press, Cambridge, MA

Davison AC, Hinkley DV (1997) Bootstrap methods and their application. Cambridge University Press, Cambridge, MA

de Boor C (1978) A practical guide to splines. Springer, New York.

de Jong M, Diekmann O, Heesterbeek H (1995) Epidemic models: their structure and relation to data. How does transmission of infection depend on population size? Press Syndicate of the University of Cambridge, Cambridge, pp 84–94

De Leeuw J, Hornik K, Mair P (2009) Isotone Optimization in R/ Pool-Adjacent-Violators Algorithm (PAVA) and Active Set Methods. J Stat Software 32(5):1–24

Del Fava E, Shkedy Z, Hens N, Aerts M, Suligoi B, Camoni L, Vallejo F, Wiessing L, and Kretzschmar M (2011) Joint modeling of HCV and HIV co-infection among injecting drug users in Italy and Spain using individual cross-sectional data. Statistical Communications in Infectious Diseases 3(1):3. Doi: 10.2202/1948-4690.1010

Diamond LD, McDonald JM (1992) Demographic application of event history analysis. Analysis of current-status data. Oxford University Press, Oxford

Diekmann O, Heesterbeek J (2000) Mathematical methodology of infectious diseases: model building, analysis and interpretation. Wiley, West Sussex

Diekmann O, Heesterbeek J, Metz J (1990) On the definition and the computation of the basic reproduction ratio R_0 in models for infectious diseases in heterogeneous populations. J Math Biol 28:65–382. doi: 10.1007/BF00178324

Dietz K (1993) The estimation of the basic reproduction number for infectious diseases. Stat Methods Med Res 2:23–41

Dietz K, Schenzle D (1985) Proportionate mixing models for age-dependent infection transmission. Math Biosci 22:117–120

Diggle P (1990) Time Series, A Biostatistical Introduction. Oxford University Press, Oxford

Dobson A (2002) An introduction to generalized linear models. Chapman and Hall, London

Duchateau L, Janssen P (2008) The frailty model. Springer, Berlin

Edmunds W, Gay N, Kretzschmar M, Pebody R, Wachmann H (2000a) The prevaccination epidemiology of measles, mumps and rubella in Europe: implications for modeling studies. Epidemiol infect 125:635–650

Edmunds W, Kafatos G, Wallinga J, Mossong J (2006) Mixing patterns and the spread of close-contact infectious diseases. Emerging Themes in Epidemiology 3(10)

Edmunds WJ, Medley GF, Nokes DJ (1993) The influence of age on the development of the hepatitis B carrier state. Proc Roy Soc Lond B Biol Sci 253:197–201

Edmunds W, O'Callaghan C, Nokes D (1997) Who mixes with whom? A method to determine the contact patterns of adults that may lead to the spread of airborne infections. Proc Roy Soc Lond B Biol Sci 264:949–957

Edmunds WJ, Pebody RG, Aggerback H, Baron S, Berbers G, Conyn-van Spaendonck MA, Hallander HO, Olander R, Maple PA, Melker HE, Olin P, Fievret-Groyne F, Rota C, Salmaso S, Tischer A, von Hunolstein C, Miller E (2000b) The sero-epidemiology of diphtheria in western europe. ESEN project. european sero-epidemiology network. Epidemiol Infect 125(1):113–125

Efromovich S (1999) Nonparametric curve estimation: methods, theory and applications. Springer, Berlin

Efron B, Tibshirani R (1993) An introduction to the bootstrap. Chapman and Hall, New York

Eichner M, Zehnder S, Dietz K (1996) Models for infectious human diseases: their structure and relation to data. An age-structured model for measles vaccination, Cambridge University Press, Cambridge, UK, pp 38–56

Eilers P, Currie I, Durban M (2006) Fast and compact smoothing on large multidimensional grids. Comput Stat Data Anal 50:61–76

Eilers PHC, Marx BD (1996) Flexible smoothing with B-splines and penalties (with discussion). Stat Sci 89:89–121

Erkanli A, Soyer R, Costello E (1999) Bayesian inference for prevalence in longitudinal two-phase studies. Biometrics 55:1145–1150

Evans R, Erlandson K (2004) Robust Bayesian prediction of subject disease status and population prevalence using several similar diagnostic tests. Stat Med 23:2227–2236

Faes C, Geys H, Aerts M, Molenberghs G (2003) On the use of fractional polynomial predictors for quantitative risk assessment in developmental toxicity studies. Stat Model 3:109–126

Fan J, Gijbels I (1996) Local polynomial modelling and its applications. Chapman and Hall, London

Farrington C (2008) Modelling epidemics. The Open University, Milton Keynes.

Farrington C, Whitaker H (2005) Contact surface models for infectious diseases: estimation from serologic survey data. J Am Stat Assoc 100:370–379

Farrington C, Kanaan M, Gay N (2001) Estimation of the basic reproduction number for infectious diseases from age-stratified serological survey data. Appl Stat 50:251–292. doi: 10.1111/1467-9876.00233

Farrington CP (1990) Modeling forces of infection for measles, mumps and rubella. Stat Med 9:953–967

Friedman J, Silverman B (1989) Flexible parsimonious smoothing and additive modelling. Technometrics 31:3–39

Friedman J, Tibshirani R (1984) The monotone smoothing of scatterplots. Technometrics 31:3–39

Gay N, Vyse A, Enquselassie F, Nigatu W, Nokes D (2003) Improving sensitivity of oral fluid testing in igg prevalence studies: application of mixture models to a rubella antibody survey. Epidemiol Infec 130:285–291

Gelfand A, Kuo L (1991) Nonparametric Bayesian bioassay including ordered polytomous response. Biometrika 78:657–666

Gelfand A, Ecker M, Christiansen C, Mclaughlin T, Soumerai S (2000) Conditional categorical response with application to treatment of acute myocardial infraction. Appl Stat 49:171–186

Gelfand A, Smith A, Lee T (1992) Bayesian analysis of constrained parameters and truncated data problems using Gibbs sampling. J Am Stat Assoc 87:523–532

Gelman A (1996) Markov chain Monte Carlo in practice. Inference and monitoring convergence. Chapman and Hall, London

Gelman A, Carlin J, Stern H, Rubin D (1995) Bayesian data analysis. Chapman & Hall, London

Gelman A, Carlin JB, Stern HS, Rubin D (2010) Bayesian Data Analysis (second edition), Chapman and Hall/CRC

Gilks WR, Richardson S, Spiegelhalter DJ (1996) Markov Chain Monte Carlo in Practice, Chapman and Hall/CRC

Gilks W, Richardson S, Spiegelhalter D (1996) Markov chain Monte Carlo in practice. Chapman and Hall, London

Goeyvaerts N, Hens N, Ogunjimi B, Aerts M, Shkedy Z, Van Damme P, Beutels P (2010) Estimating infectious disease parameters from data on social contacts and serological status. J Roy Stat Soc C 59:255–277

Goeyvaerts N, Hens N, Aerts M, Beutels P (2011) Model structure analysis to estimate basic immunological processes and maternal risk for parvovirus b19. Biostatistics 12(2):283–302. doi: 10.1093/biostatistics/kxq059

Green P, Silverman B (1994) Nonparametric regression and generalized linear models. Chapman and Hall, London

Greenhalgh D, Dietz K (1994) Some bounds on estimates for reproductive ratios derived from the age-specific force of infection. Math Biosci 124:9–57

Grenfell BT, Anderson RM (1985) The estimation of age-related rates of infection from case notifications and serological data. J Hyg 95(2):419–36

Griffiths D (1974) A catalytic model of infection for measles. Appl Stat 23:330–339

Grummer-Strawn LM (1993) Regression analysis of current status data: an application to breast feeding. Biometrika 72:527–537

Hadler S (1991) Viral hepatitis and liver disease, Global impact of hepatitis A virus infection: changing patterns, Williams & Wilkins, Baltimore, MD, pp 14–20

Hall P (1992) The bootstrap and edgeworth expansion. Springer, New York

Halloran E, Longini I, Struchiner C (2010) Design and analysis of vaccine studies. Springer, Berlin

Hamer W (1906) Epidemic disease in England—the evidence of variability and of persistency of type. Lancet 1:733–739

Hardelid P, Williams D, Dezateux C, Tookey P, Peckham C, Cubitt W, Cortina-Borja M (2008) Analysis of rubella antibody distribution from new born dried blood spots using finite mixture models. Epidemiol Infect 136:1698–1706

Hastie T, Tibshirani R (1990) Generalized additive models. Chapman and Hall, London

Healy M, Tillett H (1988) Short-term extrapolation of the AIDS epidemic. J Roy Stat Soc A 151: 50–61

Hens N, Aerts M, Shkedy Z, Kung'U Kimani P, Kojouhorova M, Van Damme P, Beutels P (2008a) Estimating the impact of vaccination using agetime-dependent incidence rates of hepatitis B. Epidemiol Infect 136(3):341–351

Hens N, Aerts M, Shkedy Z, Theeten H, Van Damme P, Beutels P (2008b) Modelling multi-sera data: the estimation of new joint and conditional epidemiological parameters. Stat Med 27: 2651–2664. doi: 10.1002/sim.3089

Hens N, Ayele GM, Goeyvaerts N, Aerts M, Mossong J, Edmunds JW, Beutels P (2009a) Estimating the impact of school closure on social mixing behaviour and the transmission of close contact infections in eight European countries. BMC Infect Dis 9:187. doi: 10.1186/1471-2334-9-187

Hens N, Goeyvaerts N, Aerts M, Shkedy Z, Damme PV, Beutels P (2009b) Mining social mixing patterns for infectious disease models based on a two-day population survey in belgium. BMC Infect Dis 9:5. doi: 10.1186/1471-2334-9-5

Hens N, Aerts M, Faes C, Shkedy Z, Lejeune O, Damme PV, Beutels P (2010a) Seventy-five years of estimating the force of infection from current status data. Epidemiol Infect 138(6):802–812. doi: 10.1017/S0950268809990781

Hens N, Kvitkovicova A, Aerts M, Hlubinka D, Beutels P (2010b) Modelling distortions in seroprevalence data using change-point fractional polynomials. Stat Model 10:159–175

Hethcote H, Van Ark J (1987) Epidemiological models for heterogeneous populations: proportionate mxing, parameter estimation and immunization programs. Math Biosci 84:85–118

Hougaard P (2000) Analysis of multivariate survival data. Springer, New York

Isham V (1988) Mathematical modeling of the transmission dynamics of HIV infection and AIDS: a review. J Roy Stat Soc A 151:50–61

Isham V, Medley G (eds) (1996) Models for infectious human diseases. Their structure and relation to data. Publications of the Newton Institute, Cambridge

Jewell NP, Van Der Laan M (1995) Generalizations of current status data with applications. Lifetime Data Anal 1:101–109

Kanaan M, Farrington C (2005) Matrix models for childhood infections: a Bayesian approach with applications to rubella and mumps. Epidemiol Infect 133:1009–1021

Keeling M, Rohani P (2008) Modeling infectious diseases in humans and animals. Princeton University Press, Princeton, NJ

Keiding N (1991) Age-specific incidence and prevalence: a statistical perspective (with discussion). J Roy Stat Soc A 154:371–412

Keiding N, Begtrup K, Scheike TH, Hasibeder G (1996) Estimation from current status data in continuous time. Lifetime Data Anal 2:119–129

Kermack WO, McKendrick AG (1927) A contribution to the mathematical theory of epidemics. Proc Roy Soc Lond A 115:700–721

Kermack WO, McKendrick AG (1932) Contributions to the mathematical theory of epidemics ii. The problem of endemicity. Proc Roy Soc Lond A 138:55–83

Kermack WO, McKendrick AG (1933) Contributions to the mathematical theory of epidemics. iii. Further studies of the problem of endemicity. Proc Roy Soc Lond A 141:94–122

Krämer A, Kretzchmar M, Krickeberg K (eds) (2010) Modern infectious disease epidemiology: concepts, methods, mathematical models, and public health. Springer, Berlin

Kretzschmar M, Teunis PFM, Pebody RG (2010) Incidence and reproduction numbers of pertussis: estimates from serological and social contact data in five european countries. PLoS Med 7(6): e1000291. doi: 10.1371/journal.pmed.1000291. URL http://dx.doi.org/10.1371/journal.pmed.1000291

Krivobokova T, Crainiceanu C, Kauermann G (2008) Fast adaptive penalized splines. J Comput Graph Stat 17(1):1–20

Leitenstorfer F, Tutz G (2007) Generalized monotonic regression based on B-splines with an application to air pollution data. Biostatistics 8:654–673

Leuridan E, Hens N, Hutse V, Ieven M, Aerts M, Van Damme P (2010) Early waning of maternal measles antibodies in the era of global measles vaccination. Br Med J 340:c1626

Leuridan E, Hens N, Hutse V, Aerts M, Damme PV (2011) Kinetics of maternal antibodies against rubella and varicella in infants. Vaccine 29(11):2222–2226. doi: 10.1016/j.vaccine.2010.06.004

Liang K, Zeger S, Qaqish B (1992) Multivariate regression analyses for categorical data. J Roy Stat Soc B 54:3–40

Lin X, Zhang D (1999) Inference in generalized additive mixed models using smoothing splines. J Roy Stat Soc B 61:381–400

Lindsey J (1997) Applying generalized linear models. Springer, Berlin

Liu L, Yu Z (2007) A likelihood reformulation method in non-normal random effects models. Stat Med 27:3105–3124. doi: 10.1002/sim.3153

Loader C (1999) Local regression and likelihood. Springer, Berlin

Longini IM, Nizam A, Xu S, Ungchusak K, Hanshaoworakul W, Cummings D, Halloran ME (2005) Containing pandemic influenza at the source. Science 309:1083–1087

Lunn, D.J., Thomas, A., Best, N., and Spiegelhalter, D. (2000) WinBUGS – a Bayesian modelling framework: concepts, structure, and extensibility. Stat Comput 10:325–337

Mammen E, Marron J, Turlach B, Wand M (2001) A general projection framework for constrained smoothing. Stat Sci 16:232–248

Marschner I (1996) Fitting a multiplicative incidence model to age- and time-specific prevalence data. Biometrics 52:492–499

Marschner I (1997) A method for assessing age-time disease incidence using serial prevalence data. Biometrics 53:1384–1398

Massad E, Burattini M, De Azevedo-Neto R, Yang H, Coutinho F, Zanetta D (1994) A model-based design of a vaccination strategy against rubella in a non-immunized community of Sao Paulo State, Brazil. Epidemiol Infect 112:579–594

Mathei C, Shkedy Z, Denis B, Kabali C, Aerts M, Molenberghs G, Van Damme P, Buntinx F (2006) Evidence for a substantial role of sharing of injecting paraphernalia other than syringes/needles to the spread of hepatitis C among injecting drug users. J Viral Hepat 13:560–570

McCullagh P, Nelder J (1989) Generalized linear models. Chapman & Hall, London

McKendrick AG (1926) Applications of mathematics to medical problems. Kapil Proc Edinb Math Soc 44:1–34

McMahon BJ, Alward WLM, Hall DB (1985) Acute hepatitis B virus infection: relation of age to the clinical expression of disease and subsequent development of the carrier state. J Infect Dis 151:604–609

Mikolajczyk R, Kretzschmar M (2008) Methodological issues in collecting data from close contact networks. Soc Network 2:127–135

Molenberghs G, Verbeke G (2005) Models for discrete longitudinal data. Springer, New York

Morgan-Capner P, Wright J, Miller C, Miller E (1988) Surveillance of antibody to measles, mumps and rubella by age. Br Med J 297:770–772

Mossong J, Hens N, Friederichs V, Davidkin I, Broman M, Litwinska B, Siennicka J, Trzcinska A, Van Damme P, Beutels P, Vyse A, Shkedy Z, Aerts M, Massari M, Gabutti G (2008a) Parvovirus B19 infection in five European countries: seroepidemiology, force of infection and maternal risk of infection. Epidemiol Infect 136:1059–1068

Mossong J, Hens N, Jit M, Beutels P, Auranen K, Mikolajczyk R, Massari M, Salmaso S, Scalia Tomba G, Wallinga J, Heijne J, Sadkowska-Todys M, Rosinska M, Edmunds J (2008b) Social contacts and mixing patterns relevant to the spread of infectious diseases. PLoS Medicine 5(3): e74. doi:10.1371/journal.pmed.0050074

Muench H (1934) Derivation of rates from summation data by the catalytic curve. J Am Stat Assoc 29(185):25–38

Muench H (1959) Catalytic models in epidemiology. Harvard University Press, Boston

Mukomolov S, Shliakhtenko L, Levakova I, Shargorodskaya E (2000) Viral hepatitis in Russian federation. An analytical overview (in Russian). Technical Report 213 (3), 3rd edn. St Petersburg Pasteur Institute, St Petersburg

Nagelkerke N, Heisterkamp S, Borgdorff M, Broekmans J, Van Houwelingen H (1999) Semiparametric estimation of age-time specific infection incidence from serial prevalence data. Stat Med 18:307–320

Namata H, Shkedy Z, Faes C, Aerts M, Molenberghs G, Theeten H, Van Damme P, Beutels P (2007) Estimation of the force of infection from current status data using gerenalized linear mixed models. J Appl Stat 34:923–939

Nelson K, Lipsitz S, Fitzmaurice G, Ibrahim JG, Parzen M, Strawderman R (2006) Use of the probability integral transformation to fit nonlinear mixed-effects models with nonnormal random effects. J Comput Graph Stat 15:39–57

Ngo L, Wand M (2004) Smoothing with mixed model software. J Stat Software 9

Nielsen S, Toft N, Jorgenson E, Bibby B (2007) Bayesian mixture models for within herd prevalence of bovine para tuberculosis based on continuous ELISA response. Prev Vet Med 81:290–305

Ogunjimi B, Hens N, Goeyvaerts N, Aerts M, Damme PV, Beutels P (2009) Using empirical social contact data to model person to person infectious disease transmission: an illustration for varicella. Math Biosci 218(2):80–87. doi: 10.1016/j.mbs.2008.12.009

O'Sullivan F (1986) A statistical perspective on ill-posed inverse problems (c/r:p519–527). Stat Sci 1:502–518

Palmgren J (1989) Regression models for bivariate binary responses. Technical Report 101, Department of Biostatistics, University of Washington, Seattle

Peel D, McLachlan G (2000) Robust mixture modelling using the t distribution. Stat Comput 10: 339–348

Rahman H, Wakfield J, Stephens D, Falcoz C (1999) The Bayesian analysis of pivotal pharmacokinetic study. Stat Meth Med Res 8:195–216

Robertson T, Wright F, Dykstra R (1988) Order restricted statistical inference. Wiley, New York

Rogan W, Gladen B (1978) Estimating prevalence from results of a screening-test. Am J Epidemiol 107:71–76

Ross R (1916) An application of the theory of probabilities to the study of a priori pathometry. In: Proceedings of the Royal Society of London. Series A, Containing Papers of a Mathematical and Physical Character., vol 92, pp 204–230

Rossini A, Tsiatis A (1996) A semiparametric proportional odds regression model for the analysis of current status data. J Am Stat Soc 91:713–721

Royston P, Altman D (1994) Regression using fractional polynomials of continuous covariates: Parsimonious parametric modelling. Appl Stat 43(3):429–467

Ruppert D, Wand MP, Carroll RJ (2003) Semiparametric regression. Cambridge University Press, Cambridge

Schenzle D (1984) An age-structured model of pre- and post-vaccination measles transmission. IMA J Math Appl Med Biol 1(2):169–191

Shapiro CN (1993) Epidemiology of hepatitis B. Pediatr Infect Dis J 12:443–447

Shau J, Tu D (1995) The Jackknife and Bootstrap. Springer series in statistics – vol. 2, New York

Shiboski S (1998) Generalized additive models for current status data. Lifetime Data Anal 4:29–50

Shkedy Z, Aerts M, Molenberghs G, Beutels P, Van Damme P (2003) Modelling forces of infection by using monotone local polynomials. Appl Stat 52(4):469–485

Silvapulle M, Sen P (2005) Constrained statistical inference. Inequality, order and shape restriction. Wiley, New York

Simonoff J (1996) Smoothing methods in statistics. Springer, New York

Soetaert K, Petzoldt T, Setzer R (2010) Solving differential equations in R: package desolve. J Stat Software 33(9):1–25

Speed T (1991) Comment on paper by Robinson. Stat Sci 6:42–44

Spiegelhalter D, Best N, Carlin B (1998) Bayesian deviance, the effective number of parameters, and the comparison of arbitrarily complex models. Technical Report 98–009, Division of Biostatistics, University of Minisota

Spiegelhalter DJ, Best NG, Carlin BP, van der Linde A (2002) Bayesian measures of model complexity and fit. J Roy Stat Soc B Stat Meth 64(4):583–639

Sturtz S, Ligges U, Gelman A (2005) R2WinBUGS: A Package for Running WinBUGS from R. J Stat Software 12(3):1–16.

Sutherland I, Bleiker MA, Meijer J, Styblo K (1984) The risk of tuberculous infection in The Netherlands from 1967 to 1979. In Selected Papers 22, Royal Netherlands Tuberculosis Asscociation, The Hague, pp 75–91

Sutton A, Gay N, Edmunds W, Hope V, Gill O, Hickman M (2006) Modelling the force of infection for hepatitis B and hepatitis C in injecting drug users in England and Wales. BMC Infect Dis 6:93

Therneau T, Grambsch P (2000) Modelling survival data. Springer, Berlin

Thiry N, Beutels P, Shkedy Z, Vranckx R, Vandermeulen C, Van Der Wielen M, Van Damme P (2002) The seroepidemiology of primary varicella-zoster virus infection in Flanders (Belgium). Eur J Pediatr 161:588–593

Tolfvenstam T, Papadogiannakis N, Norbeck O, Petersson K, Broliden K (2001) Frequency of human parvovirus B19 infection in intrauterine fetal death. Lancet 357:1494–1497

Van Effelterre T, Shkedy Z, Aerts M, Molenberghs G, Van Damme P, Beutels P (2009) Contact patterns and their implied basic reproductive numbers: an illustration for varicella-zoster virus. Epidemiol Infect 137:48–57

Vaupel J, Manton K, Stallard E (1979) The impact of heterogeneity in individual frailty in the dynamics of mortality. Demography, 16(3):439–454

Verbyla A, Cullis B, Kenward M, Welman S (1999) The analysis of designed experiments and longitudinal data by using smoothing splines. Appl Stat 48:269–311

Vynnycky E, White R (2010) An introduction to infectious disease modelling. Oxford University Press, Oxford

Vyse A, Gay N, Hesketh L, Morgan-Capner P, Miller E (2004) Seroprevalence of antibody to varicella zoster virus in england and wales in children and young adults. Epidemiol Infect 132: 1129–1134

Vyse A, Gay N, Hesketh L, Pebody R, Morgan-Capner P, Miller E (2006) Interpreting serological surveys using mixture models: the seroepidemiology of measles, mumps and rubella in England and Wales at the beginning of the 21st century. Epidemiol Infect 134:1303–1312

Wahba G (1978) Improper priors, spline smoothing and the problem of guarding against model errors in regression. J Roy Stat Soc B 40:364–372

Wallinga J, Teunis P, Kretzschmar M (2006) Using data on social contacts to estimate age-specific transmission parameters for respiratory-spread infectious agents. Am J Epidemiol 164:936–944

Wand M (2003) Smoothing and mixed models. Comput Stat 18:223–249

Wang C, Wang S, Gutierrez R, Carroll R (1998) Local linear regression for generalized linear models with missing data. Ann Stat 26:1028–50

Wolfinger R, O'Connell M (1993) Generalized linear mixed models: a pseudo-likelihood approach. J Stat Comput Simulat 48:233–243

Wood S (2006) Generalized additive models: an introduction with R. Chapman and Hall/CRC Press, London/Boca Raton

Yee T, Wild C (1996) Vector generalized additive models. J Roy Stat Soc B 58:481–493

Yee TW (2008) The VGAM package. R News 8(2):28–39. URL http://CRAN.R-project.org/doc/Rnews/

Young N, Brown K (2004) Mechanisms of disease—parvovirus B19. New Engl J Med 350: 586–597

Zaaijer H, Koppelman M, Farrington C (2004) Parvovirus B19 viraemia in Dutch blood donors. Epidemiol Infect 132:1161–1166

Zeger S, Karim M (1991) Generalized linear models with random effects: a Gibbs sampling approach. J Am Stat Assoc 86:79–102

Zhang D, Lin X, Raz J, Sowers M (1998) Semi-parametric stochastic mixed models for longitudinal data. J Am Stat Assoc 86:79–86

Index

N. Hens et al., *Modeling Infectious Disease Parameters Based on Serological and Social Contact Data*, Statistics for Biology and Health 63, DOI 10.1007/978-1-4614-4072-7, © Springer Science+Business Media New York 2012

Printed by Printforce, the Netherlands